Yulia Krasheninnikova

# INFORMAL HEALTHCARE IN CONTEMPORARY RUSSIA

Sociographic Essays on the Post-Soviet
Infrastructure for Alternative Healing Practices

With a foreword by Vasily Vlassov

*ibidem*-Verlag
Stuttgart

**Bibliografische Information der Deutschen Nationalbibliothek**
Die Deutsche Nationalbibliothek verzeichnet diese Publikation in der Deutschen Nationalbibliografie; detaillierte bibliografische Daten sind im Internet über http://dnb.d-nb.de abrufbar.

**Bibliographic information published by the Deutsche Nationalbibliothek**
Die Deutsche Nationalbibliothek lists this publication in the Deutsche Nationalbibliografie; detailed bibliographic data are available in the Internet at http://dnb.d-nb.de.

Cover picture: © copyright 2016 by N. Paramonova

Translated by Julia Kazantseva

Note: The book relies on the findings of studies supported by the Khamovniki Foundation for Social Research (Project 2013-001, The Economics of "Informal Healthcare" in Modern Russia).

∞

Gedruckt auf alterungsbeständigem, säurefreien Papier
Printed on acid-free paper

ISSN: 1614-3515

ISBN-13: 978-3-8382-0970-8

© *ibidem*-Verlag
Stuttgart 2017

Alle Rechte vorbehalten

Das Werk einschließlich aller seiner Teile ist urheberrechtlich geschützt. Jede Verwertung außerhalb der engen Grenzen des Urheberrechtsgesetzes ist ohne Zustimmung des Verlages unzulässig und strafbar. Dies gilt insbesondere für Vervielfältigungen, Übersetzungen, Mikroverfilmungen und elektronische Speicherformen sowie die Einspeicherung und Verarbeitung in elektronischen Systemen.

All rights part of this publication may be reproduced, stored in or introduced into a retrieval system, or transmitted, in any form, or by any means (electronical, mechanical, photocopying, recording or otherwise) without the prior written permission of the publisher. Any person who does any unauthorized act in relation to this publication may be liable to criminal prosecution and civil claims for damages.

Printed in the EU

# Soviet and Post-Soviet Politics and Society (SPPS)    Vol. 165
ISSN 1614-3515

**General Editor:** Andreas Umland,
*Institute for Euro-Atlantic Cooperation, Kyiv,* umland@stanfordalumni.org

**Commissioning Editor:** Max Jakob Horstmann,
London, mjh@ibidem.eu

## EDITORIAL COMMITTEE*

### DOMESTIC & COMPARATIVE POLITICS
Prof. **Ellen Bos**, *Andrássy University of Budapest*
Dr. **Ingmar Bredies**, *FH Bund, Brühl*
Dr. **Andrey Kazantsev**, *MGIMO (U) MID RF, Moscow*
Prof. **Heiko Pleines**, *University of Bremen*
Prof. **Richard Sakwa**, *University of Kent at Canterbury*
Dr. **Sarah Whitmore**, *Oxford Brookes University*
Dr. **Harald Wydra**, *University of Cambridge*

### SOCIETY, CLASS & ETHNICITY
Col. **David Glantz**, *"Journal of Slavic Military Studies"*
Dr. **Marlène Laruelle**, *George Washington University*
Dr. **Stephen Shulman**, *Southern Illinois University*
Prof. **Stefan Troebst**, *University of Leipzig*

### POLITICAL ECONOMY & PUBLIC POLICY
Prof. em. **Marshall Goldman**, *Wellesley College, Mass.*
Dr. **Andreas Goldthau**, *Central European University*
Dr. **Robert Kravchuk**, *University of North Carolina*
Dr. **David Lane**, *University of Cambridge*
Dr. **Carol Leonard**, *Higher School of Economics, Moscow*
Dr. **Maria Popova**, *McGill University, Montreal*

### FOREIGN POLICY & INTERNATIONAL AFFAIRS
Dr. **Peter Duncan**, *University College London*
Prof. **Andreas Heinemann-Grüder**, *University of Bonn*
Dr. **Taras Kuzio**, *Johns Hopkins University*
Prof. **Gerhard Mangott**, *University of Innsbruck*
Dr. **Diana Schmidt-Pfister**, *University of Konstanz*
Dr. **Lisbeth Tarlow**, *Harvard University, Cambridge*
Dr. **Christian Wipperfürth**, *N-Ost Network, Berlin*
Dr. **William Zimmerman**, *University of Michigan*

### HISTORY, CULTURE & THOUGHT
Dr. **Catherine Andreyev**, *University of Oxford*
Prof. **Mark Bassin**, *Södertörn University*
Prof. **Karsten Brüggemann**, *Tallinn University*
Dr. **Alexander Etkind**, *University of Cambridge*
Dr. **Gasan Gusejnov**, *Moscow State University*
Prof. em. **Walter Laqueur**, *Georgetown University*
Prof. **Leonid Luks**, *Catholic University of Eichstaett*
Dr. **Olga Malinova**, *Russian Academy of Sciences*
Prof. **Andrei Rogatchevski**, *University of Tromso*
Dr. **Mark Tauger**, *West Virginia University*

## ADVISORY BOARD*

Prof. **Dominique Arel**, *University of Ottawa*
Prof. **Jörg Baberowski**, *Humboldt University of Berlin*
Prof. **Margarita Balmaceda**, *Seton Hall University*
Dr. **John Barber**, *University of Cambridge*
Prof. **Timm Beichelt**, *European University Viadrina*
Dr. **Katrin Boeckh**, *University of Munich*
Prof. em. **Archie Brown**, *University of Oxford*
Dr. **Vyacheslav Bryukhovetsky**, *Kyiv-Mohyla Academy*
Prof. **Timothy Colton**, *Harvard University, Cambridge*
Prof. **Paul D'Anieri**, *University of Florida*
Dr. **Heike Dörrenbächer**, *Friedrich Naumann Foundation*
Dr. **John Dunlop**, *Hoover Institution, Stanford, California*
Dr. **Sabine Fischer**, *SWP, Berlin*
Dr. **Geir Flikke**, *NUPI, Oslo*
Prof. **David Galbreath**, *University of Aberdeen*
Prof. **Alexander Galkin**, *Russian Academy of Sciences*
Prof. **Frank Golczewski**, *University of Hamburg*
Dr. **Nikolas Gvosdev**, *Naval War College, Newport, RI*
Prof. **Mark von Hagen**, *Arizona State University*
Dr. **Guido Hausmann**, *University of Munich*
Prof. **Dale Herspring**, *Kansas State University*
Dr. **Stefani Hoffman**, *Hebrew University of Jerusalem*
Prof. **Mikhail Ilyin**, *MGIMO (U) MID RF, Moscow*
Prof. **Vladimir Kantor**, *Higher School of Economics*
Dr. **Ivan Katchanovski**, *University of Ottawa*
Prof. em. **Andrzej Korbonski**, *University of California*
Dr. **Iris Kempe**, *"Caucasus Analytical Digest"*
Prof. **Herbert Küpper**, *Institut für Ostrecht Regensburg*
Dr. **Rainer Lindner**, *CEEER, Berlin*
Dr. **Vladimir Malakhov**, *Russian Academy of Sciences*

Dr. **Luke March**, *University of Edinburgh*
Prof. **Michael McFaul**, *Stanford University, Palo Alto*
Prof. **Birgit Menzel**, *University of Mainz-Germersheim*
Prof. **Valery Mikhailenko**, *The Urals State University*
Prof. **Emil Pain**, *Higher School of Economics, Moscow*
Dr. **Oleg Podvintsev**, *Russian Academy of Sciences*
Prof. **Olga Popova**, *St. Petersburg State University*
Dr. **Alex Pravda**, *University of Oxford*
Dr. **Erik van Ree**, *University of Amsterdam*
Dr. **Joachim Rogall**, *Robert Bosch Foundation Stuttgart*
Prof. **Peter Rutland**, *Wesleyan University, Middletown*
Prof. **Marat Salikov**, *The Urals State Law Academy*
Dr. **Gwendolyn Sasse**, *University of Oxford*
Prof. **Jutta Scherrer**, *EHESS, Paris*
Prof. **Robert Service**, *University of Oxford*
Mr. **James Sherr**, *RIIA Chatham House London*
Dr. **Oxana Shevel**, *Tufts University, Medford*
Prof. **Eberhard Schneider**, *University of Siegen*
Prof. **Olexander Shnyrkov**, *Shevchenko University, Kyiv*
Prof. **Hans-Henning Schröder**, *SWP, Berlin*
Prof. **Yuri Shapoval**, *Ukrainian Academy of Sciences*
Prof. **Viktor Shnirelman**, *Russian Academy of Sciences*
Dr. **Lisa Sundstrom**, *University of British Columbia*
Dr. **Philip Walters**, *"Religion, State and Society", Oxford*
Prof. **Zenon Wasyliw**, *Ithaca College, New York State*
Dr. **Lucan Way**, *University of Toronto*
Dr. **Markus Wehner**, *"Frankfurter Allgemeine Zeitung"*
Dr. **Andrew Wilson**, *University College London*
Prof. **Jan Zielonka**, *University of Oxford*
Prof. **Andrei Zorin**, *University of Oxford*

\* While the Editorial Committee and Advisory Board support the General Editor in the choice and improvement of manuscripts for publication, responsibility for remaining errors and misinterpretations in the series' volumes lies with the books' authors.

# Soviet and Post-Soviet Politics and Society (SPPS)
ISSN 1614-3515

Founded in 2004 and refereed since 2007, SPPS makes available affordable English-, German-, and Russian-language studies on the history of the countries of the former Soviet bloc from the late Tsarist period to today. It publishes between 5 and 20 volumes per year and focuses on issues in transitions to and from democracy such as economic crisis, identity formation, civil society development, and constitutional reform in CEE and the NIS. SPPS also aims to highlight so far understudied themes in East European studies such as right-wing radicalism, religious life, higher education, or human rights protection. The authors and titles of all previously published volumes are listed at the end of this book. For a full description of the series and reviews of its books, see www.ibidem-verlag.de/red/spps.

**Editorial correspondence & manuscripts** should be sent to: Dr. Andreas Umland, c/o DAAD, German Embassy, vul. Bohdana Khmelnitskoho 25, UA-01901 Kyiv, Ukraine. e-mail: umland@stanfordalumni.org

**Business correspondence & review copy requests** should be sent to: *ibidem* Press, Leuschnerstr. 40, 30457 Hannover, Germany; tel.: +49 511 2622200; fax: +49 511 2622201; spps@ibidem.eu.

**Authors, reviewers, referees, and editors** for (as well as all other persons sympathetic to) SPPS are invited to join its networks at
www.facebook.com/group.php?gid=52638198614
www.linkedin.com/groups?about=&gid=103012
www.xing.com/net/spps-ibidem-verlag/

**Recent Volumes**

157   *Vladimir V. Karacharovskiy, Ovsey I. Shkaratan, Gordey A. Yastrebov*
      Towards a New Russian Work Culture
      Can Western Companies and Expatriates Change Russian Society?
      With a foreword by Elena N. Danilova
      Translated by Julia Kazantseva
      ISBN 978-3-8382-0902-9

158   *Edmund Griffiths*
      Aleksandr Prokhanov and Post-Soviet Esotericism
      ISBN 978-3-8382-0903-6

159   *Timm Beichelt, Susann Worschech (eds.)*
      Transnational Ukraine?
      Networks and Ties that Influence(d) Contemporary Ukraine
      ISBN 978-3-8382-0944-9

160   *Mieste Hotopp-Riecke*
      Die Tataren der Krim zwischen Assimilation und Selbstbehauptung
      Der Aufbau des krimtatarischen Bildungswesens nach Deportation und Heimkehr (1990-2005)
      Mit einem Vorwort von Swetlana Czerwonnaja
      ISBN 978-3-89821-940-2

161   *Olga Bertelsen (ed.)*
      Revolution and War in Contemporary Ukraine
      The Challenge of Change
      ISBN 978-3-8382-1016-2

162   *Natalya Ryabinska*
      Ukraine's Post-Communist Mass Media
      Between Capture and Commercialization
      With a foreword by Marta Dyczok
      ISBN 978-3-8382-1011-7

163   *Alexandra Cotofana, James M. Nyce (eds.)*
      Religion and Magic in Socialist and Post-Socialist Contexts
      Historic and Ethnographic Case Studies of Orthodoxy, Heterodoxy, and Alternative Spirituality
      With an afterword by Catherine Wanner
      ISBN 978-3-8382-0989-0

164   *Nozima Akhrarkhodjaeva*
      The Instrumentalisation of Mass Media in Electoral Authoritarian Regimes
      Evidence from Russia's Presidential Election Campaigns of 2000 and 2008
      ISBN 978-3-8382-1013-1

# Contents

Foreword by Vasily Vlassov ................................................................. VII

Author's note ........................................................................................ XI

Acknowledgements ............................................................................. XV

1   **Goals and tools of informal healthcare sociography** ......... 1
    1.1.   Problem statement ............................................................. 1
    1.2.   Description model ............................................................. 10
    1.3.   "Informal healthcare" drivers ........................................... 34

2   **Agents in the markets for health products** ....................... 51
    2.1.   "We are like Galileo—they burn us at the stake, but we continue promoting dietary supplements": Direct selling of health products ................................... 55
    2.2.   Latent functions of the healthcare institution: The case of pharmacies .................................................. 70
    2.3.   Contemporary peddlers: Itinerant trade and peddling health products ................................................................ 84

3   **Health from the garden, forest, and market: Procuring and selling gifts of nature** ................................ 95

4   **Shadow and respectable alternative medicine: From healers to "complementary" specialists** ................ 111
    4.1.   "People remember a certain Baba Vanga, so they will also remember me": Healers ....................... 112
    4.2.   Frontier zone: Ambivalent status, recognition problems and shadow practices of complementary and alternative medicine specialists .......................... 128
    4.3.   All diseases of the nerves: Psychotherapy as an alternative to orthodox medicine ................................. 168

## 5 Religious institutions: Health concerns and commerce on health problems ............ 175

- 5.1. The attitude of religious organizations to conventional and alternative medicine ............ 182
- 5.2. Treatment arsenal: Religious ceremonies, rituals, and practices to address health problems ............ 192
- 5.3. Social service as a form of religions' participation in healthcare ............ 209
- 5.4. Religious associations in the markets for health products ............ 223

## 6 The "informal healthcare" framework: Information markets ............ 233

- 6.1. Mass media ............ 234
- 6.2. Information intermediaries ............ 246

**Afterword** ............ 253

**Appendices** ............ 255

**References** ............ 269

# Foreword

Medicine, more than any other field of human activity, is surrounded by a halo of secrecy. Mutual recognition by professionals reigns here. The very notion of professionalism in the English context applies only to doctors, lawyers, and priests. Hence, besides being a reason for snobbery, this also underlies the well-known detachment that doctors demonstrate towards the problems of "others" in their everyday sense.

Social practice aimed at alleviating human suffering associated with diseases is the best definition of medicine. Professionals—doctors and nurses—identify, study, and recognize diseases, as well as diagnose their individual cases. The boundaries of this relatively specified field—medicine—are changing under the influence of forces striving to medicalize conditions that are not diseases and include practices not peculiar to physicians and not accepted by them.

Quite recently by historical standards (some 120–130 years ago), professional medicine in its present form was only emerging and was unavailable to most people. Even now, most of the population in Russia, Brazil and other BRICS countries, not to mention countries below its "lower" borders, has limited access to medical care. At the same time, health problems, or rather the suffering associated with what people understand to be diseases, are vital and daily. There is a constant and strong flow of aspirations and practices, which partially overlaps the field of competence assigned to professional medicine. It is precisely the unsatisfied demand for medical care, rather than folly, which determines the situation where "everyone understands in medicine." In a broader sense: more or less actively, people practice self and mutual treatment everywhere. This is as inevitable in life as eating.

Due to the excessive formalism of the authorities, restrictions on self-medication and mutual aid in the Soviet Union were probably harsher than anywhere else. In addition to rigorous government regulation, physicians were intolerant to self-medication and any practices not legalized in public health facilities; and there were virtually none other at the time. Hence, after 1988 there was a marked explosion of various widely circulated "medical manuals" and public practices unimaginable under Communist control.

The revolutionary health legislation enacted in 1993 could have become the most important event for the development of alternative and complementary practices in medicine. Unfortunately, as in many other spheres of public life, promises of innovations of the time were not implemented. The opportunities for healers to work legally were reduced to the extent that virtually only medical professionals could legitimately practice alternative and complementary interventions. A government institute functioning under the auspices of the Federal Ministry of Health issued national certificates authorizing doctors to practice alternative methods of treatment.

The past decade in Russia has been marked by government recognition of some alternative practices as part of medicine (osteopathy) and the expanding intervention of religious organizations in certain aspects of medical care; a reference to homeopathic remedies has appeared in the federal law on circulation of medicines. With no intention to include "energy informational practice" or "manual therapy" in the scope of scientific medicine, the government licenses such activities on the same basis as proper medical care. In contrast to the common understanding of the need for evidence-based practice in medicine, this increasingly erodes the boundaries of "normal" medical practice.

Russian healthcare has now been shrinking for more than fifteen years. This trend—most pronounced in small towns and rural areas—has brought about a massive decline in access to healthcare. Consequently, in recent years, for the first time in Russian history, the government acknowledged the need to legalize the situation when people without relevant professional training would be authorized to provide care in remote villages. Lack of access to professional medical care forces a substantial part of the population to turn to healers and other helpers.

The book *Informal Healthcare* focuses on a systematic qualitative study of health-related practices and attitudes that are not entirely within the field of professional medicine, or rather medicine institutionalized by the Russian state. It can be expected that at least part of the professional medical community and public health experts will be wary about the book. First, because qualitative research is still not widely used in medicine and healthcare. Second, because the picture painted by the author can be regarded as an unsightly image of reality in the mirror of a method which makes little sense to physicians.

A great merit of the book is a systematization of the practices of various health care actors. The perception of their methods and the selected approach to classification are sometimes paradoxical and judgmental, but the author presents them quite convincingly. The results of empirical studies are likewise clearly presented.

This book may be of interest to the English reader primarily because it gives a detailed picture of an understudied aspect of contemporary Russian life, where many elements seem archaic at first glance. The backdrop for this picture is formal Russian healthcare with its Soviet legacy, unique terminology, and specific regulations, which the author also meticulously analyzes. Offering a wealth of factual information and original classifications, the book stimulates further, including comparative, research in this area.

**Vasily Vlassov**
President of the Russian Society for Evidence Based Medicine
Professor of Public Health at the National Research University Higher School of Economics in Moscow

# Author's note

The idea for this book came from searching for an answer to a seemingly trivial question—how and with whose help are Russians today fighting diseases and maintaining health outside the scope of the formal healthcare system?

The World Health Organization (WHO) and the national legislation give extremely broad definitions of "healthcare system". They include all health-related aspects of social life. However, in public and ordinary speech in Russia, this notion is most frequently used to designate formal healthcare institutions under public administration. That is why it is possible to use regulatory measures and public financing to "reform", "develop" or "modernize" the healthcare system.

When we speak about the healthcare system in the second, narrow, meaning (and that is what I will use in this book), it is obvious that numerous substituting or complementary health maintenance practices exist beyond its scope, along with associated providers of services and goods. I believe that to understand the magnitude and functioning of this variety of activities, one has to start with routine sociographic work aimed at revealing, structuring, and providing a phenomenological description of the elements of this diversity.

For ordinary people, such health practices are a part of their everyday life. Everyone has some personal experience to share. However, we know little about this sphere in general. For state statistics, public health protection is limited to the activities of medical, pharmaceutical, and sports and fitness organizations. Therefore, they do not record anything beyond this. Social sciences focus on selected institutions and practices that substitute the healthcare system in Russia, such as healing and alternative medicine.[1] However, in general, this sphere is understudied and depicted in a rather fragmentary manner.

---

[1] Folklore-ethnographic and anthropological studies of the magical rituals and folk medicine of peoples inhabiting Russia is the most popular genre among the works focusing on various social health maintenance practices beyond the scope of the existing healthcare system. The staff of the Institute of Ethnology and Anthropology of the Russian Academy of Sciences, as well as many ethnographers in different Russian regions are working along this line of research (*e.g.,* Mazalova, 2012; Templing, 2014; Kharitonova, 1999; *Epic Heritage,* 2013).

Sociography, which includes observing and recording simple facts and their relations, is useful when it precedes theoretical constructs, goes before reasoning about habitus or transaction costs with regard to Russian realities. In this context, its findings serve as a basis for scientific problematization and the development of explanatory concepts, as well as for decision making in public administration. It also provides the necessary ground for comparative studies. On the example of alternative health maintenance practices, we shall see that the resulting picture of reality may significantly differ from the dominant public perception of the arrangement and magnitude of such practices. These considerations clearly show why it makes sense to embark on a description of those social phenomena which seem to be of no big interest either to the academic community or the state.

This book is a series of sociographic essays. They focus on agents who serve alternative health maintenance practices and substitute or complement the formal healthcare system.

The publication is based on the records and findings of a pilot research project conducted in the Perm Territory of Russia (Kama area) in 2013 and aimed at describing informal healthcare phenomena. About ten people participated with me in the fieldwork. When I write "we" in the text of the book, I mean our research team, with students of the Perm branch of the Higher School of Economics forming its core. We relied on the methodology developed under the guidance of Simon Kordonsky on the basis of the Laboratory for Local Administration at the National Research University Higher School of Economics. The methodology is intended for empirical research of local social life (Kordonsky et al., 2011).

The project continues a series of studies of health maintenance institutions and practices that were conducted in 2010-2012 with the support of the Khamovniki Foundation for Social Research (*The Health Maintenance System,* 2012). Their ultimate goal is to form an understanding of health care in Russia that would be broader than that prevailing in

---

Some works focus on the social status of alternative medicine practitioners and the ways of professionalizing their activities (*e.g.,* Volkova, 2007; Krasheninnikova, Kolonuto, 2012; Sadykov, 2013; Salo, 2008; Salo, 2009; Samarskaya, Teper, 2007; *Traditional Medicine,* 2011). We should also mention sociological studies that focus on the attitude of the population and the medical community to alternative medicine practices during different post-Soviet periods (Brown, Rusinova, 2002; Iarskaia-Smirnova, Romanov, 2008; Stickley et al., 2013).

healthcare policy and public discussions. Like the previous works, this one proceeds from the need to develop an understanding of the social environment in which the public healthcare system functions and on which it depends.

The book consists of two parts. The first chapter contains some generalizations and reflections on the subject matter in general. It explains what "informal healthcare" means and offers a methodology to describe the phenomena in this field. It also provides assumptions as to the reasons promoting their development. The following chapters focus on selected "informal healthcare" phenomena classified by the principal product offered to the customer: manufactured goods, gifts of nature, diagnostic and treatment services, ideas and information.

The book was conceived as a series of essays rather than an encyclopedia. The selected format focuses on the most interesting "informal healthcare" agents, but does not provide a comprehensive and detailed picture of this field. The activities of some agents are disclosed more fully than the others, whereas some of them are not even considered separately despite having been recorded and described during fieldwork. In particular, the book contains no special section on health movements and original doctrines of self-healing, including oriental schools (yoga, qigong, and others), though the activities of such network structures definitely contribute to maintaining the health of the population and deserve the researchers' separate attention.

The last remark concerns the period referred to in the publication. Except when explicitly specified, the text describes the situation at the time of the fieldwork. Thus, when reference is made to the present time, this means the year 2013. It is important to bear this in mind, since the described sphere is sensitive to external influences, such as the economic situation and the evolution of legislation; so, for the readers, some of the presented facts may already be in the past.

\* \* \*

This monograph was initially published in Russian in February 2016 under the title "*Neformal'noe zdravookhranenie. Sotsiograficheskie ocherki*" (Informal Healthcare. Sociographic Essays).[2] This edition is an abridged, revised, and translated version of the book. The corpus was reduced at the cost of some illustrative material (quotes from interviews with informants, examples, and description of the facts in the body text; background information and fragments of fieldnotes in appendices). However, new information was also added. The text for English-speaking readers includes an explanation of certain terminology and regulations specific for Russian healthcare, as well as the US dollar equivalent for all mentioned costs and prices. Some corrections and updates were made due to important recent changes in the rules and regulations of the Russian Federation. Finally, the bibliography was extended by adding literature relevant to the theme of research.

---

2   Its imprint is as follows: Krasheninnikova Yu. *Neformal'noe zdravookhranenie. Sotsiograficheskie ocherki,* Moscow: Strana Oz, 2016, 456 p.

# Acknowledgements

It was a great pleasure for me to work on the book, and I am sincerely grateful to everyone without whom it would not have been possible.

First and foremost, I would like to thank the participants of the fieldwork in the Kama area who engaged with me in collecting the empirical evidence. My thanks go to Olga Makarova, Andrey Maslennikov, Maria Okuneva, Marina Tsevileva, Alina Yagudina, Dmitry Subbotin, Dmitry Syuzev, Nikita Oparin, Elena Shuraleva, Artem Shavrin, and Anna Kolonuto. Many remarkable facts on the activities of "informal healthcare" agents presented in the book were obtained through their efforts. Their field notes and interview transcripts gave me an invaluable basis for analytical work. The work of our research team would not have been possible without the organizational talent and direct participation of Dr. Elena Zueva, academic supervisor of the master's program in Public Administration at the HSE campus in Perm.

I fully owe the opportunity to write and publish the book to the Khamovniki Foundation for Social Research, whose grant also covered fieldwork. I would like to express my deep appreciation to its founder Alexander Klyachin for his attention to the subject of the research. Special thanks go to Simon Kordonsky, academic supervisor of the Khamovniki Foundation, and Cholpon Beishenalieva, its director, for their moral support and for creating the best possible conditions for work on the manuscript. I appreciate the engagement of my friends (Natalya Baulina, Vladimir Gubarenko, German Gladyshev, and others), who kindly provided me with useful information on the subject of the research. Discussions with them have allowed me to clarify some important points in the work.

Finally, I would like to thank those who were engaged in preparing the English edition of the book—translator Julia Kazantseva for her professionalism, endless patience and fruitful dialogue, and photographer Natalya Paramonova for a kindly provided photo for the cover.

# 1 Goals and tools of informal healthcare sociography[3]

## 1.1. Problem statement

We should start by clarifying what "informal healthcare" means. When one describes the health maintenance institutions and practices unrelated to formal healthcare, the terminology to be used is the initial problem. The field of study cannot be called a *system*, because it is a spontaneous diversity of phenomena often unrelated and not associated with each other. Designating it as a separate *market* would be incomplete, since non-profit activities play an important role in this diversity. However, further we will show that specific markets are emerging on the basis of some methods of health maintenance. The concept of *organization field* applied quite successfully to studying healthcare (Scott, 2004) is also not the best methodological tool—in such a field the basic units are organizations that are somehow related and interact with each other. In our case, more or less structured organization fields exist within the sphere of our research, but they do not embrace it completely.

The term "alternative medicine" is most often used to designate health practices alien to mainstream medicine. However, if we look at the issues covered by the extensive body of academic papers addressing this topic, we will see that alternative medicine is mentioned either in the general context of its acceptance/rejection by conventional medicine and the public authorities, i.e. in the context of the struggle for a monopoly on expert knowledge about human health and manipulations with it, or with reference to specific cases. Researchers avoid the task of internally structuring and describing the space of alternative medicine. This may be due to the negative nature of the notion as such—being effective in analytical procedures of contraposition, it is insufficient to systematize the existing knowledge about the subject. Upon closer examination, not all agents can be classified as representatives of alternative medicine, although they

---

[3] The main ideas of this chapter have been presented earlier at the NRU HSE XV April International Academic Conference on Economic and Social Development (1-4 April 2014, Moscow) and in an article published in the *Mir Rossii* journal (Krasheninnikova, 2015).

help ill people and do not belong to the formal healthcare system. Institutions not related directly to medicine (religious organizations, mass media) play an important role there.

Given these considerations, hereinafter I will refer to alternative medicine in the narrow sense—as a specialized field of knowledge and treatment practices that the agents themselves, their patients, and competitors perceive as a special kind of medicine that differs from the Western biomedical model. In this meaning the services of alternative medicine will not be identical to health maintenance services alternative to conventional healthcare. The latter, for example, include massage in beauty salons, where skillful experts "treat the back", or religious healing ceremonies performed by priests.

Besides, the expression "alternative medicine" is politically overloaded for a scientific term. The choice of the adjective used to indicate the methods that are not included in conventional medicine depends on the shade of meaning intended by the speaker. For WHO officials and experts, folk, alternative, traditional, non-conventional, and unorthodox medicine are only synonyms, the use of which depends on national specifics. Traditional or folk medicine usually implies indigenous methods and forms of treatment, whereas alternative or complementary medicine practices that are outside the scope of conventional medicine and are not part of the country's traditional culture.[4]

However, the difference in terms is crucial for the supporters and opponents of alternative medicine. The designation "traditional" emphasizes the right to exist on a par with conventional medicine as part of the national health system. The words "alternative" or "non-conventional" place this activity on the periphery of healthcare or even in the ghetto for those who are prepared to risk their health. Mike Saks reasonably argues that the political legitimacy of certain therapies determines the scope of alternative medicine: those recognized by the state are included in orthodox medicine and the politically marginal ones—in alternative medicine (Saks, 2003). The naming in this field is an exercise in power (Gale, 2014). Regulatory acts in post-Soviet Russia contain reference to both "folk medicine" and "traditional medicine". The meaning attributed to them is differ-

---

4    See *Beijing Declaration*. Adopted by the WHO Congress on Traditional Medicine, Beijing, China, 8 November 2008; *WHO Traditional Medicine Strategy: 2014–2023*.

ent. The former refers to health promotion methods entrenched in people's experience, but not included in the arsenal of medical science. The latter notion unites methods admitted to formal medical practice and those that have no "scientific rationale or logical explanation".[5]

The history of the term "traditional medicine" in the laws and regulations of the Russian Federation has a beginning and an end. Its introduction into professional medical discourse was associated with the activity of a limited range of stakeholders (authors of draft regulations, guidelines, etc.). Mostly those were representatives of the Federal Clinical Trials Research Center for Traditional Diagnostic and Treatment Methods of the Russian Ministry of Health (hereinafter, FCTRC TDTM). Therefore, its very promotion can be regarded as a *project* of the supporters of integrating alternative methods into conventional medical practice. Respectively, it makes no sense to state that the notion of "traditional medicine" reflects any objective reality.

When interviewing physicians, we encountered various interpretations of these terms. There is no established semantic framework. In particular, "traditional medicine" can be understood as either formal methods conventional for medical institutions ("traditional medicine is the medicine which we currently practice" and "the non-traditional one belongs to the days gone by") or alternative treatment practices common in folk tradition.

Considering the above mentioned problems, I have applied the metaphor of "informal healthcare" to designate the field of our studies. Quotation marks in this case are necessary, because they emphasize that the analyzed natural diversity of institutions and practices is in itself the very opposite of any organized system and their generalization is merely an analytical tool. Of course, the use of a metaphor is not the best solution to the problem and the search for adequate terminology should be continued. However, it seems to be quite a working construct for the purposes of this study.

---

5   "Traditional medicine is based on centuries-old traditions of folk healing practices and represents the totality of disease prevention, diagnostics, treatment and medical rehabilitation methods, approved for medical use in accordance with the established procedure and taught as part of the supplemental medical curriculum, as well as attitudes, knowledge, skills and abilities relating to traditional health systems, which are passed down from generation to generation in oral or written form and not always have a current scientific rationale or logical explanation" (Karpeev, Kiseleva, 2003).

When trying to understand how and with whose help the inhabitants of present-day Russia are fighting diseases and maintaining their health outside formal healthcare, I proceed from the following assumptions:

- "Informal healthcare" is not an integral system or organizational field opposing formal healthcare. Moreover, the borderline between them is not fixed, and its very movement is of particular interest for the understanding of this sphere.
- Similar to healthcare per se, "informal healthcare" includes the activity of economic agents serving health maintenance practices of people. Accordingly, one can explore this sphere by studying the behavior of either the consumer or the suppliers of goods and services. I chose the latter option for my work.
- Such activity becomes informal in view of the standards and rules set by conventional medicine and the government. The former evaluates the validity of knowledge and the efficacy of therapies. The latter establishes the regulations for socio-economic activities and controls compliance with them. Therefore, the following criteria can be applied to include one or another activity in the scope of "informal healthcare": the therapeutic effect of the offered goods or services; the degree of recognition by conventional medicine, and the degree of recognition by the state.
- "Informal healthcare" incorporates not only alternative medicine facilities, but also non-medical social institutions that for various reasons exercise a function unusual for them, namely, substitute a patient's visit to the doctor (religious organizations, pharmacies, including veterinary ones, media, culture and leisure centers, and others).

Abstaining from any assessment of how effective treatments are is an important prerequisite for sociographic work. The evaluation approach is risky, because the researcher's personal trust or mistrust of certain alternative methods affects his or her perception of the socio-economic aspects of such practices. Consequently, the study of social phenomena turns into their apology or criticism.

I believe the very attempt to evaluate something significantly distorts perception—unintentionally, it narrows the scope of "informality" to those practices that have no actual therapeutic effects, although consumers may perceive them as useful. Discussions about efficacy are part of the strategies of interaction between representatives of orthodox medicine and non-conventional methods. Actually, the advantage of a third-party observer consists exactly in the fact that a neutral position broadens the perspective and allows detecting social practices which a stakeholder tends to ignore.

The next question is: how can one describe "informal healthcare"?

In order to get an understanding of what this sphere includes in Russia, we first collected and processed information from public sources (official statistics, media communications, laws and regulations, public registries and databases, corporate websites, etc.). In general, the first step is to record the very existence of certain health practices alternative to conventional medicine, as well as the economic agents serving them. The criteria for including various phenomena in the subject matter of the study are dealt with in Section 1.2. After that, it is necessary to determine the magnitude and nature of the described phenomena: the extent of the agents' activities; the history of their emergence; development dynamics; their interrelationships; and consumer audiences. The description also implies systematizing and classifying the recorded types of socio-economic activities.

The way the state perceives the activity of such agents is crucial to including them in the scope of "informal healthcare"; therefore, it was important to record the position of the state. We can recreate it based on the legal framework and official documents, but the approach to their analysis must differ from the standard approach of a lawyer. According to the theory of law, legislation reflects the established rules according to which people co-exist. It captures the norms prevailing in society; therefore, if laws come into conflict with human practices, they will not work. By contrast, for studying the position of the state, it does not matter whether the rules and procedures established by the authorities are violated. The picture of the world created by laws and regulations may differ from reality, which is most often the case.

Using publicly available sources of information, we somehow reconstruct the reality formed by various stakeholders working in public (the media, researchers-sociologists, law enforcement and supervisory bodies, and proponents and opponents of alternative medicine). Respectively, it inevitably contains an element of distorting and myth-making. In addition, the Russian mass media always tend to be imbalanced in favor of news stories from Moscow and the major cities.

For this reason, our next step was a series of fieldwork studies in selected localities. From the national picture painted in bold strokes we switched to studying the situation "under the microscope". The pilot attempt to record, systematize, and describe the currently existing diversity of "informal healthcare" phenomena on the level of settlements was made in 2013 in one of Russia's regions—the Perm Territory (Krai).

The geography of fieldwork included the regional center Perm—a city with over a million inhabitants, three towns with a population of 50,000–70,000 people (medium-sized towns), three administrative centers of municipal districts (up to 10,000 inhabitants), four administrative centers of rural settlements (up to 3,000 inhabitants), five villages and small settlements (up to 500 inhabitants), as well as four isolated communities (a health resort, two Orthodox monasteries and one convent). We used qualitative methods to study the selected localities—semi-structured interviews and informal conversations with experts, including local officials, journalists, doctors, public figures, "informal healthcare" agents, and the local residents. All in all, we held over 370 interviews and conversations. Mandatory elements of the research program included field observations at the locations where the "informal healthcare" goods and services were provided, search for information in the local newspapers, online forums, social networks, public places, etc. A more detailed description of the informants, observation sites, and the methodology for surveying the localities is provided in Appendix 1.

Apparently, it would be incorrect to simply extrapolate the data obtained in one region to the general situation in Russia. However, among the constituent entities of the Russian Federation, the Perm Territory is neither an obvious leader nor an outsider. In terms of socio-economic development, it can probably be classified as a rather successful area; however, the indicators depicting the state of the regional healthcare system and the health of the local population are in general lower than the national averages, but not as dramatically as in certain other regions.[6] Considering this, we can expect that "informal healthcare" on the regional level will demonstrate more national features than any local specifics.

---

[6] According to the Federal State Statistics Service (Rosstat), as at 2013, the Perm Territory ranked 18th among the Russian regions by per capita income, 21st–25th—by per capita investment in fixed assets, and 63rd—by life expectancy at birth; as at 2012, it ranked 21st by gross regional product per capita (*Regions of Russia*, 2014).

In an era when quantitative research methods are entirely dominant in social sciences, resorting to observations and in-depth interviews may seem an ill-considered choice for researchers. However, the subject of our research is within those spheres of the society's life where no measuring can bring us closer to understanding what actually is going on. Scientists have no clear picture of how these spheres function; moreover, the concepts they use are inconsistent with the language of everyday routine practices.

When it comes to describing "informal healthcare", standard research and measurement methods, such as large-scale opinion polls and official statistics, are hardly applicable. Further I will attempt to demonstrate this, referring, in particular, to our fieldwork findings.

Recourse to alternative providers of health services is an aspect of human life which questionnaires can hardly capture. It is highly probable that the obtained data will be distorted. One of the reasons for such distortions is obvious—people realize that the work of such providers is largely illegal. In the course of interviews, we often faced situations when the informants deliberately distorted facts (this could be revealed only during extended conversations) or simply refused to provide information. They justified the latter attitude, in particular, by the following apprehension, "I do not want to draw the attention of the authorities."

Social attitudes that alternative medicine is dangerous and resorting to it is improper also influence the answers. Sometimes our interlocutors stated that they were committed to conventional medicine, but then in the course of the conversation they revealed that they had personal and positive experiences of dealing with alternative health practices. Primarily this concerned taking dietary supplements and seeking the help of healers.

When comparing the results of nationwide surveys conducted at different times, we see that dominant trends and social norms have an impact on how sincere the respondents' answers are. Thus, in February 2014, the Public Opinion Foundation (FOM) asked respondents the following question: "Have you ever used the services of alternative medicine (traditional healers, herbalists, psychics, etc.)?" Nine percent of the respondents answered, "Yes, I have".[7] However, in 2002, twenty-six percent

---

7   *What Treatment Is Preferable? What Russians Think About Conventional and Non-Conventional Medicine and Self-Treatment.* Report on the opinion poll of 16 February 2014. Public Opinion Foundation (website).
    URL: http://fom.ru/Zdorove-i-sport/11379.

of those surveyed gave an affirmative answer. The sociologists then stated that "representatives of the middle generation resorted to healing practices almost twice as often as senior citizens".[8] It appears that seventeen percent of Russians *have forgotten* that at a certain point they had visited a healer. In the course of an omnibus survey held in 1990 and 2009, the Russian Public Opinion Research Center (VCIOM) asked one and the same question: "Please recollect whether you have ever watched Anatoly Kashpirovsky's televised psychic healing sessions? If yes, how closely did you watch?" In 1990, fifty-seven percent answered that they put aside whatever they were doing and tuned in to watch, whereas two decades later only thirteen percent of the respondents gave this answer. The share of those who thought that these sessions had been more useful than harmful also experienced a dramatic fall (from fifty-two percent to six percent).[9]

Due to the vagueness and political preconceptions of the basic notions used to designate alternative health practices, the respondents may differently interpret the wording of the questions, and this may undermine the representativeness of the answers. One the same issue can be designated as "folk", "traditional" or "non-conventional" medicine—and the answers will differ (Iarskaia-Smirnova, Romanov, 2008; Stickley et al., 2013). It is also possible that the respondents will attribute a different meaning to these concepts than the sociologists processing the results of the questionnaire.

Let us now take a look at the official statistics in Russia. Most activities of "informal healthcare" agents are in no way reflected in such statistics. There are two reasons for this. First, the overwhelming majority of "informal healthcare" markets is in the shadow sector of the economy, which means that the agents themselves evade public records or submit distorted information, since their activity is illegal and they pay no taxes. These include direct sellers of dietary supplements operating without incorporating a legal entity; alternative medicine specialists practicing at home; fly-by-night sole proprietorships; religious organizations charging

---

8   *Conventional and Non-Conventional Medicine*. Report on the opinion poll of 25 July 2002. Public Opinion Foundation (website).
    URL: http://bd.fom.ru/report/cat/beruf/doc/dd022932.
9   *TV Wonderworkers Yesterday and Today*. 10.01.2010. Russian Public Opinion Research Center (website). URL: http://wciom.ru/index.php?id=236&uid=13020.

fees for healing services under the guise of donations; and peasants engaged in unauthorized trade and underreporting the size of their assets (including apiaries) in income books.

Second, even if entities provide financial statements and statistical reports to the authorities, it is impossible to single out and analyze the statistical data on their activities, because the classifiers and reporting forms do not envisage such analyses and products. In particular, wellness services are sometimes classified as medical services, but most often as trade or consumer services.

We should mention separately that the municipal authorities demonstrate low awareness of the situation in the field of our research. In most cases we were unable to obtain any information from the local officials about the number and key economic indicators of the entities that were of interest to us. For example, the municipalities had no knowledge about the number of locally registered massage practices or private medical centers simply because the licensing of medical organizations falls under the competence of the regional health ministry. Many "informal healthcare" agents are not locals and may be registered in other municipalities or even regions, which also objectively limits the possibility to collect data on the municipal level. It turned out that the municipal authorities had generally no idea that their subordinate establishments (libraries, clinics, community cultural centers) leased out their premises to visiting vendors of medicinal herbal balms and hearing aids, psychotherapists and specialists in "computer-aided diagnosis".

In the absence of reliable quantitative data, we can only make assumptions as to the size and diversity of "informal healthcare" markets based on the number of identified agents, their business activity and service prices. Due to its informality, it is currently impracticable to assess precisely the extent of "informal healthcare" (the number of people involved in this field, financial expenditures, etc.).

## 1.2. Description model

We assessed various activities along three lines to determine whether they were associated with the subject of our research:
- Therapeutic effect of the goods and services offered to the consumers
- Extent of their integration into official medicine (science-related rating)
- Compliance with the effective Russian legislation (legality rating)

*Therapeutic effect*

The importance of the first criterion is determined by the fact that the therapeutic effect is what makes a patient decide in favor of seeking treatment in a medical establishment or elsewhere, where he is promised recovery through faith, specific energy, natural resources, mental attitude, exercise, and much more.

Whether this will help depends on many factors, and not least on the expectations of the patient who counts on the efficacy of such methods. According to Jonathan C. Smith, American psychologist and author of the popular science bestseller *Pseudoscience and Extraordinary Claims of the Paranormal: A Critical Thinker's Toolkit* (Smith 2010), such expectations underlie the therapeutic effect of any placebo, which does not necessarily have to be a pill, but can include any intervention, be it in the form of psychotherapy, ritual, dietary prescription, etc.

However, in our case we are talking not only about placebos. A therapeutic effect recognized by orthodox medicine can actually take place and be considered proven. Such goods and services are also present in "informal healthcare" markets. For example, some gifts of nature are grown and picked primarily for their taste. However, they also possess certain medicinal properties due to the high content of biologically active substances (cranberries, seaberries, honey, rowan berries, viburnum berries, mint, etc.). This triggers such social practices as harvesting them to use as drugs. For example, viburnum berries are used in Russia to prepare infusions to lower the blood pressure, cranberries and honey—as a home remedy against colds, and so on.

The situational factor is also important. Standard religious practices (prayers and others) become an "informal healthcare" phenomenon when they address health problems. Another example is trampoline jumping so fancied by children. It can be included in "informal healthcare" when the trampoline owner claims that his services promote health, and pediatricians advise parents to exercise their children on the trampoline to strengthen their immune system, improve blood circulation and resolve orthopedic problems.

The borderline that separates medical goods and services from those that have no formal relationship to medicine is constantly crossed under the pressure of consumer demands and advertising aspirations of the suppliers. For example, dietary supplements, like fortified foods, are formally intended to make up for the deficiency of certain vitamins and minerals in the body, and the small dosage of vitamins in the dietary supplements excludes any possible therapeutic effect. However, the advertising of dietary supplements often turns into a display of their healing properties even with regard to ailments currently incurable by conventional medicine. Virtually every direct seller of health products we contacted during our research had a personal or family story to tell of recovering from a serious chronic disease.

As for the two other "informal healthcare" criteria, the simplest case concerns those phenomena that the medics consider quackery, and the state—an offense. Russian media generally associates such practices—witch doctors, phone sales of "wonder devices" to gullible elderly ladies, etc.—with alternative medicine. However, there are other widespread services in Russia where the contemporary medical science recognizes their therapeutic effect, but they are administered in violation of the law. Other practices, on the contrary, are within the legal framework, but outside medical competence and influence—magazines containing "popular advice" on fighting diseases, religious healing ceremonies, etc. In addition, the degree of recognition can be different, thus allowing to construct a complex, multidimensional picture of this field. Let us take a closer look at the diversity of these cases.

*The attitude of official medicine*
By official medicine we mean mainstream Western biomedicine as a system of specialized knowledge and associated practices distinguished by a purely materialistic approach to human nature and focus on physiology. Robert A. Hahn and Arthur Kleinman note that biomedicine is perceived by its practitioners and patients as medicine per se, whereas all other socio-cultural models of medicine are identified by adjectives—Chinese

medicine, Eastern medicine, etc. (Hahn, Kleinman, 1983, p. 312). In professional medical discourse it is also referred to as "conventional medicine". This word combination reflects the notion that the employed knowledge and treatment practices have been recognized by the entire medical professional community and are generally accepted. English-speakers also extensively use the term "orthodox medicine".

In recent decades, *evidence-based medicine* (EBM) has assumed the task of enhancing the scientific credibility of Western biomedicine. EBM focuses on proving the efficacy of various medical interventions. Medical practice is being standardized and priority in knowledge is attributed to the results of randomized controlled clinical trials (e.g., Timmermans, Kolker, 2004; Sackett et al., 1996). Such an emphasis on scientific knowledge reduces the opportunities for the legitimate existence of alternative medical practices with their holistic approach to the human being, especially their chances to be integrated into national healthcare systems (e.g., Barry, 2006; Villanueva-Russell, 2005).

Russian (as previously Soviet) medicine has developed in the same direction as the Western one; therefore, the biomedical model is also dominant in national healthcare (*Traditional Medicine*, 2011). In recent years, the evidence-based approach has also been actively implemented into national health policies. Certainly, in generally accepted medical practice (i.e., in conventional medicine), many methods also do not meet the criteria of evidence-based medicine, but in this paper we are addressing only those of them that originate outside of Western biomedicine.

In the Russian context, a ranking of various treatment methods based on their recognition by conventional medicine would produce a scale with complete rejection on one end and approval by evidence-based medicine substantiated by scientific research on the other end. Some alternative practices are assessed as clearly harmful to health (treatment by hydrogen peroxide, urine therapy, prolonged fasting, etc.). Healing ceremonies practiced by religious organizations are perceived primarily as psychotherapeutic actions that have a placebo effect. Some of the methods are recognized as useful; they have received "scientific upgrading" and are partially integrated into regular medical practice (Yoga, herbal therapy, etc.). Some services have been monopolized by the medical community (leech therapy, homeopathy and others), although they do not meet the criteria of evidence-based medicine, and not all physicians accept them. Those methods that have been proven effective by statistically valid research are not a topic of our discussion.

Professional medical discourse applies the term "complementary" to methods borrowed from traditional/alternative medicine. This designation captures their secondary, complementary, marginal role as related to medicinal or surgical treatment, on which orthodox medicine relies. According to one of the definitions, which I encountered in the Russian professional publication *Practicing Physician (Lechashchiy Vrach)*, complementary medicine includes "all types of non-conventional medicine used for healthcare purposes in combination with conventional medicine" (Astafieva, Kobzev, 2012).

We would like to emphasize that the same methods can be either alternative or complementary depending on the intention of the physicians applying them. In the former case, they replace standard treatment—for example, a patient is prescribed herbal therapy instead of chemical drugs. This contradicts the approach of orthodox medicine. In the latter case, they complement the principal methods, mainly at the stage of recovery. In Russia, complementary methods are primarily practiced at health resorts, where doctors engage in the rehabilitation and health promotion of people without acute illnesses, and the guests require no scientific evidence of the treatment's efficacy.

Speaking about recognition by conventional medicine, we must bear in mind one of its important features, namely, the corporate professional logic of the medical community based on the statutory monopoly on knowledge about the human body and manipulations with it (Saks, Allsop, 2003; Saks, 2003; Larkin, 1983; Berlant, 1975). This monopoly provides control over the resources allocated to fight diseases. Only trained professionals with respective proficiency levels are authorized to cure people. Individual corporations by medical specialty are emerging within the medical profession. They have monopolized the fight against specific diseases. Only oncologists may fight cancer, TB specialists—tuberculosis and so on.

Historically, the medical profession established itself by segregating from other treatment practices which were declared illegal or quack. Later, professional medical corporations adopted, among others, the strategy of taking over these practices. In such cases, the corporations acknowledge that alternative treatment methods are based on common sense, provide respective scientific rationale, and incorporate them into conventional medical practice. Since the medical sector in Russia is strictly regulated by the state and the professional medical community has virtually no functioning self-regulatory organizations, this process can be mainly traced by the regulatory acts of the federal health authorities.

In a study conducted in 2012 (*The Health Maintenance System*, 2012) I described the emergence of medical specialties as a natural form of the existence of medical corporations. Due to the corporate nature of Russian medicine, alternative treatment practices at the final stage of recognition are inevitably formalized as a medical specialty and in this new capacity fall under government licensing requirements. Thus, acupuncture as a practice of alternative medicine is replaced by a newly emerged medical specialty—"reflexology". After that, only specially trained physicians may practice acupuncture. No one else, be it a healer, a nurse, or a qualified pediatrician, is authorized to apply this treatment. Only a professional reflex therapist in a respectively licensed clinic may since then engage in this medical activity. The work of alternative healers who do not comply with these requirements becomes illegal (details are provided in the next section and in Chapter Four that focuses on diagnostic and treatment services).

Thus, *recognition* of alternative treatment methods by official medicine takes place in the form of a *take-over*, which, at first glance, should be disadvantageous to those who practice such methods. However, professional medical corporations are the best framework for utilizing public resources allocated for healthcare. For this reason, the agents of complementary and alternative medicine (CAM), struggling to be recognized, focus their efforts on formalizing their activities as separate medical specialties. This is evidenced by the public lobbying of their professional associations.

The medical community considers diagnostic or treatment methods not recognized by medical science to be quackery. If a method is recognized, then its application without the participation or supervision of a physician becomes quackery. For example, phytotherapy is widely used as a complementary treatment for many diseases in conventional medicine. However, herbalism that substitutes medication is not approved, especially if the patient takes herbal teas or without consulting a physician relies on popular advice published in various health magazines. Interviews with physicians held under this study demonstrate that this position is one of the basic professional attitudes.

In the process of being recognized by medical science alternative methods of health maintenance undergo a substantial metamorphosis. Their philosophy is diluted. Many non-conventional treatment practices are based on the idea of the holistic nature of the human being, where the spiritual component is as important as physical, chemical or biological parameters. This is where they oppose the orthodox medicine, which treats a human being as a biological organism. However, when such methods are admitted to authorized medical practice, the holistic approach has to be abandoned—their scientific rationale may not extend beyond the biological paradigm underlying contemporary medical science.

To study the borderline between formal and informal healthcare, it is important to understand the procedure of one or another method being integrated into conventional medicine. When can we say that such methods have become part of it? Common formal criteria are references in scientific publications, but judgments based on them can be misleading in Russia.

The fact is, marketing strategies for promoting non-conventional therapies are largely based on establishing in-house systems for generating knowledge and training personnel, which are identical to standard scientific procedures. Such systems are closed; their reputation is high only among their supporters, but not in the scientific community in general. An important role here is played by professional associations, independent institutions, departments in public medical schools, scientific journals, academic conferences, academic degrees, and patents. Such systems are sustainable and viable, since all ideas are discussed only "among themselves", i.e., by the proponents of a certain theory.

In post-Soviet Russia, the FCTRC TDTM (earlier—the Research Institute for Traditional Therapies; the Research and Development Center for Traditional Therapies and Homeopathy of the Russian Ministry of Health) used to be the main platform for evaluating the scientific validity of alternative therapies. It issued expert opinions and developed guidelines for the application of traditional therapies and licensing of associated medical services. Therefore, when the Center was closed in 2009, the professional complementary and alternative medicine community took it as a serious blow to its positions in the healthcare system. Beside the

Center, there were and still are many small independent entities generating formally scientific knowledge about non-conventional methods in medicine.

Thus, the Russian market of technical devices with dubious health-promoting effects (from Pankov's glasses and Kuznetsov's applicator to energy-informational protection and live blood analysis devices) has a standard procedure for their legitimation. A self-contained set of intellectual products developed by the author and his/her relatives or followers (patent for the invention, thesis, presentations at conferences organized with their participation, articles and books) provide the required scientific rationale and evidence of the device's efficacy.

Such techniques and inventions are vulnerable to external, independent scrutiny. However, in Russia internal scientific mechanisms of purging the academic community of pseudo-scientific concepts and sciolists often fail. The agencies whose function is to block unscrupulous research and erroneous theories (dissertation councils, editorial boards of academic journals, and others) do not always work properly. Like in other academic fields, this also happens in medicine (Aleksandrov, 2006; Vlassov, 2014).

An illustrative example is eLIBRARY.RU—a scientific electronic library integrated with the Russian Science Citation Index (RSCI). The availability of publications in this database is currently one of the principal tools for assessing the performance of publicly funded scientists in Russia. In response to a search query with the keyword "healer", the library displays over 300 publications (337 as at 13 August 2015). Of these, about two-thirds concern religious, esoteric and similar literature, which cannot be called scientific even with great reserve.

Determining whether certain therapies are recognized by conventional medicine or not, one must also take into account that on the individual level the attitude of Russian medical professionals to various non-conventional healing practices can be polar—from absolute rejection to approval and active participation.

So, the mere reference to a method of treatment in academic literature or the opinion of individual practicing physicians, who deem it to be "good", cannot be relied upon to determine the extent to which this method is integrated into orthodox medicine. Therefore, we are forced to use poorly measurable characteristics, such as a "footprint" in widespread medical practice and clinical guidelines, and the absence of an image of a marginal field of medical knowledge. Given that the state sets the standards of medical practice in Russia rather than the self-regulated professional community, reference to such therapies in the laws and regulations governing the work of physicians is also an important indicator. Finally, the position of the proponents of various therapies—whether they oppose them to the contemporary mainstream medicine or not—also matters.

*The attitude of the state*

In applying the third "informal healthcare" criterion (recognition by the state) we cannot restrict ourselves to two assessments only—legal/illegal, since this conceals the difference in the regulations governing particular activities. Certain practices associated with healthcare are prohibited in Russia, certain others are permitted subject to special conditions, and some are allowed under general requirements for business or social activities. Accordingly, the violations of these statutory provisions also differ, entailing different penalties and terms of punishment.

National specifics are also fundamentally important. The situation in different countries varies significantly depending on the economic model of healthcare, policies governing the provision of medical care, the status of the medical community, etc. For example, in Southeast Asia traditional Chinese medicine is integrated into the health system; it is recognized and taken into account wherever healthcare is provided. Even in countries with similar parameters, such as the UK and the US, the official status of alternative medicine professionals differs markedly (Saks, 2003).

The Russian legal framework identifies medicine with orthodox biomedicine. A clear evidence thereof is the definition of "health" provided in the Law *On the Fundamentals of Public Healthcare in the Russian Federation* (No. 323-FZ, Art. 2): health is "a state of physical, mental and social well-being of an individual characterized by the absence of disease or disorder of the functions of the body's organs and systems." Besides medical care, the notion of "health protection" also implies a complex of other measures undertaken by various authorities, organizations and the individuals themselves; however, other definitions of basic concepts (such as medical service or medical intervention) reduce any health maintenance activity to biomedicine.

Medical services and the market for medical products in Russia are strictly regulated—here, it is necessary to obtain a license (permission to engage in a certain activity), comply with specific premise and staff qualification requirements,[10] restrict advertising one's goods and services,[11] etc. The more regulatory requirements, the harder it is to comply with them. Therefore, very few alternative agents work legally and without violations.

As healthcare practices become professional and commercial, non-compliance with the legislation grows. There is a significant non-market segment in "informal healthcare", where these practices are either free of charge on a reciprocal basis or against small monetary or in-kind contributions. For instance, medical workers and witch doctors consult their neighbors in the villages in such a way. Often, they do not perceive such work as a separate service. However, as the client base expands and prices are set, the potential for violating the rules set by the state increases.

The principal business conflict here is the following: if certain services are advertised as therapeutic, they should be provided by certified health practitioners and the respective legal entity must be licensed to engage in medical activities. Where the services are not medical, advertising them as therapeutic misleads the consumer. The situation is similar with

---

10  For readers who are not familiar with Russian medical education, it makes sense to clarify that the basic education of physicians consists of three stages: medical school; obtaining a core medical specialty (internship or residency); obtaining a specialty requiring additional training, such as reflexology (as part of retraining, residency or postgraduate program). Physicians who have completed all these stages must confirm their qualifications and receive a respective certificate; moreover, they must do it on a regular basis throughout their career. Professional development courses are mandatory every five years. Therefore, the services of a doctor with specialized education, but *expired* certificate, are also a violation of the licensing requirements, as well as the work of a doctor without a diploma. Certification requirements also apply to nursing staff. Recently, the Russian system of medical education has been amended. With effect from 2016, internship has been abolished and certification has been replaced by accreditation of medical staff; however, the general principle of confirming regularly one's right to engage in medical practice remains.

11  Pursuant to Federal Law No. 38-FZ *On Advertising*, any advertisement of drugs, medical services (including methods of treatment) or medical equipment must contain a warning about the existing contraindications for their use or application and inform about the need to read carefully the patient information leaflet or consult a specialist (Art. 24, part 7). Since 2014, no prescription drugs, medical services or medical products, the use of which requires special training, may be advertised in the lay media (Art. 24, part 8).

health products. Medical products (drugs and medical devices) must undergo state registration and comply with particular provisions governing trade in such goods; promoting non-medical products as remedies against diseases is a violation of the law on advertising.

Due to the specifics of medical activity licensing in Russia, many suppliers of complementary health services (massage, for example) are forced out of the legal field. The problem is that the license is issued to a medical institution (a legal entity or a sole proprietor) rather than to an individual physician. Licensing requirements contain provisions as to the professional experience and educational background of the entity's head that can be hardly met by any private practice. Moreover, the license is issued to perform certain work or provide particular services in accordance with medical specialties. Therefore, the work of a reflex therapist in an organization holding a license, but for other services (e.g., neurology or general practice), will be a violation.

Another licensing requirement is the conformity of the declared premises to the stipulated area, condition, and equipment. As a result, the provision of authorized medical services is tied to a specific location. The list of "locations where medical activities will be performed" is included in the mandatory information package to be provided by the applicant for a license; any change in address necessitates renewal of the license. Accordingly, medical services provided at home or out of the office are considered to be administrative offenses, except in expressly stipulated cases.

In the regulatory framework, however, a license for medical activities is just the final step in assessing whether healthcare agents meet the statutory requirements for staff structure and qualifications, equipment, premises, and the scope of medical services. Those requirements that concern the integration of non-conventional therapies into medical practice are of key significance for our discussion about "informal healthcare". In the previous section we mentioned that recognition of alternative therapies by orthodox medicine is also reflected in the position of the state and is stipulated in laws and regulations. The bulk of them are departmental regulations (orders), primarily those that allow using certain methods in medical practice and establish medical specialties.

When analyzing how the state recognizes non-conventional medicine, it is important to bear in mind the time factor and the fact that the legislative work of any authority is far from the ideal picture where laws and regulations only capture the objective reality. The very authorization or banning (there were such precedents also) of such methods result from stakeholder lobbying or opposition. Therefore, with time, the state can change its attitude to certain alternative practices; their official status will change accordingly. A vivid example is the story of Scientology's detoxification method first admitted to Russian healthcare practice and then banned from it.[12]

In post-Soviet Russian history, two periods are identifiable in the state's attitude to non-conventional medicine. The first period lasted until the mid-2000s. At that time, alternative methods were extensively recognized as "traditional" and integrated into the official medical practice. Subsequently, the state strove to dissociate gradually such methods from conventional medicine. This can be traced by the regulations governing licensing of medical activities.

As can be seen from Table 1, the first post-Soviet list of medical activities subject to licensing (1996) contained a separate section *Traditional Medical Activities*. It was appended by *Recommended Criteria for Licensing Traditional Medical Activities* and a *Commentary to the List of Traditional Medical Activities* defining various methods and setting the requirements for the professionals who were applying them. The document is interesting by the fact that it classified most of the diagnostic and treatment methods then known by alternative medicine, including "treatment by 'concentrators' and 'transformers' of cosmic energy". This list threw open the doors of medical institutions to alternative therapies, barring only healing by prayers and magic. Since then, only graduates of medical and nursing schools were authorized to provide such services (in the case of phytotherapy—also certified pharmacists, and in the case of massage—

---

[12] The method of detoxification intended to treat drug addiction, exposure to radiation, and to purify the mind and body was developed by L. Ron Hubbard as part of his Dianetics theory. His followers from the Church of Scientology promoted it in Russia. On 5 August 1994, Vasily Agapov, Deputy Minister of Health and Medical Industry of the Russian Federation, approved the *Detoxification Program Guidelines*. Under these guidelines, detoxification programs were introduced at certain Russian health resort institutions and Scientology rehabilitation clinics were opened. However, two years later Agapov was dismissed from office and the Health Minister canceled the Guidelines by a special Order No. 254 of 19 June 1996. Pursuant to the Order, the heads of subordinated medical organizations were instructed to prevent the promotion and use of the Scientology and Dianetics methods.

also holders of diplomas of higher education in sports and fitness). The activities of healers without medical diplomas who had mastered Ayurveda, for example, at some private courses became illegal.

However, two years later, the Supreme Court of the Russian Federation declared the order null and void in respect of healing. The Ministry of Health had to amend it. In the new list of medical activities subject to licensing, alternative medicine was presented as "folk (traditional) medicine". The list of its specific types was further adjusted, but in general a license was required to engage in it.

Since 2002, regulations on licensing medical activities already distinguished manual therapy, reflexology (both activities were recognized as separate medical specialties in 1997), medical massage, classified within predoctor care, and "traditional medicine methods" without any internal differentiation. Finally, the latest list of works (services) pertaining to medical activities (2012) contains no reference whatsoever to "traditional medicine". The indication of traditional medicine as a separate branch of medical knowledge and practices disappeared from other regulatory acts as well.

Table 1. The evolution of the approach to licensing traditional medicine activities in the Russian legal framework

| Regulation | Quote with reference to traditional medicine in the list of licensed medical activities |
| --- | --- |
| Order of the Russian Ministry of Health and Medical Industry No. 270 of 1 July 1996<br><br>*On Approving the Tentative List of Medical Activities Subject to Licensing in the Russian Federation* | "1.9. Traditional medical activities:<br>- Acupuncture<br>- Homeopathy<br>- Manual therapy<br>- Traditional diagnostics<br>- Traditional healing systems<br>- Phytotherapy and treatment by other natural remedies<br>- Energy informational practice" |

| Regulation | Quote with reference to traditional medicine in the list of licensed medical activities |
|---|---|
| **Order of the Russian Ministry of Health No. 142 of 29 April 1998** *On the List of Medical Activities Subject to Licensing* | "8. Folk (traditional) medicine:<br>8.1. Leech therapy<br>8.2. Homeopathy<br>8.3. Manual therapy<br>8.4. Medical massage<br>8.5. Reflexology<br>8.6. Traditional diagnostics (authorized for use according to the legally established procedure)<br>8.7. Traditional healing systems (authorized for use according to the legally established procedure)" |
| **Decree of the Government of the Russian Federation No. 402 of 21 May 2001** *On Approving the Regulation on Licensing Medical Activities*<br><br>The list of works and services included in licensed medical activities | "Traditional medicine:<br>Bioresonance therapy<br>Homeopathy<br>Manual therapy<br>Medical massage<br>Natural therapies (phytotherapy, leech therapy and other methods authorized for use by the Russian Ministry of Health)<br>Reflexology<br>Traditional diagnostic methods authorized for use by the Russian Ministry of Health<br>Traditional healing systems authorized for use by the Russian Ministry of Health" |
| **Decree of the Government of the Russian Federation No. 499 of 4 July 2002** (as amended on 1 February 2005) *On Approving the Regulation on Licensing Medical Activities* | "3. Medical activities include medical work and services on providing predoctor, ambulance and emergency, outpatient, wellness, and inpatient (including expensive specialized) medical care in line with respective medical specialties, including preventive medical, diagnostic and therapeutic measures and medical examinations, **applying methods of traditional medicine**, and procuring organs and tissues for medical purposes." |

# GOALS AND TOOLS 23

| Regulation | Quote with reference to traditional medicine in the list of licensed medical activities |
|---|---|
| **Order of the Ministry of Health of the Russian Federation No. 238 of 26 July 2002** (as amended on 10 March 2006) *On the Procedure of Licensing Medical Activities* (with the *Nomenclature of Works and Services for Providing Appropriate Medical Care* and the *Regulation on the Central Commission for Licensing Medical Activities of the Ministry of Health of the Russian Federation*) | "In accordance with the Nomenclature of Works and Services for Providing Appropriate Medical Care (Appendix No. 1 to the Order of the Ministry of Health of the Russian Federation No. 238 of 26 July 2002), manual therapy shall be licensed under Sections 03.021, 04.014, and 05.012 ('work and services under the manual therapy specialty'), reflexology—under Sections 03.022, 04.026, and 05.013, and medical massage—under Section 01.006. Bioresonance therapy, homeopathy, natural therapies, and traditional diagnostics shall be licensed under Section 06.019—'work and services related to applying methods of traditional medicine'." <br><br> Already in 2006, the item "work and services related to applying methods of traditional medicine" was removed from the list of licensed medical activities along with several other activities (Order of the Russian Ministry of Health and Social Development No. 141 of 10 March 2006). |
| **Decree of the Government of the Russian Federation No. 30 of 22 January 2007** (as amended on 24 September 2010) *On Approving the Regulation on Licensing Medical Activities* List of works (services) when exercising medical activities | "Work (services): <br> Manual therapy <br> Medical massage <br> Methods of traditional medicine <br> Reflexology" <br> *(the types of works (services) are listed in the document in alphabetical order, without classifying "traditional medicine" in a separate section)* |
| **Decree of the Government of the Russian Federation No. 291 of 16 April 2012** (as amended on 17 January 2013) *On Licensing Medical Activities...* List of works (services) included in medical activities | "Work (services): <br> Manual therapy <br> Medical massage <br> Reflexology" <br> *(the types of works (services) are listed in the document in alphabetical order)* |

Thus, by 2013 the situation was as follows. "Traditional Medicine" as a legal concept had disappeared from the legal framework. Three activities that previously pertained to traditional medicine were fully integrated into formal healthcare: medical massage, manual therapy, and reflexology. Only medical professionals holding a valid certificate were authorized to engage in them. In the first case, a diploma of secondary medical education was sufficient, whereas in the two others—a diploma of higher medical education. An organization must obtain a license to provide services in this field. Accordingly, illegal massage, reflexology, and manual therapy practices include: work at home on a private basis with fees paid under the table; work in wellness centers and clinics that are not appropriately licensed to engage in such medical activities; work of service providers without medical diplomas or physicians without specialized training who hold no valid certificate of a massage therapist, reflex therapist or manual therapist; services of foreign specialists who hold no diploma of a Russian medical school or college (Chinese acupuncturists and Thai masseuses and masseurs).

The status of other activities that were previously included in the wording "applying methods of traditional medicine" remains unclear. Leech therapy, apitherapy, bioresonance therapy, and homeopathy services continue to be provided in clinics under licenses issued prior to 2012. At the same time, such services are stipulated by a relatively recent document regulating the procedure of medical rehabilitation (Order of the Russian Ministry of Health No. 1705n of 29 December 2012). According to the new rules, a clinic may provide such services if it holds a medical rehabilitation license.

Let us now look at the regulations governing the services of healers who have no established medical specialties and whose methods have not been integrated into the conventional medical practice in Russia. To begin with, the state acknowledges their existence for accounting and statistical research purposes. In the *Russian Classifier of Occupations* there is a sub-group within nursing staff *Folk Medicine Practitioners and Healers*. Furthermore, since 2015 the group *Physicians* includes a separate sub-group *Highly Skilled Healers and Alternative and Folk Medicine Practitioners*, such as Ayurveda practitioner, acupuncturist or naturopath.

The state recognizes folk medicine practice as part of healthcare and sets respective requirements for it. The very appearance of this term in legislation allowed distinguishing diagnostic and treatment services not backed by scientific evidence from conventional medical practice. It allowed putting them under control to prevent the potential risk of harming patients. I believe that the evolution of legal provisions in this sphere demonstrates the intention of the state to segregate folk medicine from healthcare services interpreted in the spirit of biomedicine and reduce it to nothing by making illegal.

The *Fundamental Principles of the Legislation of the Russian Federation on National Healthcare* adopted in 1993 referred to folk medicine and healing as synonyms.[13] Pursuant to this law, only certified healers were authorized to practice folk medicine. The Law stipulated that public clinics were allowed to use methods of folk medicine upon decision of hospital chief executives and according to the procedure established for unregistered diagnosis, prevention and treatment methods. In addition, the Law expressly prohibited healers to hold mass sessions, including through the media.

The authors of the new Law *On the Fundamentals of Public Healthcare in the Russian Federation* (No. 323–FZ), effective as of 2012, attempted to narrow down the scope of folk medicine and disassociate healing from official medicine, which is subject to the regulatory framework of healthcare. The word "healing" as such disappeared. Only Article 50 refers to folk medicine, and it expressly clarifies that folk medicine does not include "occult magic services or religious rituals". Since healing has ceased to be subject to regulation, the ban on mass healing sessions has also lost validity. The Law also states that folk medicine services are not covered by universal health insurance, and folk medicine practitioners are liable under the legislation of the Russian Federation for any damage to the life or health of their patients. Permits to engage in folk medicine replaced healer certificates, but the power to issue them remained with the regional authorities.

It is safe to assume that most healers and folk medicine practitioners used to work and are working in Russia illegally. First, there is no clear procedure for issuing permits by the regional authorities. Second, in most

---

13 The Law provided the following definition: "Folk medicine means wellness, prevention, diagnosis and treatment methods based on the experience of many generations, entrenched in national traditions and not registered according to the procedure established by the legislation of the Russian Federation" (Article 57).

cases practicing healers cannot comply with the requirements that the authorities impose on the applicants for permits (medical education, work as a legal entity or sole proprietor, dedicated premises, etc.).

In addition to diagnostic and treatment services provided by alternative medicine practitioners, "informal healthcare" includes a variety of other services and goods not associated with medicine (according to the authorities), which are nevertheless offered to the consumers as having a therapeutic effect. How legal are they? Activities in these areas should also be subject to certain legal provisions, but this is not always the case. The more extensive the regulations, the greater the scope of violations.

For example, dietary supplements are not medicines; however, sellers often attribute therapeutic properties to them in violation of the law on advertising. In Russia, the requirements for such products are less stringent than for drugs—they are also subject to state registration, but the procedure is easier, they must comply with the Sanitary Rules and Regulations (SanPiNs) and pass certification. Accordingly, the sale of unregistered dietary supplements is illegal. Trade regulations also create an extensive shadow market for dietary supplements. The Federal Service for Protecting Consumer Rights and Public Health (Rospotrebnadzor), the functions of which include registering and controlling the circulation of dietary supplements, relies on a departmental regulation—SanPiN 2.3.2.1290–03 *Requirements for the Circulation of Dietary Supplements*. The Regulation contains an exhaustive list of places authorized to sell such supplements: "pharmaceutical establishments (pharmacies, drug stores, pharmacy outlets, etc.), shops specializing in dietary products, food stores (specialized departments, sections, booths)". All other options—e-trade, direct selling, sale to acquaintances, at fairs, at consumer goods stores or even in supermarkets without a specialized section or department—are an offense.

Production and sales of health products for external use are much less regulated, if only they are not registered as medical products. Such "healing" goods are formally classified as cosmetics, household appliances, etc. They are of interest to the state only in terms of protecting consumer rights in general and controlling advertising. As a result, situations emerge when law enforcement bodies cannot hold liable the seller of a "healing wonder device" who had sold it to an elderly person for a fortune, even if the disappointed buyer did not experience any therapeutic effect and filed a complaint with the police.

No specific restrictions apply to harvesting gifts of nature for their subsequent use or sale as medicine. The *Forest Code of the Russian Federation* differentiates harvesting of medicinal plants and non-timber forest products for commercial purposes and for personal needs. The former case requires formal lease of forest land parcels; in the latter case, harvesting is free of charge and requires no formal permits. Since 2007, harvesting rules for personal needs are established by the legislation of the constituent entities of the Russian Federation. In particular, the Perm Territory allows picking wild plants only during specified periods and "in a way excluding the depletion of natural resources"; however, it sets no harvesting limits. Therefore, gathering is a legal side job for the rural population, and for some low-income or jobless people it is the main seasonal occupation, even though the amounts harvested may significantly exceed "personal needs". An exception is gathering plants listed in the *Red Data Book* of endangered species, as well as those that are recognized as narcotics.

Hunters run a much higher risk of breaking the law than gatherers. According to the *Law on Hunting and Preserving Hunting Resources* (No. 209–FZ), hunting requires a hunting ticket, a registered weapon, licenses to kill specified animal species, and compliance with rigid hunting seasons and bag and size limits. Moreover, completely legal hunting is nowadays quite a costly affair. So, to procure any valuable health products for sale, with the proceeds becoming a substantial item of income, the hunter is forced to poach. Further, some animals are especially valued for health purposes, and this is the cause of their extermination. They are generally protected by the state as endangered species—their hunting is restricted or even prohibited, just as trade in their derivatives. This applies primarily to those animals whose derivatives are used in traditional Chinese medicine. There is always high demand for them in East Asia. Their export is prohibited or subject to quotas under CITES. This has triggered the emergence of extensive black markets for products of poaching and smuggling (Homes, 2004; Burgess, Stoner, Foley, 2014).

On the contrary, private beekeeping is not subject to any serious restrictions. Like gathering for personal needs and individual hunting, beekeeping on the household level is not classified as a business activity. But the situation changes as soon as the beekeeper, hunter or herbalist bring their products to the market. Here they face two regulatory requirements: the veterinary-sanitary inspection must certify that their goods are safe for consumers, and the goods must be sold in designated places. Both requirements mean additional work and expenses. Sellers with no legal business status try to evade these requirements and join the ranks of those engaged in unauthorized trader, i.e. trade outside the established market places and sites designated by the local authorities. In Russia, peddling most foodstuffs from door to door, vending them in public transport or in the street is forbidden on a par with drugs and medical devices.

The procedure for legalizing occult services, which currently include treatment by magic or psychic therapy, is different from that stipulated for practicing folk medicine. The only requirements are to incorporate a legal entity for business purposes and register with the tax authorities and the statistics service. No special education, qualifications or compliance with established standards for premises are needed in this case. The only restriction meaningful in the context of our study is that individuals not authorized to practice folk medicine may not advertise their activity as health services.[14] However, most psychics in Russia do not register their activity and pay no taxes, thus joining the ranks of shadow sector agents.

"Informal healthcare" agents have even more freedom of action, if they offer patients ideas and rituals of treatment and are registered as NPOs rather than business entities. In accordance with the freedom of conscience principle, dissemination of spiritual teachings is regulated in the Russian Federation only by laws on nonprofit and religious organizations. The substance of these teachings, except for propaganda of extremism, may not be censored. Complaints regarding the health practices of such NPOs may be filed only in the following cases: 1) religious organizations openly advertise their activities as treatment, i.e. as medical services that require a license; 2) their activities threaten the health of their followers, thus falling under the definition of extremism; 3) they engage in illegal business. For this reason, church shops are forced to call their price

---

14 For example, in 2012 a commission of one of the regional antimonopoly service offices found the following ad inappropriate: "ALL KINDS OF MAGIC. Breaking hex spells, evil eye and other curses. PROTECTION. Alternative medicine. Talismans. Amulets. Clairvoyance. Tarot cards. Runes....". The decision was based on the grounds that "the list of advertised services includes alternative medicine, a reference to which may mislead the consumers into believing that they are offered services pertaining to traditional medicine".
URL: http://www.regionfas.ru/39/9124.

tags "recommended donations". In general, state control over this segment of "informal healthcare" is minimal, and this determines its significant impact on health practices in Russia.

Finally, the state imposes no special requirements on the media offering its audience information that is used for self-treatment. This market is subject only to the general requirements for the publishing business, the media, advertising and so on. At best, the information provider makes a disclaimer as when advertising drugs: "You are recommended to consult your doctor" or "This information is not a handbook on self-treatment".

The evolution of regulatory requirements has a serious impact on the expansion of the shadow segment of "informal healthcare". This is the case when legislative changes force formerly legal suppliers of goods and services either to abandon their occupation or move into the shadow.

In the context of improving the system of training health professionals, since 2000, doctor subspecialties in Russia are rigidly mapped to particular major specialties. Only a neurologist by training may engage in reflexology and only a psychiatrist may work as narcologist. Therefore, many professionals who complied with the previous requirements and worked in the market legally, now lost their formal status.

Another example is state control over medical products. Many health devices with dubious efficacy had been previously registered as medical devices in Russia. Hence, methods based on controversial scientific theories penetrated medical practice. Since 2013, the requirements for the pre-registration safety and efficacy appraisal of medical products have become more stringent. Eventually, this will have the same effect as that from excluding traditional medicine from licensed medical activities—non-conventional diagnostic and treatment methods will be eliminated from medical practice. In addition, the Russian government explicitly banned peddling of medical products in January 2015. Consequently, not only widespread direct selling of therapeutic massagers, portable physiotherapy devices, and bioenergy shields became illegal, but also itinerant markets for hearing aids.

In view of all these legal provisions and requirements the reader may very well wonder: if some practices are prohibited and thus illegal, why are they nevertheless flourishing in Russia? After all, the society does not even perceive many of them as something reprehensible.

Here we are dealing with the paradox of public administration in ensuring people's safety. The regulatory requirements and prohibitions are intended to serve the good cause of protecting the life and health of the population. Theoretically, a person without medical training and certified skills can harm the patient in the process of treatment, even if it is only massage; unknown herbs bought from an elderly woman on the roadside can cause food poisoning, etc. However, the supervisory authorities do not have the adequate resources to reveal and stop such activities. Therefore, in the absence of direct complaints from consumers, obvious crimes (death or serious harm to the patient or consumer) or the need for show trials, they prefer to turn a blind eye to the violations.

The role of the state in prosecuting illegal activity manifests itself there, where a governing body can easily realize its control and supervisory function, rather than there, where the violations are serious and numerous. When it comes to medical activities, regulation primarily concerns public health and social care facilities subject to regular inspections by the Federal Service for the Supervision of Public Health and Social Development (Roszdravnadzor) for compliance with licensing terms. It is easier to prove their guilt than to expose the illegal medical services of a masseur or healer quietly practicing at home. In the case of dietary supplements, Rospotrebnadzor regularly inspects pharmacies, but this has absolutely no impact on shadow trade. Another tool is performing inspections following people's complaints. Their number is negligible because people rarely complain to the supervisory authorities, even if they have a claim to the suppliers of "informal healthcare" goods and services. Thus, Rospotrebnadzor's regional office for the Perm Territory annually receives only two-three complaints against vendors of dietary supplements, and usually such complaints are filed by residents of the regional capital. No complaints ever come from the branch offices located throughout the Territory.

The last nuance pertaining to the legality/illegality of the activities in the field of research is as follows. Besides non-compliance with health legislation and other special requirements, shadow practices common for Russian business in general are also widespread here: tax evasion, failure to prepare and submit financial statements and statistical reports; business without incorporating a legal entity or work through fly-by-night entities and so on. Note that in addition to the commercial activities of market agents that violate legal provisions, the scope of "informal healthcare" also embraces healing practices that can be attributed to the gift or household economy (besides the above mentioned gratuitous aid of rural healers, it includes sharing recipes and tips, harvesting medicinal plants for personal needs, activities of informal health groups and representatives of various self-healing doctrines, etc.). In view of the above, we can safely say that "informal healthcare" is largely a part of the informal economy. In this context, informal economy means "the diversity of qualitatively different types of activity united by their distance (total or partial) from state regulation and statistics" (Barsukova, 2003, p. 23).

The diversity of health management methods within the scope of "informal healthcare" is expressed in time, money and other costs. Their extent is concealed from the authorities, since they are not reflected in official statistical records. Accordingly, they are not considered when developing and implementing the national health policy, although in fact "informal healthcare" covers part of the state's unfulfilled social obligations and to a certain extent contributes to maintaining the health of the population.

\* \* \*

Applying the selected criteria for including certain phenomena in "informal healthcare", we can distinguish the core of illegal and dangerous practices, as perceived by orthodox medicine, as well as interim areas more or less close to the officially recognized medical or recreational activities. The borderline between this sphere and conventional healthcare is flexible and often depends on the situation, including legislative developments and the life circumstances of individual providers of health goods and services. Therefore, no description of "informal healthcare" will be complete without a review of the border zones.

A certain systematization is also needed to depict "informal healthcare" phenomena. I believe that due to the above nuances in determining the boundaries of this sphere, any streamlining will serve the sole purpose of facilitating research. In any case, a classification is an artificial, analytical construct applied to the diversity of human practices.

Here we should clarify why the generally accepted approach to the classification of non-conventional health practices by treatment method is not applicable in this case. It is essentially based on the logic inherent in orthodox medicine. It is common to distinguish acupuncture, naturopathy, manual therapy and faith healing (healing by prayer) within alternative/traditional/folk medicine. People use this classification most often with reference to the WHO, emphasizing that complementary and alternative medicine fields are largely heteronomous, and each country may have its own unique internal structure of this sphere. Researchers that undertake quantitative measurements face a variety of interpretations and are forced to introduce their own typologies. Several examples of different classifications are provided below.

- The guidelines on licensing works and services related to applying methods of traditional medicine in Russia included the following fields: bioresonance therapy, homeopathy, manual therapy, medical massage, natural therapies (phytotherapy, leech therapy, apitherapy and other methods of treatment by natural remedies authorized for use by the Russian Ministry of Health), reflexology, traditional diagnostic methods authorized for use by the Russian Ministry of Health, traditional healing systems (Karpeev, Kiseleva, 2003).
- In 1990, a sociological survey was held in the USA on non-conventional therapy preferences. The survey used the following classification: relaxation techniques, chiropractic, massage, imagery, spiritual healing, commercial weight-loss programs, lifestyle diets (e.g., macrobiotics), herbal medicine, megavitamin therapy, self-help groups, energy healing, biofeedback, hypnosis, homeopathy, acupuncture, folk remedies, exercise, and prayer (Eisenberg et al., 1993).
- The classification used for another widely known sociological survey of CAM use among the U.S. public included twenty-seven CAM therapies, of them ten types of provider-based therapies and seventeen therapies for which the services of a provider are not necessary. All these types were classified into groups based on the method of treatment: biologically based therapies (diets, natural products, folk medicine and others); manipulative and body-based therapies (chiropractic care, massage and others); and mind-body therapies (hypnosis, yoga, prayer, meditation, deep breathing exercises and others). However, the researchers had to add separately "alternative medical systems" that did not fit into this classification: Ayurveda, acupuncture, homeopathic treatment, and naturopathy (Barnes et al., 2004).

- Brian Hughes performed a regression analysis of the correlation between CAM availability and religious affiliation of the Irish public. He distinguished the following CAM types: traditional Chinese medicine, acupuncture, shiatsu, kinesiology, Reiki, yoga, aromatherapy, reflexology, alternative chiropody, spiritual healing, colonic irrigation, meditative healing, and hypnotherapeutic healing (Hughes, 2006).

The trouble with this biomedical approach is that in real life the adherents and providers of such services combine different methods (massage plus prayer plus herbs and so on). The logic of the scientific classification of knowledge underlying biomedicine may be alien to them and they may not see the need to follow it. Another problem is the competition among providers of goods and services, which stimulates the ongoing production of new therapies isolated from their parent field.

In an effort to circumvent these difficulties, anthropologists and sociologists turned to medical systems that are defined as historically established systems of knowledge and practices, which combine different methods of diagnosis and treatment (traditional Chinese medicine, Ayurveda, Arabic medicine, ancient Slavic medicine, etc.). However, classifying nonconventional medicine by health system can be useful for the analysis of traditional societies. In the contemporary multicultural world, different health systems not only coexist in one country, but are also constantly developed and compiled.

Another reason why such classifications do not serve the purpose of this work is that our description focuses not on health practices but on the associated providers of goods and services. In this context, we decided to classify "informal healthcare" agents by the principal product they offer to the consumers: manufactured goods, natural products, ideas/doctrines, services, and information. Thus, we can distinguish five major segments within "informal healthcare":

- Production and distribution of health products
- Harvesting and distribution of medicinal gifts of nature
- Treatment services
- Religious practices and health doctrines
- Provision of information for alternative treatment

This segmentation is largely relative, since "informal healthcare" agents often offer products of different nature. However, it allows identifying a general trend. Successful players in these markets seek to diversify their activities to meet all the demands of their customers and thus prevent them from turning to formal healthcare or other agents.

This is clearly visible on the example of companies engaged in direct sales of health products. Such vendors of goods strive to build a comprehensive health system alternative to public healthcare with their own concepts of human health, diagnostics, health services and their own periodicals. For their part, spiritual movements and religious organizations, in addition to the main function of disseminating ideas and rituals, establish their own production and distribution networks for health products. Russian authors of treatment techniques and health appliances open their own clinics and offer training courses for doctors. Famous healers, in addition to treating patients, write books, sell branded herbal remedies or healing amulets, hold seminars all over the country, and establish regional communities of their followers and disciples.

Thus, we can see that the activities of agents from different segments reproduce one and the same framework consisting of a variety of businesses and social activities. We should emphasize that such multidisciplinary agents are the most conspicuous and noticeable, but by far not the only providers in "informal healthcare" markets.

## 1.3. "Informal healthcare" drivers

*Assumptions*
It is widely believed that the main reason for the development of alternative healthcare is dissatisfaction with conventional medicine. This correlation is so obvious that it tends to be banal. However, what is actually meant by dissatisfaction? The popularity of non-conventional techniques in present-day Russia coincided with a sharp decline in public funding of healthcare. In the public sphere this was perceived as a direct consequence of reduced availability of high quality medical care for the population.

In 2010-2012, together with colleagues from the NRU HSE Laboratory for Local Administration we studied healthcare in rural areas and small towns of Russia (Kordonsky et al., 2011; *The Health Maintenance System,* 2012). The findings of the studies supported this opinion. It seems only logical for alternative practices to substitute conventional healthcare in response to a permanently shrinking scope of public healthcare services in small localities.

During fieldwork in the Kama area in 2013, we aimed to test this correlation by comparing the extent and diversity of "informal healthcare" phenomena in various localities—from small villages to a million-plus city.

Apart from the size, the administrative status of the locality is of significance (administrative center of a constituent entity of the Russian Federation, urban district, center of a municipal district, center of a rural settlement).[15] It matters primarily because the allocation of public healthcare resources traditionally depends on the status of the settlement.

So, we tentatively assumed that the development of "informal healthcare" is driven by the poor availability of high quality medical care due to the geographical remoteness of the settlement and/or inadequate infrastructure of formal healthcare. Based on common sense, the following factors also matter:

- Health problems of the population
- Susceptibility of the people to spiritual and non-scientific ideas
- Adequate income levels that allow people to invest time and money in health
- Availability of specific natural and other resources, which can serve as a basis for health services

The size and status of the localities were the main parameters for comparison during fieldwork. In general, all the listed factors depend on them: in major cities, personal income levels are higher, formal healthcare is more available, and the social infrastructure for maintaining a healthy lifestyle is better developed. However, certain external factors can distort this typical picture. We strove to minimize such factors when determining the geography of research.[16]

Besides Perm (the administrative center of the Perm Territory), we selected areas with relatively average indicators in terms of economic development, social sphere and public health, as well as with average distances to Perm: an agricultural area in the southeast and an industrial one

---

15 Russian legislation stipulated the following territorial organization of local government in 2013. Urban and rural settlements form the lower level of a municipality. The territory of one settlement may include several localities. The upper level of the municipality consists of municipal and urban districts.

16 Therefore, we initially excluded from the list remote depressive districts in the north and the north-east of the Perm Territory where even in the district centers the living standards are markedly lower than in the villages in the central part of the region. We also excluded Perm's dacha suburbs where the inhabitants extensively use the resources and infrastructure of the million–plus city.

in the northeast of the region. In the first case, it is the town of Kungur, where the food industry, manufacturing, and trade are the main sectors of the economy, and four surrounding agricultural areas—the Kungur, Suksun, Orda, and Kishert districts. In the second case, we chose the towns of Lysva and Chusovoy—two centers of the iron and steel industry located 13 km apart—and their respective districts[17], where agriculture is less developed and the density of the population is lower than in the first case. Selected statistical data on the situation in the surveyed municipalities is provided in Table 2.

---

17  In 2012, the Lysva municipal district received the status of urban district.

Table 2. Selected socio-economic and healthcare indicators in the surveyed municipalities of the Perm Territory[18]

| Municipality | Population (persons, at 01.01.2014)[19] | Retail trade turnover, RUB mln, 2013 | Volume of paid services to the population, RUB mln, 2013 | Average monthly salary of employees (without small businesses), RUB, 2013 | Number of hospital beds per 10,000 people, 2013 | Number of doctors per 10,000 people, 2013 | Mortality rate of the working population from all causes per 100,000 people, 2012 | Total score in the regional rating of healthcare performance indicators, 2012[20] |
|---|---|---|---|---|---|---|---|---|
| Perm urban district | 1,026,481 | 304,920.3 | 93,518.6 | 33,156.5 | 117.6 | 70.4 | 496.2 | 54 |
| Kungur urban district | 66,765 | 8,730.5 | 2,189.8 | 24,258.5 | 64.4 | 32.7 | 494.9 | 51 |
| Lysva urban district | 75,586 (64,038) | 8,847.7 | 962.5 | 20,089.2 | 88.8 | 34.1 | 671.5 | 34 |
| Chusovoy district | 69,524 (50,451) | 5,895.3 | 2,337.7 | 21,829.0 | 49.2 | 30.6 | 664.5 | 35 |
| Kungur district | 43,088 | 1,227.7 | 245.4 | 16,969.4 | 29.0 | 22.5 | 636.0 | 42 |
| Suksun district | 19,760 | 1,181.1 | 648 | 18,190.1 | 41.0 | 29.9 | 675.0 | 40 |
| Kishert district | 12,330 | 469.9 | 76.2 | 17,691.7 | 45.4 | 28.4 | 851.4 | 28 |
| Orda district | 15,248 | 639.2 | 103.3 | 19,739.1 | 44.6 | 23.6 | 844.7 | 41 |
| *Perm Territory (total)* | 2,636,154 | 453,294.5 | 124,279.1 | 28,020.3 | 86.3 | 49.9 | 667.0 | 36 |

18 Sources: the Rosstat *Municipality Indicators* database; *The Statistical Yearbook of the Perm Territory—2014*; the official website of the Ministry of Health of the Perm Territory.
19 The figures in parentheses indicate the population of the cities Lysva and Chusovoy (with Lyamino suburb).
20 The latest rating of healthcare performance indicators by Perm Territory municipality is available on the website of the regional Health Ministry only for 2012.

*The state of healthcare and the availability of medical care*
It is common knowledge that the smaller the locality in Russia, the less opportunities its inhabitants have to receive specialized care, including consultations of specialist physicians and diagnostic tests (Burdyak, Selezneva, Shishkin, 2008; Cherkashina, 2014). Moreover, in order to consult the required doctor, villagers have to bear the expenses of traveling to the district or regional center. On site, only primary medical care is available either at the local hospital, rural outpatient clinic, or health post (feldsher-midwife post, or FAP in Russian). A village or small settlement may even have no FAP.

For example, in one of the surveyed villages the FAP was closed back in 1975. Once a week a feldsher (i.e., a paramedical practitioner) comes from the neighboring village to treat the locals. These villagers used to have no access to the district health center without a referral from the feldsher; now "everyone shows understanding", and they are admitted without any referral. Drugs can be purchased also only in the district center. In another village, the FAP had also been closed. However, a representative of the local administration claims that the residents are experiencing no healthcare problems. Following is his view of a normal availability of healthcare services:

> The locals do not resort to non-conventional medicine. I believe that only outsiders do. They want to get cured as soon as possible, whereas the locals go to doctors. At present, we have no FAP. There is the building, of course, but no specialist; so, the situation is not very good. Once per month our assigned therapist comes to receive patients. When there is an opportunity, he refers the patients to specialist physicians; when there is none, consults them himself. That's it.[21]

In turn, municipal district centers offer less health care opportunities than towns with the status of an urban district. In recent years, inter-district specialized medical care centers are being established on the basis of town hospitals. This means that additional funding is channeled there, whereas resources in the rural areas are shrinking. In addition, such towns have some private medical providers, so patients can pay out of their pocket for services unavailable under compulsory medical insurance.

However, a full-scale system of specialized medical care, including treatment of complex cases, exists only in the regional center. Although

---

21   Informant: male, 55–60 years old, official of the rural administration, village.

the above mentioned inter-district centers concentrate human resources and equipment, in fact they do not provide comprehensive specialized care to the residents of the neighboring rural areas.

The difference in the resource provisioning of urban and rural healthcare is visible not only in absolute but also in relative terms. According to the office of the Federal State Statistics Service for the Perm Territory (Permstat), as at 2013, the regional capital's inpatient capacity per 10,000 residents was from two and a half to three times higher than that in the surveyed rural areas. A similar difference was registered for the number of doctors per 10,000 people. This difference could be attributed to the fact that medical centers serving the population of the entire region are located in Perm. However, better staffing and inpatient care capacities, albeit with a lesser gap, are noticeable when comparing rural districts with urban municipalities. It is therefore not surprising that Perm's urban healthcare system scores higher in the rating of municipalities drawn up by the regional Ministry of Health (see Table 2).

*Health problems of the population*
Hypothetically, the poor health of the population raises the demand for all kinds of therapeutic services, including alternative ones, especially if it concerns chronic or terminal illnesses. Although the ecology in the countryside is better than in the towns, low availability of quality medical care and timely diagnostics, as well as hard manual labor determine the increased need in treatment and the higher rate of chronic diseases. The very lifestyle also negatively affects the health of the population in rural areas. As one of our informants—a doctor—noted,

> The health of the rural population is always poorer than that of the urban population, because the villagers have no time for themselves and no time to take care of their own health.[22]

It hardly makes sense to rely on the official statistics on morbidity and disability. It reflects the performance of medical institutions rather than the actual number of sick people, because it is formed on the basis of patients' visits to healthcare facilities (Krasheninnikova, 2011).

---

22  Informant: female, 30–40 years old, otolaryngologist, medium-sized town.

We should also bear in mind that the morbidity statistics is generated on the level of the central district hospital (CDH) serving the population of the municipal district. As a result, on paper the differences between the localities are leveled off. Actually, the share of seriously ill people in remote villages, which the doctor visits once a month and where elderly residents prevail, may be higher than in the district center.

According to demographic indicators, villagers in general live less and more often die before reaching retirement age. In the Russian Federation, urban residents have a higher life expectancy at birth than the rural ones. According to Rosstat, the difference in the recent decade exceeded two years. In the Perm Territory, this difference is even more pronounced: as at 2012—3 years (for Russia—2.22). The mortality rate of the working population per 100,000 people (as per available statistics for the surveyed municipalities) also shows a significant difference between a major city and rural areas (see Table 2).

*Personal income levels*

Why can the income level be a sensitive "informal healthcare" driver? It affects personal healthcare behavior in general, allowing individuals to satisfy needs not covered by public healthcare out of their pocket. The Russian public opinion combines a Soviet attitude to health as subject to the care of the State and a capitalist perception of the need to invest personally in health. The second strategy implies the availability of time and money for this. Therefore, nowadays people with higher incomes pay more attention to their health. Our physician informants also mentioned this as a trend of the recent decade. One of them noted:

> Especially the rich people have started taking care of their own health, because they have the money. People with modest incomes have no means to follow the recommendations of modern medicine.[23]

Dependence of income levels on the size of the locality is also clearly traceable in the surveyed areas. In 2012, the contrast between rural areas and the administrative center of the Perm Territory was striking—there was approximately a two-fold difference in the average nominal monthly salaries of employees (exclusive of small businesses). In 2013, the gap slightly narrowed, but was still considerable. Judging by the official statis-

---

23   Informant: female, about 50 years old, neurologist, medium-sized town.

tics, without taking into account informal employment and shadow incomes, Perm leads by the business activity of the population, the volume of paid services, and retail trade turnovers, i.e. by the parameters that are an indirect evidence of income (see Table 2).

*Specific natural and other resources, which can serve as a basis for health services*

If the previous factors are expected to increase the demand for goods and services of "informal healthcare" agents, here we are speaking about the natural capacity to generate supply. By capacity we mean both unique natural resources known to have healing properties (mineral waters, etc.) and the simple local availability of premises for a healthy lifestyle business. Here, the correlation with the size and status of the locality is not as clear-cut as for the previous factors.

Sports and recreation facilities, which can serve as a basis for the promotion of "informal healthcare" services, are more developed in urban than in rural areas. This is particularly true for private fitness centers, beauty parlors, sports clubs, swimming pools, and with certain exceptions, public resources such as municipal sports and recreation centers. For example, over 70 fitness centers (independent or as part of a sports facility) function in Perm. For a fee, anyone may train there. The surveyed medium-sized towns have no more than a dozen of them. In rural areas, a private fitness industry, which is not tourist-focused, is lacking altogether. There, promotion of a healthy lifestyle is solely the responsibility of the local authorities, and they perform this function to the extent of their financial capacity.

Certain specific resources do not depend on the size or status of the locality. We therefore selected for our fieldwork localities of a similar size with and without such resources. In the first case these were:

- Local peloids and mineral springs (two spa facilities in the Suksun and Kishert districts)
- Religious symbols, which are attributed healing powers (two Orthodox monasteries and a convent in the Kungur and Chusovoy districts)
- Natural anomalies (the Perm anomalous zone near Molebka village and the Kungur ice cave)

*Susceptibility of the people to spiritual and non-scientific ideas*
Orthodox medicine does not accept treatment methods that do not survive the scrutiny of rational thinking and scientific reasoning. Accordingly, if people resort to such methods, this may be due to certain features of their world view: piety, reliance on esoteric knowledge, and a skeptical attitude to modern science.

It is, however, difficult to identify the relation between the type of settlement and such features of the people's mindset. Available data of Russian national opinion polls give no indication that rural and urban residents have a substantially different attitude to religion.[24] Neither is there any clear evidence that the size of the locality determines the trend for a weaker or stronger faith in paranormal phenomena.[25]

There are differences in the average educational level of the population. According to the Russian population census of 2010, the proportion of people with higher education is substantially greater in urban areas than in the rural ones: 22.4% against 9.2%, respectively. However, higher education does not in itself generate skepticism towards methods of treatment that are not evidence based. On the contrary, our communication with adherents of self-healing doctrines and distributors of dubious (according to official medicine) devices demonstrated that there were many professionals in science and technology, teachers, and medical workers among them. Obviously, the total number of people potentially interested in alternative methods of treatment will certainly be higher in a large city than in a small village, but that is a different story.

---

24  For example, a survey conducted by the Levada Center in 2009 produced the following percentages of respondents who do not consider themselves religious: 21.8% in Moscow; 17.6% in cities with a population of over 500,000; 19.8% in cities with a population from 100,000 to 500,000; 18.2% in towns with a population under 100,000; and 18% in the rural areas. See *Courier 2009–07*. United Archive of Economic and Sociological Data. URL: http://sophist.hse.ru.

25  According to a 2011 survey of the Levada Center, the larger the city, the more people believe in the predictions of astrologers. No apparent correlation was revealed with regard to other paranormal phenomena, such as prophetic dreams, omens, or "eternal life". See *Courier 2011–03*. United Archive of Economic and Sociological Data. URL: http://sophist.hse.ru.

*The situation in localities of different size and status: comparison results*
In general, based on empirical data obtained in the Kama area we can state that the magnitude of "informal healthcare" and the diversity of activities on providing health goods and services is higher in the urban environment than in the countryside. Primarily this concerns commercial practices. This refutes the initial hypothesis that poor availability of formal medical care is one of the main incentives for the development of the environment that is the subject of our study.

Table 3 illustrates the above by providing the average numbers of certain "informal healthcare" agents and sites for their activities which we observed in the course of fieldwork in the surveyed localities.

Table 3. The average number of "informal healthcare" agents and sites for their work in the surveyed localities (2013)

| Suppliers of "informal healthcare" goods and services | Perm (1 million inhabitants) | Towns (<50,000) | District centers (>10,000) | Center of a rural settlement (>3,000) | Village within a rural settlement (>500) |
|---|---|---|---|---|---|
| Direct sellers of health products (number of companies) | ≥35 | 7–10 | 3–5 | 0–1 | 0 |
| Alternative medicine clinics | ≥10 | 1–2 | 0 | 0 | 0 |
| People using paranormal abilities/phenomena for treatment (healers, bonesetters, psychics) | < 35 | 4–7 | 2–5 | 0–2 | 0–2 |
| Massage parlors | About 30 | 5–7 | 0–1 | 0–1 | 0 |
| Yoga studios | ≥55 | 2–4 | 0 | 0 | 0 |
| Followers of self-healing and esoteric doctrines, number of groups | ≥15 | 2–5 | 0–2 | 0 | 0 |
| Health literature and press sales outlets | <200 newsstands; <60 book shops; 65 post offices | 8 post offices; up to 15 newsstands; 3–5 book shops | 1 shop; 1–3 newsstands; 1–2 post offices | 1 post office | 0 |

The most extensive and diversified commercial practices are observed in the regional center where public healthcare is significantly better developed than in any other locality of the Perm Territory. This applies to all segments of "informal healthcare" that we distinguish.

Thus, Perm has considerably more agents dealing in non-medicinal goods, which are deemed to have healing properties, than the other surveyed localities. We identified over fifty continuously operating companies, of them thirty-five engaged in direct selling. In addition to a network of independent distributors, many of them have dealerships, consulting offices, exhibition halls, and permanent specialized departments in large shopping centers. In the city, such companies can have from seven-eight to over ten sales outlets each.

The sales channels are also most diversified in big cities. Besides the sales outlets of network marketing companies, there are local online stores and small shops offering health products from different manufacturers—all of them serving the urban fashion for a healthy lifestyle in its different variations. Itinerant trade is also available—in some palaces of culture, at the central city market or at organized trade fairs.

In rural areas, the range of vendors selling dietary supplements and other health products shrinks dramatically. In district centers, itinerant traders—vendors of various remedies, therapeutic devices, and hearing aids—play an important role. They visit the towns on a weekly, monthly or semi-annual basis. They do not appear regularly in small settlements and villages, apparently because there are too few consumers of their goods and services.

In large cities, health services based on paranormal abilities and phenomena, as well as on methods of traditional (alternative) medicine, are also better developed. A monitoring of commercial ads revealed that at least thirty-five psychics, healers, and magicians were providing fee-based services in Perm. There are also at least a dozen witch doctors who do not advertise their services. In all the surveyed medium-sized towns and district centers, we located from two to seven well-known witch doctors, who use spells, magical rituals or their own original manual therapy or osteopathy techniques to treat patients. Some types of alternative medicine services, like homeopathic consultations, exist only in Perm. We found no homeopaths in any other surveyed locality. Those very rare rural residents who are particularly interested in their health and do not trust orthodox medicine travel to district centers to consult with a homeopath.

A fancy for oriental health practices is also a purely urban phenomenon. We will illustrate this on the example of yoga. In 2013, Perm had at least thirty fitness centers and sports clubs with yoga classes. In addition, about twenty specialized studios were offering advanced courses of yoga or other oriental health practices. At least six organizations and informal movements related to certain spiritual teachings also promoted yoga as a healthy lifestyle. This data pertains only to agents that advertise their services without taking into account informal activities which are conducted in private. For comparison: in Lysva we managed to detect only two trainers, who were offering their services in four sports and recreation centers; in Kungur—three, of whom two left the town the same year (2013); and in Chusovoy—only one. If such services exist in other localities, they are not advertised.

Due to TV and the Internet, the market for information on self-treatment has become nationwide, thus mitigating the difference between the city and the village. However, judging by the number of sales outlets and the choice of literature in book stores and church shops, the segment of printed matter is more developed in the cities. In rural areas, the lack of information is compensated by municipal libraries that house health clubs and groups for socializing. This is where the local residents (primarily retired women) learn about original self-healing techniques, look up and share folk medicine recipes.

Perhaps the only thing that is more developed in the countryside is gathering natural remedies. However, the distribution and consumption of medicinal herbs and other gifts of nature here is largely situational. In a municipal district, only a handful of people are professionally engaged in herbalism, treatment with bee products or animal derivatives.

The situation turned out to be the most interesting in towns with a population of 50,000-70,000 people (Kungur, Lysva, and Chusovoy). Such places become centers of "informal healthcare" markets serving nearby rural areas. For example, vendors of dietary supplements from Kungur travel to neighboring district centers to sell their products at local marketplaces or though acquaintances. On the other hand, rural residents go to Kungur to sell bee products and other natural remedies at unauthorized sales points. Besides, traveling alternative medicine specialists, propagators of doctrines and ideas, and vendors of medicinal balms and devices include such towns in their itineraries. Usually they place advertisements not only in the local newspaper, but also in the press of the neighboring areas to draw the attention of rural residents. Finally, these places attract solitary representatives of practices and services exported from major cities. They attempt to establish branches of esoteric centers from Perm, organize seminars of Indian astrologers or lectures of Protestant preaching healers, and so forth.

So, the initial assumption that the worse the situation with formal healthcare, the more people turn to substituting agents of "informal healthcare" was not confirmed.

In the process of gathering empirical data, we did not intentionally clarify the motivation driving the consumers of "informal healthcare" goods and services, since we originally focused our attention on the activities of the suppliers. Nevertheless, although the question about the reason for resorting to alternative agents and self-treatment was not included in the guide, it constantly emerged during the interviews. Villagers and townspeople alike complained to us about the local medical facilities. However, their discontent was more often caused by the feeling that the doctors were incompetent and the service in the clinics awful rather than by the unavailability of professional care. The lack of healthcare resources was not the determining factor for those consumers of "informal healthcare" goods and services with whom we communicated. Rather, they were dissatisfied with how official medicine managed their health.

An analysis of the situation in the surveyed localities allows stating that the health of the population has a minor effect on the development of "informal healthcare". The only exception is alcohol and drug abuse. Here the market is extremely responsive to the needs of the population and lack of high-quality medical care. Different agents offer a variety of options for getting rid of alcoholism and drug addiction. One of the reasons for this can be the inadequacy of the domestic addiction treatment system (lack of resources, underdeveloped rehabilitation facilities, etc.). Besides, registering for substance abuse treatment is fraught with a restriction in rights and stigma, which potential patients want to avoid.

The demand for anonymous dependence treatment generates supply from the state-founded addiction hospitals which open fee-based facilities, from psychotherapists, as well as agents that have no medical training. Healers operate in rural areas, where alcoholism is an acute problem; the geography of their clients is not limited to one locality or district. It should be noted that working with alcoholics is not the most common specialization among traditional healers. Few witch doctors undertake such treatment and virtually none of them work with drug addicts. In the towns, alcohol abuse is also treated by visiting psychotherapists, who once per month rent premises in local cultural or educational establishments. Non-profit rehabilitation centers (in the surveyed localities most of them were founded by Pentecostal or Neo-Pentecostal religious communities) promise recovery from drug addiction.

Healing springs, shrines, and natural anomalies that attract tourists and are located in or near a settlement significantly promote the development of "informal healthcare".

This was most noticeable in the village of Klyuchi in Suksun district, where there is a rather large resort with mineral springs and peloids. Here, various goods and services "wrapped up" as health products acquire added value and an extra price. However, the resources of the resort, as well as the "informal healthcare" facilities are meant for holiday-makers. Due to high prices, local residents do not use them.

Where there is a steady stream of incoming tourists, markets for health services also emerge on the basis of natural resources not directly related to medicine. A good example is the Kungur ice cave. Besides hotel accommodation, a restaurant, and a tour desk, the Stalagmite Tourist Complex also offers a fitness center with a swimming pool and a salt chamber. Speleotherapy sessions are held in the cave. On the one hand, the owners of the tourist infrastructure thus try to develop wellness tourism here. They engage the assistance of official medicine—research in the cave is conducted jointly with the Perm Medical Academy. On the other hand, the cave is a favorite "power place" in the Perm Territory for people interested in esoteric knowledge. Clubs and movements from other cities (Perm, Ufa, Chelyabinsk, and others) organize tours here "to replenish their energy". Given the susceptibility of some Stalagmite personnel to such ideas, the tourist center also becomes an information hub where wellness ideas and techniques are collected and disseminated. According to a staff member, "I have things to learn from people who come here".

It is noteworthy that the neighboring Orda district also has a large karst cave. However, it is hard to reach, so only professional speleologists and extreme athletes ever go there. Mass tourism to the cave is not developed; consequently, no wellness businesses emerge and no one mentions the potential therapeutic effect of cave air.

Another curious example is the village of Molebka in the Kishert district, which since the 1990s has been attracting the attention of ufologists and people interested in paranormal phenomena. There, a local stalker for a fee arranges trekking and hiking tours to the Perm anomalous zone. Besides, the fame of a power place attracts people keen on esoteric doctrines and those who practice oriental and energy healing methods. Some of them take up permanent residence in the area. These methods are alien to the everyday culture of the local villagers, but when necessary, they resort to them.

The demand for religious miracles as a way to address health problems is met mainly by Orthodox monasteries and convents housing sacred objects (relics, etc.) which attract pilgrims. In addition, virtually every surveyed Orthodox parish has a local natural attraction or artefact that are revered as sacred. Most often it is a water source. For example, the Plakun Waterfall on the Sylva River in Suksun district is a natural hydrological landmark, as well as a popular leisure destination for local residents and tourists. For esoterics, this is a "power place". In Orthodox tradition, the waterfall is revered as the sacred Elijah spring. It is the final destination of the annual Procession of the Cross and a must for all pilgrimage tours.

In general, observations in the Perm Territory showed that the urban environment is more favorable for the development of "informal healthcare" than the rural one. Settlements with special resources that provide a constant inflow of visitors are an exception. In rural areas, the lack or mistrust of "informal healthcare" services and agents results in the fact that a considerable number of local residents prefer to ignore their health problems. Partially, they compensate the local unavailability of high-quality medical care by self-medication using pharmacy drugs and recipes of traditional medicine found in the popular press. They also turn to witch doctors and religious organizations. In the cities, the options for improving one's health without visiting a doctor are much more extensive and can suit every taste (including ideological and religious beliefs) and budget.

However, we cannot assert that personal income levels and the size of the locality directly promote the development of the field of our study. We can assume that such development depends on the availability of a critical mass of people with a certain world view and lifestyle, who are confronted with the inefficiency of the healthcare system, value their health, independently seek some secret knowledge, and are interested in esoteric doctrines and practices. They are at the same time active consumers and suppliers of "informal healthcare" goods and services. One can find such people everywhere. In a small village, for example, they are united in a health group at the local club or library. However, it is only logical that in a large city they are more numerous.

# 2  Agents in the markets for health products

This chapter opens the second part of the book, which focuses on describing selected "informal healthcare" agents and practices in present-day Russia. Here we will deal with suppliers of such consumer goods that customers buy at their own initiative, beyond the control of formal healthcare, to improve their health and fight diseases. During fieldwork, our research group recorded all observable forms of selling such goods. This chapter addresses three trade practices, which I believe to be most interesting: direct selling; pharmacy services; itinerant trade and peddling. A brief overview of the traded goods precedes the description of each practice.

The total market for health products can be presented in the form of a sphere with the core integrated into the healthcare system and a periphery, which is actively developing due to the expanding philosophy of healthy nutrition and healthy living. The core consists of medical products, the production and distribution of which is strictly regulated (drugs and medical devices). The periphery contains goods, which people can use (along with exercises) to manage their body and improve their health: organic foods; functional nutrition, including fortified and dietary products; dietary supplements; massagers; and many others. The regulations for their production and sales in Russia are much less stringent.

The attitude of official medicine to "peripheral" goods varies. At one end of the spectrum are fully accepted products that are included in a doctor's arsenal (mineral water, dietary foods, etc.); at the other—products that are not supported by scientific evidence and are declared fraudulent and even harmful. Somewhere in between are registered dietary supplements with label statements warning to "consult your physician before use". In other words, doctors explicitly recommend their patients to use some products as a supplement to medication or for the prevention of diseases. At the same time, contrary to the position of medical science, the producers of health products often promote them, and the consumers use them as an alternative to medication.

The "informal healthcare" segment considered in this chapter serves extensive self-treatment practices or helps alternative specialists provide their services. The offered products—extremely diverse in origin,

purpose, and method of use—can be classified into two large groups based on their formal status:
- Medical goods (drugs and medical devices) that are applied by official medicine, but are also used for alternative therapies and self-medication
- Non-medical goods that are bought and used to improve health without the approval of orthodox medicine

The first group includes not only conventional drugs extensively used without prescription, but also veterinary medicinal products, which their buyers believe to be perfectly suited to treat human diseases, and some medical devices. The latter form a specific Russian market of medical equipment applied by CAM specialists or used for self-treatment. Usually such devices are based on techniques that evidence-based medicine considers dubious: electro-, magnetic, color and other acupuncture therapy and diagnostics; bioresonance therapy; quantum and low-level laser therapy. Their state registration as medical devices was an element of recognition by official medicine and the state, thus allowing to integrate them into conventional medical practice. For this reason, manufacturers sought to pass this procedure.

Such industry players can be considered "informal healthcare" agents not only because they serve complementary and alternative medicine. Manufacturers and suppliers of physiotherapy devices are a significant and quite legitimate part of the Russian industry for medical devices procured for hospitals and wellness resorts. However, most of them also offer portable devices intended for individual customers and their respective budgets. They are classified "for home use", although the wording is misleading for two reasons. First, if the equipment is intended for therapy, the process should be controlled by a physician, whereas home use encourages self-treatment.[26] Second, it is logical that a portable, ten times cheaper version of the physiotherapy device used by clinics, is much less powerful (and therefore harmless and permitted for use outside medical

---

26   Here is how one of our informants—a doctor—formulated her negative attitude to such devices: "It happens that visiting vendors walk the streets advertising devices which they claim are physiotherapy ones. They tell people: apply this to your source of pain, and everything will be fine. I am definitely against such things, because this can trigger cardiac arrhythmia. It is inadmissible to prescribe a person magnets without any prior examination" (female, 30–40 years old, general physician, district center).

institutions). In other words, there is absolutely no guarantee that it will be of any use at all.

The second group of goods consists of foodstuffs, cosmetic products, clothing, household appliances, and souvenirs, which are sold and purchased for therapeutic purposes. Such goods include:
- Dietary supplements
- Other food products (tinctures, herbal infusions, etc.)
- Health products for external application, including but not limited to:
    - Clothing, accessories, and household appliances with therapeutic metals and minerals: magnets, tourmaline, zircon, sylvinite and others
    - Consumer goods with reference to nanotechnology ("therapeutic nano socks", "nano underwear with bio-photons", etc.)
    - Massagers, the therapeutic effect of which is based on stimulating acupressure points
    - Devices for regulating radiated emissions, energy, and information flows: "electromagnetic anomaly neutralizers" (*neitralizatory electromagnitnykh anomaliy*); "biofield correction" and "energo-informational protection" devices (*apparaty korrektsii biopolya i energo-informatsionnoi zashchity*); "functional regulators" (*korrektory funktsional'nogo sostoyaniya*), etc.
    - Cosmetics and care products on the basis of traditional medicine recipes and natural remedies—medicinal herbs, bee products, peloids, animal derivatives, and minerals

A comparison of regulatory acts and commercial ads clearly shows that state regulation aims to draw a line between medical and non-medical products,[27] whereas manufacturers of the latter base their advertising on the desire to erase this distinction. Information booklets, leaflets and unit

---

27 Thus, Resolution No. 2 of Russia's Chief Sanitary Inspector dated 17 January 2013 *On Supervising Dietary Supplements* ordered not to register supplements that contain ingredients included in the National Pharmacopoeia and are therefore medicines, as well as those that have no "tradition of food use". This was done to curtail the promotion of dietary supplements as an alternative to medicine.

packs demonstrate rich imagination and methods typical of marketing professionals promoting health products.[28] Despite the diversity of such products and devices, there are similar, reproducible features in the way they are presented to the buyer: myths about the therapeutic effect; claims about unique properties and versatility at the same time; outward mimicry of medical products.

Myths extend to the healing properties of the product or the material from which it was made. For example, besides the products, a manufacturer of multi-purpose birch hand and foot massagers advertises the healing properties of the birch tree: "Everything in it—from the roots to the branch tips, from buds to pollen, from birch sap to birch tar, leaves, aments, and coal—is healing to people". The therapeutic effect is generally exaggerated, and the product is presented as a universal remedy for a broad range of diseases. Thus, an advertisement for a physiotherapy machine reads as follows: "This complex allows treating all principal types of diseases without wasting time on visits to the physiotherapist... The OptiDom Complex is a home doctor, which you can use to treat the whole family, including pets." Finally, the wording of the indications (uses) imitates the stylistic of instructions for the use of drugs. The manufacturer describes the therapeutic effect of the product and indicates what specific diseases and symptoms it is intended to cure.

An emphasis on the relation to folk medicine is indispensable when promoting goods for internal use (reference to the "healing power of Altai herbs", "the wonderful gifts of mother nature", etc.). Here we should mention the mythologized and widespread image of Altai's natural cures. At present, Altai herbs as a regional brand may likely have the same effect on the mind of the average Russian consumer as Japanese electronics. The records of our observations and interviews in the Perm Territory show that this brand is not only present in the advertising media, but is also reproduced in routine communications of "informal healthcare" consumers and providers. The image of unique plants picked in Altai's pristine nature that have particularly powerful therapeutic properties exists despite

---

28  Here I refer to the advertising samples collected at sales outlets during fieldwork. Naturally, they do not cover the entire diversity; however, they provide an overall picture.

evidence of the environmental situation in the area and the poor health of the local population.[29]

Concluding this brief introduction to the description of "informal healthcare" trade practices, I would like to mention one more aspect of the domestic production of health products. In many cases, we can observe here how research and technology is commercialized in Russian reality.

Companies, the names of which contain abbreviations like NPO (*nauchno-proizvodstvennoye ob'edinenie*—research and development association) and NII (*nauchno-issledovatel'skij institut*—research institute), implement inventions at minimum costs and generate massive demand for innovative consumer products: "therapeutic nano socks"; dietary supplements "produced under a unique technology"; devices to protect a person's biofield; hardware and software systems for treating with "charged" water, etc. Many of these manufacturers are residents of technopoles (*naukograds*) and industrial parks or have spun off from enterprises of the military-industrial complex. It is this segment that for many ordinary Russian consumers is the real showcase of domestic industrial innovations, no matter how much the officials or myself would like to see something else in its place—for example, the electronic, aerospace or pharmaceutical industry.

## 2.1. "We are like Galileo—they burn us at the stake, but we continue promoting dietary supplements": Direct selling of health products

The phrase quoted in the header is taken from an interview with an independent distributor of a direct selling organization marketing dietary supplements and other health products in many Russian localities. Although this statement confuses historical facts, it perfectly well illustrates the perception of the special social mission that such "informal healthcare" agents attribute themselves.

---

29  In Soviet times, part of the Altai Territory and the Altai Republic had been exposed to radiation as a result of nuclear tests at the Semipalatinsk test site. This had a negative impact on the health of the local population. Besides, some areas are still exposed to adverse environmental conditions caused by the launching of space ships from Baikonur: fragments of missiles, toxic components of rocket propellants and their derivatives land on their territory.

I will make no distinction between direct selling organizations (DSOs) and network marketing or MLM (multi-level marketing) companies, although some researchers insist that these notions are not synonymous and it is important to distinguish two models of organizational structure: a single-level and a multi-level one (e.g., Brodie, Stanworth, Wotruba, 2002; Zuyeva, 2005). Direct selling means direct interaction with the customer away from a fixed retail location. In a multi-level organization, the salespeople are also involved in recruiting other direct salespeople and earn on this (Peterson, Wotruba, 1996). According to the World Federation of Direct Selling Associations (WFDSA), direct selling

> takes place through independent sales representatives who are sometimes also referred to as direct sellers, consultants, distributors or other titles. Direct sales often occur in a one-to-one, small group or party plan environment, often in the consumer's home. Direct sales also may take place in a branded shop or retail location, online via e-commerce or social media, or by subscription/automatic delivery.[30]

Most DSOs operating in Russia have a multi-level structure and use all the sales channels mentioned above. For us, therefore, the distinction between these notions is insignificant. What is important is that the traditional segregation of buyer and seller roles is eroded in this field. The rank-and-file network members—the sellers-distributors—are themselves the principal consumers of the company's products. It is this main feature of such a business model that is relevant for the purposes of this work.

It is also important that salespeople are not employees—under the slogan of free partnership, they are independent entrepreneurs united only by the product brand, general motivational techniques (training, seminars, workshops, competition, leisure), and a single network hierarchy. Describing direct selling organizations in the USA, Nicole Biggart notes that "every distributor is legally the owner of a business run under the direction of an often revered corporate leadership to which the distributor is morally, but not legally, subordinate" (Biggart, 1989, p. 8).

The company as a legal entity has no significant impact on the activities of its distributors and is not liable for their actions. This circumstance is a powerful incentive for distributors to market health products as

---

30 *WFDSA Annual Report 2015*, p. 4. WFDSA (website).
URL: www.wfdsa.org/.../annual-report-2015.pdf.

medicinal remedies. At least, this is the case in Russia.[31] Even if the brand owners and MLM company founders state that their products are to be used exclusively for preventive purposes,[32] independent distributors resort to a more successful sales strategy—direct competition with conventional medicine. In particular, as we have seen in the Perm Territory, sometimes they invent original methods of using their products to treat various diseases (including cancer, diabetes and other serious illnesses); moreover, they market these methods, and even fear that their know-how can be stolen by their colleagues.

The transformation of goods into remedies is one of the reasons why network marketing is of particular interest among the sales channels for health products. The other reason is that DSOs are similar to civic associations. Besides a job, they offer their members a particular lifestyle, a special approach to health management as part of network control. They base their sales training sessions on motivational techniques that are designed to transform an individual completely and build a closed system of socialization. In addition to managing their career, time and education, distributors must also manage their body, appearance, and mood (Lan, 2002; Savelieva, 2013b). In this sense, the distributors are not only agents selling the products of MLM companies; they themselves become *products* of these companies (Gu, 2004).

The third reason is that some network marketing companies directly criticize orthodox medicine and promote specific health practices based on traditional medicine or pseudo-scientific theories, such as concepts of "structured water", "parasitic" nature of diseases, the human biofield, and torsion fields.

In Russia, network marketing is a stigmatizing occupation. It is generally not considered to be an adequate alternative to normal employment and is associated with fraud (Savelieva, 2013a). In the public opinion, it is firmly associated with dietary supplements, although independent representatives actually offer a much broader range of health products. Besides, pharmacies also sell dietary supplements. A negative attitude to dietary supplements is a social norm—they are rarely a topic of discussion. People generally mention them in association with Herbalife's aggressive

---

31 Researchers of direct selling organizations in other countries also capture this feature (*see* Cahn, 2009; Droney, 2016).
32 With wording, such as: "improves health", "restores the balance of essential mineral nutrients", "healthy food for healthy people", etc.

marketing policy in Russia. Stories of fraud based on personal experience and newspaper articles, pushy distributors, cases of damage to health, consumer addiction—such is the average set of negative associations expressed by the informants in association with direct selling of health products.

At the same time, some of our respondents demonstrated a negative attitude to dietary supplements despite having a positive or neutral experience of using such products. This may be a psychological trick—people convince themselves that what they are taking has nothing to do with dietary supplements and their negative image. Direct selling companies use this feature of consumer psychology. According to one of the distributors, he avoids mentioning "dietary supplements" altogether, because people fear them "as the devil fears holy water". He refers to his products as *tinctures* and *infusions. Preparations* and *nutritional dragees* are some other substitutions used by direct sellers. In particular, Tentorium domiciled in Perm applies this technique, and even formally does not register its products as dietary supplements. Consequently, its customers—even with a medical background—sometimes do not realize that this is not medication. With people demonstrating such an ambivalent attitude to health products distributed through network marketing, it is understandable why MLM companies are still active in the Russian health market despite their sustainable negative image in society.

*Direct selling companies: geography and business processes*
Herbalife was the first MLM company promoting health products in Russia. In fact, it imported direct selling techniques to post-Soviet Russia, and its name became a household word in modern Russian. Subsequently, Russian companies producing dietary supplements and other health products on the basis of Soviet pharmaceutical and biotechnology developments successfully adopted these techniques. Such companies include Siberian Health Corporation (*Sibirskoye Zdorovye*), Art Life, Tentorium, Coral Club International, DENAS MS, and many others.

Health products are a major type of goods for DSOs. Of the 133 such companies operating in Russia in 2012, about 73.7% sold health products. Slightly over half of them were firms of Russian origin. These proportions are taken from the industry journal *Network Marketing and*

*Direct Selling.*[33] However, the picture will be different if we judge by the sales volumes rather than the variety of offers. Cosmetics and personal care items account for the lion's share of Russia's direct selling market. According to the Direct Selling Association (DSA),[34] the share of wellness products in 2013 was only 13.8% of RUB 141.5 billion; in 2014, it was 16% of RUB 141.9 billion ($4.45 billion).[35] For comparison: in 2011, the share of wellness products in the total sales of DSA members in Russia amounted to 9%. According to the WFDSA, it was substantially lower than the share of wellness products in the global direct selling market (25%), the national markets in the USA (24%), Great Britain (38%), South Korea (38%), and Taiwan (59%), and comparable with France (8%) and Germany (11%).[36]

During fieldwork in the Perm Territory, we recorded at least thirty-five direct selling companies dealing in health products; of them, foreign businesses account for about a third. The remaining are Russian entities, although sometimes they position themselves as international companies referring to offices in other countries. Most of them appeared in the late 1990s—early 2000s, i.e. relatively recently (e.g., NL International—in 2000; Coral Club—in 1998).

All direct selling companies marketing health products in Russia may be tentatively divided into four groups:
- Network marketing giants (Amway, Avon, and Oriflame), which have their own line of vitamins and dietary supplements
- Companies specializing primarily in dietary supplements: Siberian Health (*Sibirskoye Zdorovye*), Tentorium, Art Life, Altera Holding, Spring of Health (*Rodnik Zdorovya*), Argo, Coral Club, and others

---

33   SINAMATI. *Network Marketing and Direct Selling.* Special Issue: Twenty Years of Network Marketing in Russia. 2012.
URL: mlm-gazeta.ru›upload/journals/spec_2012.pdf.
34   The Association unites major DSOs operating in Russia: Amway, Avon, Herbalife, Mary Kay, Nikken, Oriflame, Tupperware, CIEL Parfum, Coral Club, Faberlic, Florange, Jafra Cosmetics, LR Health & Beauty, MIRRA, Morinda, Nu Skin, and Tentorium (as at November 2014).
35   Here and further, prices and amounts in Russian rubles are followed in brackets by rounded amounts in US dollars. Calculations are based on the average weighted USD/RUB exchange rate for 2013 (USD 1 = RUB 31.848).
36   *Fact Sheets. Global Direct Selling. 2012.* WFDSA (website).
URL: http://www.wfdsa.org/files/pdf/global-stats/Fact_Sheets_Final_6-20-2012.pdf.

- Distributors of health appliances and devices, as well as products for external use: Center-Region (*Zentr-region*), DENAS MS, DETA-ELIS, Nuga Best, Tiens, Gamma7, Healthy Joy, and others
- Club networks uniting under their "umbrella" health products from different manufacturers, e.g., The Joy of Life (*Schastie Zhizni*) Philosophical Recreational Movement

Companies of the first group were of least interest to us, since wellness products for them are only a supplement to the core goods—cosmetics, personal and home care. Due to this, they differ by the sociodemographic profile and motivation of their distributors from companies that specialize in health products.

The distinction between the second and third groups is quite relative: the product lines of some companies include goods of various types—from dietary supplements and products for external use to massagers and clothing with a specified therapeutic effect. Many networkers rely on a wide range of goods that form a comprehensive set of everything that a person needs for a healthy lifestyle. However, a certain type of product will nevertheless dominate.

There is an essential difference between the distribution of dietary supplements and health devices. The former allows maintaining active customers for lengthy periods because of the need to take dietary supplements regularly. The latter requires an ongoing search for new buyers. On average, the price of health devices is significantly higher than that of dietary supplements, and their target audience often consists of entrepreneurs (rather than ordinary people) who use the purchased devices to provide health and diagnostic services to others.

Along with DSOs offering everything that may be required for a lifestyle of *wellness*, some firms operating in Russia specialize in a single product or technology, which they replicate in similar devices. The Tree of Life (*Derevo Zhizni*) is such a company in the Perm Territory. It sells Oleksin dietary supplements, which are advertised as a strong immunomodulator and antitumor agent.

MLM companies occasionally include goods produced by other manufacturers in their product mix; however, generally they combine them with their own brands. Club systems, on the contrary, are built on establishing a network of people regularly consuming health products rather than advancing their own brands. For example, the above mentioned The

Joy of Life (*Schastie Zhizni*) Philosophical Recreational Movement promotes the goods of over fifty small-scale manufacturers, primarily from St. Petersburg, but also from other cities.

How many active DSOs were there in the surveyed settlements? Local residents noted that people were less interested in distributing health products than five or ten years ago. Rather than learning about current experience, we more often heard stories that someone in the locality used to do it, but had by now quit it. However, outdoor observations and a review of the local press show that the attempts to expand the networks dealing in health products are ongoing—some wind down their activities, others open new offices or engage in distribution. In other words, the cooperation of local residents with MLM companies is usually short-lived, but new companies and proposals emerge regularly.

In general, the networkers are more active in urban areas. In the villages, the number of new regular customers is insignificant in terms of business prospects. The visual presence and operating methods of MLM companies differ accordingly. In the towns, they open offices—dealer/advisory centers with their own retail outlets. Here, distribution activities are generally formalized as the local residents' small-scale but more or less legitimate and independent business. In the villages, such activities are more often carried out by visiting networkers from neighboring towns. They hold sales presentations in public places, knock on the doors of offices, and sell their products in the marketplace. This tactic is not always successful. The events attract very few people, usually, no more than a dozen. The venue varies depending on the distributor's persuasion skills, acquaintances, or arrangements with premise owners. Thus, presentations can be held in a local club, library, children's art school, etc. In one case, potential buyers were invited to a veterinary station.

Summarizing the methods direct salespeople use to familiarize customers with their health products in the surveyed localities, distribution through acquaintances, or word-of-mouth marketing, definitely leads. In small settlements, this means the process may virtually involve a distributor's entire social environment: distant relatives, friends, neighbors, fellow patients in a hospital, and colleagues in the main job. The network of client acquaintances includes the parents of a child's classmates or kindergarten pals, or, if the distributor is a social service provider—the elderly people they serve. In recent years, the distributors have also been extensively using the free of charge communication opportunities provided by online social networks, primarily, VKontakte.

To attract the attention of people beyond their circle of contacts, distributors use various stationary and temporary retail outlets (offices and specialty shops, marketplaces and trade fairs).

Online and mail order shopping also serve to expand the client base of MLM businesses—sometimes because there are no permanent representatives or offices in the locality; sometimes because the buyers believe this will be better and cheaper. Distance selling is currently typical for many DSOs. Usually online shops are opened by distributors operating as sole proprietors. This means that the company bears no liability for their activity. This allows using online opportunities even to trade in dietary supplements, although their distance selling is illegal in Russia.

Finally, a method popular in the 1990s still exists—a door-to-door round of offices during working hours. For the merchants this is the least convenient sales method, because they generally encounter irritation, displeasure or even face a "Distributors are requested not to disturb" sign. No wonder many distributors emphasized during interviews that they made no round of various establishments. They considered this as evidence of the respectable nature of their business.

Judging by the number of active customers, how extensive can be the presence of individual direct selling companies specializing in health products in the localities? The only figures at our disposal have been provided by some of the distributors (by far not all of them). It hardly makes sense to rely on them for estimations, since the respondents might have attempted to embellish the reality, make an impression, or, on the contrary, conceal the scale of the business. In general, we can say that the client base is very limited. Thus, the office of one MLM company in Chusovoy has altogether 400 clients in three municipalities, including Lysva and the Chusovoy and Gornozavodsky districts, and this is considered an apparent success. The office of another MLM company in Perm serves about twenty regular customers. Deta Elis Holding, which sells portable wellness devices, acquired about ten regular clients over several months of operating in Chusovoy.

*Distributors: portrait and motivation*
Communication with ordinary distributors of health products gives the impression that their key motivation is neither poverty driving people to engage in unpopular work stigmatized by society, nor the naive desire to get rich by shamelessly advertising goods of dubious efficacy, but the lifestyle they choose focused on improving their health.

The overwhelming majority of such distributors are women—retired and of pre-retirement age.[37] This is to be expected, as this is the age when many chronic health problems emerge, and women are more likely to take care of their health than men. According to an informant—office director of an MLM company in Perm,—this segment of network marketing attracts "people, who begin to realize that the best part of their life is already in the past, and who want to go on living". Everyone with whom we communicated told us a personal story of health problems which made them turn to network marketing. The interviewees, sometimes with tears in their eyes, gave accounts of wonderful recovery, either their own or that of close relatives. They mentioned the broadest range of diseases—from chronic problems with blood pressure and allergy to cancer and sight problems. Moreover, another important feature typical of distributors of health products is a passion for alternative medicine in general. Many of them are involved in various "informal healthcare" practices.

As to the financial costs and benefits of health products distribution, it is not a particularly profitable occupation for people at the foot of the network pyramid. This activity was not the main source of income for the majority of our respondents. They had a principal job, pension, or a parallel business associated with health or related subjects (gift shop, beauty parlor or alternative medicine center). The only exception was some office (dealer center) directors, for whom networking was the main income. But they also did not give an impression of high earners and participated in this business primarily to maintain their health. In interviews, distributors

---

37 Since we focused on DSOs specializing in health products, our observations of the distributors' age characteristics and the respective evidence provided by experts differ from the results of sociological surveys of Russian network marketing in general. Thus, according to a survey conducted in 2001, over half of the distributors (58.8%) were of middle age (31–50 years old), and only 25.6 % were of pre-retirement and early retirement age (51–60 years old) (Kamushkina, 2003).

either concealed information about actual incomes or, on the contrary, exaggerated earnings. Nevertheless, we obtained some figures. Thus, an ordinary distributor in one company earned from three to ten thousand rubles per month ($94–$314). An office director in another company claimed to receive up to seventy thousand rubles monthly (about $2,200).

For ordinary distributors, purchases of their company's products constitute a significant part of everyday expenses; however, in interviews they emphasized that buying even a complete set of dietary supplements is cheaper for them than buying drugs in pharmacies. Sometimes they spoke about the ultimate benefit ("not cheaper than in a pharmacy, but much more effective").

To a large extent, the success of network marketing is based on the distributors' loyalty to their firm. This is achieved through a robust system of rewards, which besides discounts includes gifts and special offers. Tourism is an important incentive: trips to Moscow and St. Petersburg or even Turkey and Egypt to attend workshops, congresses of distributors, and the company's anniversaries. MLM companies give their customers the opportunity to escape from the provincial routine. Although the participants generally cover travel expenses themselves, the distributors often mention such trips among the bonuses of their work.

*Integration of physicians into network marketing*
Participation of physicians from the public health system in direct sales of health products, the efficacy of which is dubious in terms of medical science, gives a fresh perspective of the relationship between official medicine and "informal healthcare".

For MLM companies, the medical community is doubtlessly an ideal distribution channel, so they actively seek to engage physicians. The principal technique of major direct sellers is to organize training courses, which are presented as professional development. Upon completing the courses, the physicians are awarded new qualifications, such as *Nutritionist* or *DENS-therapist,* which are not included in the approved list of medical specialties. When the company has sufficient resources, the courses take place under the auspices of conventional medical schools. A simpler version is to train distributors under a system completely alternative to medical education:

Our personnel attend professional development courses in nutrition. Physicians get credits for continuing education, and we obtain general knowledge. Valentina is a rural feldsher, and in the countryside, a feldsher is everything—a gynecologist, oncologist, and ophthalmologist. She was promoted to a doctor here and was awarded a certificate.[38]

In our opinion, medical workers cooperate with DSOs not only for financial reasons. Some other factors are a low educational level and awareness of the problems facing the therapeutic process in the national healthcare system, such as poor preventive work or ineffective drugs. I suppose that the professional community does not seriously oppose participation in network marketing. It is widely believed that physicians join the ranks of distributors because of the meager incomes they receive at their principal place of work; therefore, the medical community is indulgent when it comes to such practices.

In general, we can distinguish three ways in which healthcare professionals participate in network marketing. First, MLM companies attract people with higher or secondary medical and pharmaceutical education who are not satisfied with the salaries and working conditions in public healthcare and want to change the job. This employment option is more relevant in the countryside than in a large city. In a city, a physician has more opportunities to find a new job (e.g., in a private clinic or as medical representative in a pharmaceutical company).

Second, there is the formally persecuted but ineradicable practice of engaging in network marketing while being employed in healthcare institutions. The following pattern is widespread: rather than selling the products at the workplace, a doctor only advertises them. For example, an informant working as physiotherapist recommends her patients to purchase devices for home use manufactured by DENAS MS and gives them the contact details of the respective distribution center in Perm. She has been cooperating with this center for the past ten years.

Third, doctors are extensively involved in direct selling as external experts for fees. They give lectures to potential buyers; perform diagnostic examinations at company premises and prescribe dietary supplements based on the results; and train ordinary distributors. This is what allows direct selling of health products to mimic the healthcare system. Notably, the specialty of the expert often does not match the topic of his or her

---

38    Informant: female, about 40 years old, office director of an MLM company, medium-sized town.

consultations. For example, a TB-specialist lectures on healthy eating. Here, the only thing that matters is the certificate of medical education, but the general healthcare principle stipulating that a physician may treat only in line with professional qualifications does not work.

Our research team encountered situations when consulting physicians were not residents but came regularly from other localities. The Perm Territory was mostly "served" by doctors from the regional capital, whereas Perm itself was a destination for physicians from other regions—Ekaterinburg, for example. This way of making money on the side mitigates potential reputational risks for the physicians.

*DSOs as an alternative to the healthcare system*
The vast majority of DSOs we encountered during fieldwork win customers by diagnosing their health problems using devices generally based on a combination of Chinese acupuncture and computer technologies. This procedure reveals pathologies which require taking or applying the company's products. "Computer-aided diagnosis" services are also provided on a fee basis without prescribing dietary supplements. In the Perm Territory, such diagnosis cost anywhere from RUB 200 ($6) to RUB 2,000 ($63). In-house diagnosis with a subsequent personalized prescription of remedies based on the specific characteristics of each client is becoming a key advantage of direct selling companies, which allows them to compete with pharmacies.

Moreover, mutually beneficial cooperation is widespread in this sphere. In some cases, distributors of electronic devices (diagnostic and therapeutic appliances) deliver equipment to vendors of dietary supplements. In other cases, they themselves perform a "comprehensive diagnosis" of the patient and then prescribe products of certain friendly companies.

Such companies train in-house health consultants who do not necessarily have to be physicians. Some of them have no medical certificate, but believe they are competent in medicine because they "know the stuff inside out". A distributor who has attended specialized training courses and read "tons of literature on the subject" becomes an expert for friends and neighbors—a consultant they turn to just as they would to a pharmacist or a doctor. Should the distributor assume the role of a healer, he or she can even "provide some treatment" to the clients, even in violation of the principles established by the manufacturer of the health products. Healing others becomes more important than selling the goods:

> A label on the jar warns against buying the product if the seal had been broken. But if my acquaintances need only 30 capsules, I open the jar in their presence and sell them the requested amount. Why should they buy the remaining 70 capsules? Such an effect and so cheap. <...> The doctor says to me: But you are not a physician. And I reply: But I can perfectly well treat myself.[39]

Further, the distributors of wellness products substitute by their promotional activity the preventive work of medical institutions. For example, they hold public lectures on healthy living.

Thus, Spring of Health organizes healthy eating courses on a fee basis.[40] In one of the surveyed towns such courses have been conducted since 2010. According to the organizers, over 800 people have attended them in three years. Most of them are women—retired and of pre-retirement age. The group consists of about ten people. Sessions are held on a weekly basis and last one hour. Invited physicians explain the basics of human physiology, tell about the properties of different foodstuffs and sensible nutrition and advertise weight loss supplements.

Other companies emphasize the gratuitous nature of their outreach to the public, for example:

> Our company holds free lectures throughout the country devoted to health issues. Absolutely free of charge. Here we also worked for six years. We were allowed to use premises free of charge. Lots of people attended. The lecturer was a doctor.[41]

Besides a free lecture on the functioning of the spine, anyone visiting Nuga Best showrooms can enjoy a free session on a massage bed. Pensioners are frequent visitors of such showrooms, and many of them take advantage of this opportunity. In Lysva, for example, visitors could test a massage bed for free, whereas in Kungur RUB 50 ($1.6) were charged per session. According to a local resident, some people in Lysva enjoy this opportunity on a regular basis: "I heard about Nuga Best. I know an

---

[39] Informant: female, 60–70 years old, distributor of health products, medium-sized town.
[40] A three-month course costs RUB 1,500 ($47).
[41] Informant: female, about 50 years old, distributor of health products, medium-sized town.

old lady who went there regularly during a whole year and was very satisfied."

Besides reaching out to potential customers, DSOs widely practice various group leisure activities where people exchange wellness ideas and adopt healthy lifestyle principles. Formats can be different—from purely informal local activities, such as tea parties, hiking in the forest or pilgrimages to holy places, to healthy lifestyle festivals for the youth promoted throughout the entire MLM company.

In addition, major companies create their own market for printed matter devoted to health issues. They publish books about health doctrines developed by the companies' founders and leaders, brochures about the benefits of their products as well as their own magazines. Many of the publications are periodicals and are registered as mass media under Russian legislation. The circulation of such publications ranges from a modest 990 copies for *The Art of Living* (*Iskusstvo Zhit'*—issued by Art Life) to 200,000 copies for *Nuga News* (issued by Nuga Medical). Usually they are handed out for free and help independent distributors integrate into a single network and maintain the corporate spirit. As can be anticipated, such magazines contain 'advertorials' promoting the products, the distributors' success stories, and corporate news. Besides, they also publish popular science articles written by doctors and psychologists, practical tips on treatment, and other content typical of ordinary glossy health periodicals.

Earlier we already mentioned that many MLM companies attempt to establish in-house training systems alternative to medical education. Corporate units simulating the institutional environment for transfer of scientific medical knowledge are an important component of such systems. DENAS MS has a medical center, which provides training for medical professionals and ordinary distributors, conducts clinical research of the products, and publishes its own scientific journal—*Medical Bulletin*. Coral Club International has established a Health Academy which "professionally" trains Club members to apply "effective methods and techniques for maintaining health and use the products appropriately".[42]

Finally, some active distributors, usually with a medical background, turn their offices into alternative medicine clinics offering a variety

---

42   Coral Club Wellness (website of an independent distributor of Coral Club International). URL: http://coralmarket.com/olgabutakova.

of methods—from leech therapy to massage and osteopathy. The most ambitious project of this kind in Perm is the API-SPA Health Retreat established by Tentorium on the basis of a municipal balneary acquired by the company. The facility offers over a dozen various alternative medicine and rehabilitation treatment services. Most of the guests are rank-and-file female distributors of Tentorium products who come here for vacation twice a year.

Let us now consider two examples of smaller clinics. A medical diagnostic center called *Alternative* operates in one of the surveyed medium-sized towns. It is located on the ground floor of an apartment house. The owner of the facility lives in the same building. She is registered as a sole proprietor. In addition to local residents, the center serves clients who come from neighboring rural areas. The list of services includes visceral massage of internal organs, leech therapy, valeo diagnostics (comprehensive examination of the body), and bioresonance therapy. The owner—a doctor in the past—distributes wellness goods produced by Art Life, a company registered in Tomsk. She performs bioresonance valeo diagnostics and based on the results prescribes respective dietary supplements. The other treatments (massage, leech therapy) are performed by invited specialists, who are also registered as sole proprietors and actually rent premises from Alternative. In fact, network marketing in this case is the core around which a medical center offering alternative medicine services is built. The owner of Alternative ranks rather high in the hierarchy of the MLM company. Consequently, the distributors she had recruited to Art Life form the majority of the medical center's regular clients. On the contrary, the Perm office of Coral Club International (according to its director) joined the already existing center of alternative medicine approximately five years earlier. Currently the clinic employs several specialists, including a qigong instructor (who also works as psychologist), a bioresonance therapist, and craniosacral therapists. Besides providing core services, all of them prescribe Coral Club products.

Specific advertising methods and promotion patterns used to market health products reflect the tendency to build an alternative health maintenance system based on direct selling. These methods and patterns are firmly embedded in the distributors' everyday practice and have become part of their philosophy.

On the one hand, they emphasize the weaknesses of public healthcare and orthodox medicine which they believe determine the very existence of MLM companies: "We are in any case the last resort; when doctors are helpless, people turn to herbs and dietary supplements."[43] On the other hand, direct sellers often refer to a certain public health policy which they allegedly follow. Using the logo of the National Priority Health Project in advertising, making references to government programs and resolutions—all this is designed to emphasize that the distributors' activity is of specific social significance and is on a par with the work of medical institutions. For example, "We are fulfilling the 1998 government program on selenization of the population. It is the same as salt iodization and fluoridation of toothpaste..."[44]

In general, MLM companies are much more than just suppliers of health products, since they seek to build a coherent health maintenance system alternative to public healthcare. We believe that reducing the activity of such "informal healthcare" agents to shameless advertising of goods with dubious properties and intended misleading of potential buyers would be an erroneous oversimplification. An important aspect of network marketing is that it offers ordinary distributors a particular lifestyle, specific health maintenance principles, and a network of associates.

Although involvement in direct selling of health products is not a widespread practice in Russia, the diversity of options in this field, the viability of the business even in an adverse environment (such as an unfavorable public image, low incomes of the population, and illegal or semi-legal nature of the business) makes network marketing an alternative that anyone can resort to when not satisfied with formal healthcare services.

## 2.2. Latent functions of the healthcare institution: The case of pharmacies

Pharmacies are integrated into formal healthcare and constitute an integral part thereof. They facilitate the treatment process, which, according to orthodox medicine, consists mainly in taking medication prescribed by a physician. However, when people have health problems but for whatever reason do not want to contact a doctor, pharmacies are among the first places they would turn to.

---

43 Informant: male, about 50 years old, distributor of health products, district center.
44 Informant: female, about 65 years old, distributor of health products, medium-sized town.

In order to understand how these trade organizations currently work against the healthcare system in Russia, we should clarify the role assigned to them by the state.

According to law, pharmacies are providers of certain goods which have been recognized by the state as remedies for humans. This means that these agents have been registered as drugs and may be sold in Russia. The Law *On the Fundamentals of Public Healthcare in the Russian Federation* No. 323–FZ lists pharmaceutical entities among the structural elements of public, municipal, and private healthcare (Art. 29.35). The Law *On Circulation of Medicines* No. 61–FZ associates pharmacy (a type of pharmaceutical entity) activities with sales of drugs for medical use. In other words, although the range goods sold through pharmacies is not limited to drugs,[45] everything else is an immaterial extension of the core function.

Besides, although pharmacies may also sell over-the-counter drugs, the law assigns them a supporting role in the treatment of patients. Retail trade in drugs implies their sale in quantities prescribed by physicians (feldshers) (Art. 55.1). Thus, the existence of pharmacies is determined by the fact that a medical practitioner prescribes medication. This also provides for stringent state regulation and supervision of pharmacists' activities. Advising customers is among the duties of pharmacists, but the area of their competence is limited to information about drug effects, dosage and administration.

Such a vision of the role and place of pharmacies enshrined in law reflects the classic healthcare model. Worldwide, this position is successfully challenged by the pharmaceutical lobby. This is reflected in the concept of responsible self-medication according to which pharmacists become leading advisors to patients in their everyday health practices and key providers of medicines (Bradley, Blenkinsopp, 1996). Although this concept is gradually gaining the recognition of health professionals and governments, in Russia responsible self-medication is not yet a healthcare strategy stipulated by law.

---

45   Pursuant to Art. 55.7 of Law No. 61–FZ, in addition to drugs, pharmacies are entitled to sell medical devices; disinfectants; personal care products and means for taking care of the sick and newborn; glasses; mineral water; health food, baby food, and dietetic food; dietary supplements; cosmetics; and publications promoting a healthy lifestyle.

Besides being an element of the healthcare system designed to provide medicines (and associated goods) on prescription of a physician or other qualified health professional, pharmacies are also business entities that inevitably adapt to customer demands. Consequently, they assume functions not envisaged by the state, and this becomes a significant, albeit not core part of their activity. In the terminology of sociologist Robert K. Merton these are the pharmacies' latent functions, i.e. the unconscious and unintended consequences of their operation (Merton, 1957). First, they facilitate self-medication practices, including self-medication by dietary supplements substituting drugs and traditional remedies. Second, they replace the diagnosis and prescription of a physician by consultations of a pharmacist. In contrast to proper self-medication, the patient in this case shifts the decision-making about the treatment to the pharmacist. Finally, they meet the demand of people dependent on psychoactive substances for products to maintain these addictions. The pharmacies' latent functions are not limited to the above, as the household use of medicines and associated products is wider than pure health maintenance (from cosmetic procedures and child care to agriculture and animal health); however, the listed range is of primary importance to our research.

Publicly these functions are referred to as problems, violations, something outrageous that has to be terminated and eliminated. Therefore, publicly available information reflecting the situation nationwide is fragmentary and overloaded with negative assessments. These issues are generally discussed only in order to justify some regulatory changes, as was the case with the ban on OTC sales of codeine-containing medicines. We did not manage to piece together the full picture in the course of fieldwork (obviously, this requires a special study involving the administrative resource of pharmacies and pharmacy chains), however we believe to have captured certain general trends.

Pharmacy personnel became one of the most represented categories among our informants, although their sample is unevenly distributed across the field. In small localities, we surveyed all the available pharmacies; in Kungur, Lysva, and Chusovoy—only centrally located ones. For Perm we chose another technique due to the considerable size of the city.

Rather than interviewing and surveying, we arranged by way of experiment for the personnel of a pharmacy to monitor client behavior.[46] During a work shift pharmacists recorded the requests and purchases of every customer. Monitoring was conducted twice—on a workday and on the weekend. Selected aggregate data about the percentage of certain customer categories is presented in Table 4.

---

[46] The pharmacy operates round the clock. It is located on the ground floor of an apartment building (in a former one-room flat) in a residential area of Perm, near public transport and a medical facility.

**Table 4. Results of monitoring customer requests in a pharmacy in Perm**

| Customers | Weekend day (Saturday) | | Workday (Monday) |
|---|---|---|---|
| | Total (%) | Of them regular customers (%) | Total (%)[47] |
| Total customers over 14 hours | 100 % (92 people) | 43 | 100 % (61 person) |
| Alcoholics and drug addicts (as assessed by the pharmacist) | 42 | 73 | 33 |
| Buyers of dietary supplements | 2 | 50 | 3 |
| Customers who requested the advice of the pharmacist | 25 | 16 | 13 |
| Buyers of prescription drugs without a medical prescription | 11 | 45 | 10 |

[47] Different pharmacists monitored client behavior on Saturday and Monday. In the second case, the pharmacist failed to record whether the customer was a regular one; therefore, we provide no respective figures.

Below we summarize the opinions of pharmacists and physicians, results of the monitoring, observations of our work team, and nationwide secondary data.

It is considered that Russia experiences no shortage in pharmacies. They are even more numerous than is required to serve the needs of the healthcare system, although there is an obvious disproportion between the cities where pharmacies mushroom and small rural settlements where the pharmaceutical business is not profitable. This is particularly noticeable in the Perm Territory, which has its own higher education institution for training pharmaceutical professionals (The Perm Pharmaceutical Academy). According to Rosstat, 813 pharmacies and drug stores, as well as 258 smaller drug shops operated in the Kama area as at 2013. Rural areas account for about 20 percent of all pharmacy outlets (22 percent across the Russian Federation). About half of all the pharmacies are located in the regional center. Even compared to other Russian million-plus cities Perm stands out by numerous drug retail outlets.[48] The regional office of the Federal Antimonopoly Service proceeds from the figure of four to five thousand residents per one pharmacy. Consequently, it considers that retail trade services with regard to drugs, medical devices, and associated goods are highly available in the Perm Territory.[49] This availability would be excessive if we were to apply the standards for the development of pharmacy chains proposed by the Russian Ministry of Health in 1997: 6,200 people per pharmacy for rural areas; 10,000 people—for small towns; 12,000 people—for medium-sized towns (50,000—100,000 inhabitants); and 20,000 people—for million-plus cities. In Perm this figure is approximately 1,600 people per pharmacy, and, for example, in Orda (a surveyed rural settlement)—1,800 people.

---

48  According to 2GIS Geo Service, in 2014 Perm had 6.2 pharmacies per 10,000 residents, thus topping the list of Russian million-plus cities; it also had the largest number of 24 hour pharmacies. See 2GIS (website). URL: http://info.2gis.ru/moscow/company/news/2gis-viyasnil-v-kakih-gorodah-proshche-zashchititsya-ot-prostudy.

49  *Memorandum on reviewing and assessing the competitive environment in the retail market for medicines, medical devices, and associated products in the Perm Territory (by urban and municipal districts).* Office of the Federal Antimonopoly Service for the Perm Territory (website). 12 September 2012. URL: http://perm.fas.gov.ru/sites/perm.f.isfb.ru/files/analytic/2012/09/12/analiz_rynka_lekarstva_roznica_2012_ispr.doc.

A study of the situation at the micro level reveals certain features of the distribution of drug retail outlets across the territory. In small and medium-sized towns the pharmacies are concentrated in several central streets. Sometimes two-three outlets are located in neighboring buildings or even in one residential building with several entrances, whereas on the outskirts a pharmacy can hardly be found. In terms of market logic such a distribution would seem irrational, since it increases competition. However, pharmacists say that they do not face much competition for the customers. Regional centers generally have from two to four drug retail outlets. The surveyed villages that are centers of rural settlements also have a pharmacy or a branch thereof. Residents of smaller localities buy drugs in district centers or order them. FAPs, which were allowed to sell medicines only recently, have only the most common drugs in stock.

Besides, if almost a quarter of pharmacies in Perm are open at night, in rural areas 24 hour sales outlets are virtually nonexistent. For example, twenty thousand inhabitants of the Suksun district had no opportunity whatsoever to purchase medicines in the evening or during the night. Earlier there was one private pharmacy, which operated round the clock, but that did not last long, since personnel, security, and maintenance costs exceeded profits from night sales. However, neither the local authorities, nor the residents themselves perceive this as a problem with the availability of medications.

In general, the pharmacy professionals we spoke to were very careful in their pronouncements, since we were talking about practices that did not fit into the official paradigm of the pharmacies' mission. In those cases, when the interviewees were inclined to be critical and frank, they pointed out that Russians tended to over-consume pharmaceutical products. Thus, one informant was convinced that people often buy something in a pharmacy not because they really need it. Rather, they are used to self-medication and lack the skills of maintaining a healthy lifestyle. According to her, the pharmaceutical business is thriving because "people are accustomed to having health problems, buying medicines, and undergoing treatment."

Most people seeking the advice of pharmacists do not want to go to a doctor for whatever reason but in general believe in conventional medicine, i.e., they rely on standard medications rather than alternative methods. The customers describe (or show) the symptoms of their health problems, ask the pharmacist to recommend a drug, and rely on the suggested solution.

Pharmacists estimated that from a quarter to half of their customers were those who turned for medical advice to pharmacies rather than clinics.[50] According to the monitoring in Perm, the share of such clients on the weekend was about 25 percent, whereas on the workday it was less than 15 percent. However, if we consider only those buyers who visited the pharmacy because of health problems, almost half of them (43%) sought advice on the weekend and about a third (32%) on the workday.[51] On the weekend, about 30 percent of the customers who asked the pharmacist to recommend a drug had previously received a prescription from a doctor, but believed the prescribed medicine to be ineffective or having undesirable side effects. Rather than repeatedly visiting a doctor, they prefer seeking the advice of a pharmacist who appears to be more professional than the physician who did not meet the patient's expectations.

Pharmacists explain the significant flow of customers seeking advice by the fact that it is faster and easier than getting an appointment with a doctor. Most of them emphasized that such consumer behavior was a consequence of the problems inherent in domestic healthcare institutions (such as shortage of resources, limited time allocated for each patient, negligence, and professional errors of physicians), and pharmacists were forced to adapt to customer demands using their professional knowledge. However, when the issue of self-medication was raised in discussions with doctors, they voiced completely different opinions, as was to be expected. Physicians emphasized not only the lack of professionalism, but also the vested interests of pharmacies recommending one or another drug.

In a situation when, on the one hand, there is a formal ban on therapeutic recommendations and on the other—constant client pressure plus business considerations (which encourage the emergence of opportunities for self-diagnosis in pharmacies, such as installation of devices to

---

50    When our pharmacist informants said "all the time", "every second customer", "every fourth customer", this reflected their subjective perception, so it hardly makes sense to rely on such estimates for calculations. However, on the whole, they indicated that providing advice in pharmacies was a widespread practice.

51    Buyers of alcohol-containing drugs, syringes, and pipettes, whom the pharmacist clearly classified as people dependent on psychoactive substances, were deducted from the total number of customers.

measure blood pressure or weight free of charge), pharmacists develop an informal but generally accepted formula of ethical compromise for themselves. Our informants said they preferred recommending OTC medicines that can inflict no particular harm and urged the customers to contact a physician. The monitoring of pharmacies in Perm revealed a similar pattern of behavior typical of pharmacists. Some informants mentioned that if a customer asked to recommend a drug, they offered dietary supplements as the safest option.

I would like to emphasize that by far not all customers seek the recommendations of pharmacists. Many choose drugs for self-medication based on the advice of friends and their own knowledge. Such requests serve as a basis for the emergence of another widespread practice, which is illegal—sale of prescription drugs over the counter. Pharmacists take what their customers (especially the regular ones) say on trust, show understanding, and yield to pressure. Monitoring of the pharmacy in Perm showed that about every tenth customer asked for prescription-only medicines without providing a medical prescription.

People who in general trust conventional medicine but have no time to visit a clinic or have negative recollections of contacting a doctor are not the only ones who procure drugs for self-medication in pharmacies. People keen on alternative medicine also drop in to buy components (medicinal herbs, iodine, hydrogen peroxide, etc.) for a potion using recipes from the *Healthy Lifestyle Bulletin (HLS Bulletin, or Vestnik ZOZh)* or for a wellness course based on some doctrine of self-healing. They do not seek the pharmacist's advice; moreover, they take no heed of his professional instructions.

It is noteworthy that along with ordinary pharmacies, veterinary pharmacies also serve the needs of followers of alternative therapies. Self-medicating with drugs for animal use is another phenomenon typical of healthcare behavior in present-day Russia. Birch oil, creolin (coal tar), and Dorogov's antiseptic stimulant (ASD-2F and ASD-3F) used as a remedy against all diseases are widely known examples of such medications. Several enterprises produce ASD as a veterinary preparation, but proponents of alternative therapies favor products manufactured by Areal Medical—a company related to the drug inventor's daughter. Over the past fifteen years ASD has been steadily gaining popularity in folk medicine. It vividly illustrates the influence of conspiracy theories about the existence of super drugs which corrupt officials and the pharmaceutical business keep from the people.

A visit to a Russian pharmacy sometimes gives the feeling that locals receive treatment mainly in the form of dietary supplements and balms for external application, none of which are drugs. An extremely wide display of these products contributes to this impression. However, their visual dominance is rather a way to promote customer interest than a reflection of actual preferences. In the Kama area, cosmetics and dietary supplements occupied from one-third to half of the display area in the surveyed pharmacies; the Perm pharmacy where monitoring was conducted allocated about 90 percent of its shop windows for parapharmaceutical products. According to informants, however, dietary supplements constitute only from ten to twenty percent of the product range (in one case the pharmacist roughly estimated the share of dietary supplements to be about thirty percent).

Pharmacies are the main legitimate distribution channel for dietary supplements. According to IMS Health, in 2013 sales of dietary supplements through pharmacies in Russia amounted to RUB 37.295 billion ($ 1,171 million) in retail prices, or 321.7 million packages. Although the figures are impressive, they look insignificant when compared to pharmacy sales of medicines (about 15 times less in value and 13 times less in volume).[52] Our pharmacy informants emphasized that customer demand for dietary supplements lagged far behind that for medicines (leading position) and health care products (baby food, cosmetics, personal care items, and other associated products). Moreover, when people find out that the product they came for is a dietary supplement, they sometimes refuse to purchase it. In the course of monitoring the pharmacy in Perm, only several people came with the purpose of buying supplements.

Unlike some other countries, Russia has no developed culture of consuming dietary supplements as part of a healthy lifestyle.[53] This is partly due to their unfavorable public image as fraudulent goods, as was

---

52  According to IMS Health, in 2013 Russian pharmacies sold 4,234 billion packages of finished pharmaceutical products for the amount of about RUB 570 billion ($18 billion). *See* Remedium.ru. 04.04.2014. URL: http://www.remedium.ru/analytics/detail.php?ID=61295.

53  For comparison: national surveys in the US show that about half of the adult population regularly take dietary supplements and vitamins (Bailey et al., 2013); in 2010 their sales amounted to $28 billion (Guallar et al., 2013).

mentioned in the previous section. Moreover, for ordinary rural inhabitants they are expensive and therefore not in demand. In contrast to network marketing, pharmacies do not apply aggressive techniques to persuade their customers. How do Russian pharmacies nevertheless manage to make about a billion US dollars annually in sales of dietary supplements?

Advertising through mass media is the most obvious and trivial driver. OTC drugs and health products are generally some of the most publicized goods in the Russian media. Although law explicitly stipulates that dietary supplements and food additives may not be advertised as medicines, and any commercial ad must contain a respective notice to that effect, the skill of the promoters is aimed at convincing potential buyers that dietary supplements are essential in addressing health problems. Promotion of drugs, medical services, and dietary supplements accounts for the largest share of violations of the law on advertising (21.38% of all violations in 2013 and 12.57% in 2012).[54] Virtually all informants from among the pharmacists noted that the growth in demand for one or another supplement was directly linked with overt or covert advertising in the media.

The second driver—less visible but probably more instrumental in eroding healthcare boundaries—consists in the fact that not only ordinary citizens, but also pharmacists cease to perceive any big difference between medicines and dietary supplements. Two factors contribute to this situation. Complex and costly regulatory requirements for the registration of medicines urge pharmaceutical companies to apply a tactical maneuver. In recent years, manufacturers have started extensively producing vitamins and some other OTC drugs in the form of dietary supplements, since the total cost of obtaining a marketing authorization for supplements is significantly lower than that for drugs. Thus, for example, the familiar ascorbic acid becomes a dietary supplement. In addition, Russian drug developers practice registering new products as dietary supplements when they lack funds for clinical trials. Hence, the opinion shared also by some of our pharmacy informants: dietary supplements are in fact medicines; they only lack formal recognition and are cheaper, because their

---

54  *The results of government control and supervision of compliance with the legislation of the Russian Federation on advertising for the year 2013.* The Federal Antimonopoly Service of the Russian Federation (website).
URL:http://www.fas.gov.ru/analytical-materials/analytical-materials_31090.html.

price does not include research costs. In view of this, customers themselves sometimes ask to replace drugs with cheaper supplements of a similar composition or pharmacists offer them such options to save money.

Finally, people deliberately come to the pharmacy for dietary supplements prescribed by a physician. This is the third driver. According to an estimate of one of our informants (employee of a pharmacy outlet in a clinic of a medium-sized town), their pharmacy dispenses about 30 percent of all supplements against prescription, which means that they are recommended by doctors. Ophthalmologists lead in terms of such prescriptions; however, other medical professionals also recommend supplements based on their own preferences.

For their part, the few physician informants who openly told us about prescribing their patients dietary supplements, justified their position by the fact that such supplements are sold through pharmacies ("there are drugs which are still pending certification, and they are called dietary supplements") or that they "have passed clinical trials", and "medical schools teach" how to apply them.

So, mass media advertising, medical prescriptions, and the tactics applied by drug producers to facilitate marketing authorization contribute to eroding the boundaries between medicines and dietary supplements. I believe none of these factors alone would have triggered such a demand for dietary supplements sold through pharmacies, but together they "do the trick".

Besides serving proponents of self-medication and treatment by dietary supplements, pharmacies also meet the demands of alcoholics and drug addicts in maintaining their dependencies. This is the most dubious of all latent functions performed by the pharmacies. On the one hand, in most cases everything is done legally, i.e., within the scope of the legal framework. On the other hand, this activity of the pharmacists is most exposed to criticism in terms of morality.

In the first half of the 2000s, a plain alcohol hawthorn tincture was among the leaders of pharmacy sales by value. The reason was its popularity with alcoholics, who also extensively consumed any other cheap pharmacy remedies containing alcohol. Medicine as a surrogate drink, and pharmacy as a substitute for a wine and liquor shop—this metamorphosis is well known to the Russian people and the officials (Gil at al.,

2009). In recent years, hawthorn tincture has been replaced in the Russian list of top ten medicines with the highest share of retail sales by much more expensive popular self-medication drugs (hepatoprotectors and cartilage protectors; immunomodulators; analgesics; remedies for colds, dysbiosis, fungal infections, and to increase potency).

However, alcohol tinctures remain in high demand, at least in the places where we conducted our fieldwork. In Perm, according to AIPM and Remedium Group, the topical antiseptic Aseptolin ranked sixth by value of drug sales in 2012, and fourth in 2013.[55] Aseptolin is the direct successor of Antiseptin—the infamous solution for cleaning hands, which used to be a popular surrogate alcohol until it was banned following a wave of poisoning from consuming it in the Sverdlovsk Region in 2005. Aseptolin is produced by the same manufacturer. In 2014, the list of Top-10 products sold by Perm pharmacies included also capsicum tincture; in 2007–2008 it topped (!) the list by sales volume. It would be fair to say that in recent years, medicines used as surrogate alcohol do not make it to the Top-10 in other major Russian cities; therefore, the situation in Perm is somewhat specific. However, in Chelyabinsk, for example, the year 2013 was marked by a 58 percent growth in the sales of Lyrica (pregabalin)—a medicine popular with drug addicts. In that year Lyrica became the overall sales leader.[56]

How did the records of our fieldwork in the Perm Territory capture the services that pharmacies provide to alcoholics and drug addicts? To begin with, this practice is obviously more developed in the cities. In rural areas, there are in any case fewer drug addicts than in the cities, and drinkers prefer homemade alcoholic beverages prepared from whatever grows in the garden (home-brewed beer and moonshine). In the cities, pharmacies acquire regular customers whose needs the pharmacists can often determine at a glance without exchanging a word with them. Some come for alcohol tinctures, others—for components to prepare and consume narcotic drugs at home. Besides syringes, such components include pipettes, cotton wool, tincture of iodine, some prescription drugs (primarily

---

55 *The Drugs Retail Market of Perm in 2013*. AIPM—Remedium Market Bulletin. Remedium.ru. 07.07.2014.
URL: http://www.remedium.ru/analytics/detail.php?ID=62399.
56 *The Drugs Retail Market of Chelyabinsk in 2013*. AIPM—Remedium Market Bulletin. Remedium.ru. 09.07.2014.
URL: http://www.remedium.ru/analytics/detail.php?ID=62408.

containing codeine), and finally Naphthyzinum, where addicts use both the solution and the glass container.

Monitoring of the pharmacy in Perm showed that 42 percent of the customers on a weekend day and 33 percent on a workday were people whom the pharmacists clearly classified as individuals dependent on psychoactive substances. According to the pharmacists, such customers usually show up in the evening or during the night, as well as on Fridays and Saturdays.

The prevailing majority of such buyers were regular customers of the pharmacy (73 percent of the 39 visitors on Saturday, with six of them coming twice during the day; and 90 percent of the 20 visitors on Monday). Most of them were men (over 80 percent on Saturday and more than 90 percent on Monday). Such clients formed two distinct age groups: those who bought components to prepare homemade drugs were generally from twenty to thirty years old; and those who purchased surrogate alcohol were mainly from fifty to sixty years old. The breakdown of their purchases was as follows: on Saturday seventeen people bought capsicum tincture (on Monday—seven); ten customers purchased Aseptolin (four); three acquired hawthorn tincture (two); and eight procured syringes, pipettes, iodine and other products from the "drug addict's kit" (seven).

Regular buyers of surrogate alcohol are generally degraded individuals for whom a visit to the pharmacy has become a daily ritual. The pharmacists' comments in the monitoring records sometimes reveal their life stories:

> Man, about 50 years old. Aseptolin—two bottles (already came in the morning). Works at a plant; heavy drinker; often comes beaten up and inadequate.
> Woman, about 50 years old. Capsicum tincture—two bottles. Lives in the same building as the pharmacy; together with her son drinks away the pension of her disabled father.
> Man, 28 years old. Capsicum tincture—two bottles. Regular customer; ex-convict. Violent; threatens the staff if they refuse to sell him the tincture on trust. Beats up the local alcoholics and takes away their money if he is short of cash for "booze".
> Elderly woman, 60 years old. Bought five bottles of capsicum tincture. Always asks to put her purchase in a bag; hesitates when there are other people around.
> Female alcoholic, about 30–40 years old. Aseptolin—two bottles. Lives nearby; earns a living by removing garbage and empty boxes from stores. Tries to look well. Always comes wearing new clothes, which she seems to obtain from social services. Comes two-three times per day.

Such dismal customer behavior monitoring results may be due to the location of the pharmacy (not the most prosperous residential district; proletarian social composition of the population; nearby factory dormitories) and the specific features of Perm (it stands out even among other large cities by the rapid development of the retail segment of the pharmaceutical business). Nevertheless, we believe that these results are an exaggerated reflection of the nationwide situation, where assisting alcoholics and drug addicts to maintain their dependencies has become a noticeable social function performed by pharmacies.

At first glance, considering pharmacies in the context of "informal healthcare" might have raised doubts, but as we see, this approach is reasonable in view of the latent social functions of these commercial entities. We observed no shortage of pharmacy services in the Kama area where we conducted our fieldwork. Substituting medical consultations, providing remedies for self-medication and alternative self-treatment, supplying products that maintain alcoholism and drug addiction—all this partly explains the rapid development of the retail pharmaceutical business in an environment where by medical standards the availability of pharmacies is excessive.

## 2.3. Contemporary peddlers: Itinerant trade and peddling health products

Judging by newspaper ads, vendors of hearing aids are the apparent leaders among itinerant traders of health products. Every district center and medium-sized town hosts itinerant markets for hearing aids from one to four times a month. In one of Kungur's cultural centers, for example, such sales are organized on a weekly basis.

Following is a typical picture of the business. A notice is published in advance in the local newspaper. Premises are rented for an hour in a pharmacy, library, cultural center, club or newspaper editorial office. Usually, renting premises means the permission to use a chair and table in the lobby. The vendors—bold and stress-resistant young men who had arrived in a shabby car—offer devices from different manufacturers in a wide price range: from Russian-made behind-the-ear hearing aids for RUB 2,000 ($63) to imported digital instruments for RUB 30,000–40,000 ($940–$1,255), as well as components for them. They also help select the appropriate device, although they hold no license for medical activities.

Despite the above, ads often emphasize that the consultant is a certified specialist.

The vendors declare that they work under contracts with the manufacturers and issue a factory warranty for the product. However, in the event of failure, the unfortunate buyer has to wait for the next visit of the vendors to lodge a claim and send the device for repairs. Besides, the hearing aid can be inappropriate for the patient, because it was selected without a doctor. However, medical equipment is non-exchangeable and non-refundable in Russia, so the money can be wasted. In general, such purchases are obviously risky for the buyers.

However, this does not stop elderly people from the provinces, because in fact they have no other option to restore hearing loss. The official way of dealing with deafness is difficult and tortuous. Disabled people may receive a hearing aid free of charge, but first they must secure an appointment with an audiologist, get a prescription from him, and then travel several times to the regional center to order and pick up the device. According to Rosstat, in 2013 there were only 462 specialists in Audiology-Otorhinolaryngology throughout Russia; of them, only five were occupied in the Perm Territory. Ordinary otolaryngologists that could provide an appointment with a more highly specialized physician in Perm are also rare in rural areas. Against this background, enterprising traveling merchants that are prepared to pay a personal visit to the client upon request are a welcome opportunity for elderly people.

More or less the same contingent of vendors sells hearing aids in all the municipalities our team surveyed in the Perm Territory. The largest business belongs to sole proprietor Ekaterina Korobeinikova from Izhevsk. This businesswoman publishes ads in local newspapers throughout Central Russia, the Volga Region and the Urals. According to the Integrum regional media database,[57] in 2010—2014, sole proprietor Korobeinikova published ads in the local press of at least fourteen constituent entities of the Russian Federation—from the Volgograd and Leningrad Regions in the European part of Russia to the Omsk Region in Siberia. She combined a wide geographic spread of activities with extensive

---

57 The Integrum database (integrum.ru) covers a rather limited range of regional media where advertisements about itinerant sales of hearing aids are placed. Therefore, we can assume that sole proprietor Ekaterina Korobeinikova has a much more extensive scope of activities.

sales promotion events. For example, commercial ads show that in October 2013 vendors spent six days in the Perm Territory exhibiting and selling their products under the motto *For the Home, Everyday Life and Health*. They visited different parts of the region—from Berezniki and Solikamsk in the north to Chernushka in the south. In only two of the seventeen localities they rented space for an hour in pharmacies. In the remaining fifteen localities they used the premises of cultural institutions and leisure facilities—mainly palaces of culture, but also a library and a cinema.

Based on observations in the Perm Territory and a review of the local media in that and other regions, we can assume that a specific mobile market for hearing aids has emerged in Russia. A lack of interest from the regulatory authorities made it look legitimate for the time being. This market serves the interests of manufacturers and importers of such devices, but it is also relevant for customers outside of major cities. The fact that it commercializes the sphere within the scope of social obligations of the state makes it dubious. Besides, it offers hardly any opportunities to protect consumer rights. By Decree No. 6 of 5 January 2015 *On Amending Regulations for the Sale of Certain Products*, the Russian Government prohibited from 2015 all sales of medical products outside the established sales outlets.

For the state, the very functioning of this market is a grey area, because it is not reflected in the official statistics of providing technical devices to disabled people. If we were to extrapolate the estimated sales figures obtained from fieldwork in the Kama area to Russia in general, the annual volume of the market would be in the range from RUB 500 million to RUB 2 billion ($15.7–$62.8 million). This exceeds the amounts allocated from the state budget for hearing aids for the disabled.[58]

This market is not isolated from the rest of the "informal healthcare". Besides hearing aids, peddlers representing the above mentioned sole proprietor Korobeinikova occasionally have other health products or devices for home application in stock: Samozdrav Breathing Stimulators; Living-Dead Water Activators; ice studs for boots to prevent from slipping and falling in winter; ultrasonic washing machines; Mountain Air

---

58  According to the Federal Social Insurance Fund, in 2013 this amount was approximately RUB 555 million ($17.6 million).

Ionizers; seed sprouting kits; massagers, Coprinus mushroom against alcohol dependence; and Pankov's glasses. In short, a selection of relatively useful things customized for retired elderly people.

Summarizing we can say that itinerant trade is relevant for those health products which cannot be sold through pharmacies or other legitimate established outlets, because this is either difficult, unprofitable or forbidden. In particular, physiotherapy devices for home use under the brand name Almag used to be sold this way through intermediaries registered as sole proprietors. At the time of the fieldwork (2013), products manufactured by the Elatma Instrument Plant were allowed to be sold through pharmacies, so they disappeared from the stock of visiting vendors.

Besides hearing aids, peddlers specialize in other top-selling items, such as various wonder balms, ointments, and dietary supplements which they present as remedies against different diseases, even serious ones and those that mainstream medicine considers incurable. The product range may be limited to one item, which at the time of sale is still unknown to the buyers and therefore seems unique and exceptional (shilajit, red palm oil, the Coprinus mushroom, etc.), or include several items from one or two producers.

Trade practices are absolutely similar: the vendors rent premises for an hour; cover several localities in a day; and announce the events through advertisements in the local media.[59] Advertising follows a uniform pattern. Ads are placed either on a separate newspaper page, newspaper insert or a leaflet looking like an official publication (but without the required publisher's imprint and information about registration as mass media), which is dropped into private letterboxes. The leaflet contains information on the time and place of the event, an expert opinion of some distinguished doctor about the therapeutic properties of the product, and "extracts from the letters" of grateful cured customers. Such letters are the main argument of the advertising message and are meant to prove the case through the evidence of witnesses—a method contrary to science-based approach. In fact, advertising is the only way to communicate the therapeutic effect of the goods—their packaging and labels generally comply with the regulatory requirements for dietary supplements and

---

59 By contrast, sale notices for hearing aids contain only information about the seller and its services. The devices themselves are not advertised.

other non-medical products. For this reason, customers can hardly prove afterwards that they had been cheated.

The findings of our fieldwork in the Kama area indicate that such visiting trade fairs are specific for the urban environment. Unlike vendors of hearing aids, health product merchants rarely (twice a year or even less frequently, irregularly) appear in district centers, whereas they visit the cities routinely several times per month. Although the regional capital has numerous established sales outlets for health products, peddlers also operate here on a recurring basis. They usually rent premises in palaces of culture on the outskirts of the city.

Unlike network marketers, itinerant vendors of health products are young people. They are not proponents of a healthy lifestyle and obviously do not use regularly the products they sell. When dealing with customers, they emphasize that they work directly with the manufacturers[60] "under exclusive agreements"; therefore, they can offer better prices than the pharmacies.

Besides the above selling practice, which appears dubious even to inexperienced buyers, there are more civilized patterns of itinerant trade in non-medical products with advertised therapeutic properties that imply more emphasis on the medical aspect and extra efforts to win the customer's confidence. For example, a cultural center of the All-Russian Association of the Blind leases part of its lobby to a company from Udmurtia (a neighboring region). The company sells dietary supplements that are intended to treat a wide range of diseases. The sales consultant has a medical degree and is dressed in a white medical gown. She listens to the health problems of the potential buyers and then recommends certain supplements, thus acting as a medical consultant.

Peddlers arrange their work in such a way as to minimize the potential claims of disappointed buyers and the supervisory authorities. Most often they come from other Russian regions. The sole proprietors, on whose behalf they rent premises and trade, regularly change.

As in the case of hearing aids, such vendors can cover vast territories. For example, according to media ads, in 2010–2011 sole proprietor E.A. Mosheva from Krasnodar sold some exceptional shilajit from Kyrgyzstan throughout Russia (in the Moscow Region, in the Perm Territory, and

---

60 However, any attempt to find publicly available information about the manufacturers indicated on the packages leads to new traders, revealing a chain of intermediaries.

in Vladivostok). Prior to that, the same sole proprietor specialized in distance and itinerant sales of the "Bioactivator Health Amulet, which saves life and preserves health". The Federal Antimonopoly Service repeatedly declared its advertising to be inappropriate.

According to the staff of the institutions that rent out premises to visiting vendors of balms and other wellness products, some customers are satisfied with their purchases, whereas others are unhappy ("a woman bought some stuff here and she liked it"; "they come for an hour, and we have to listen to complaints afterwards"). Employees of Rospotrebnadzor's regional office for the Perm Territory mentioned receiving complaints about the inefficacy of the dietary supplements purchased at such visiting fairs or through distance selling. Nevertheless, such vendors quickly establish a network of regular customers. Clients pass by or call the organization where the sales took place enquiring about the next visit of the vendors.

Itinerant trade makes it easier to avoid claims and liability, but it also has another advantage. Clients perceive goods brought from afar and sold only occasionally, at a strictly defined time, as something exceptional. Consequently, according to an informant from among the pharmacists, local inhabitants readily buy remedies, which are not only of a dubious quality and therapeutic effect, but also overpriced.

Generally, such visiting trade events take place at the premises of cultural institutions and leisure facilities (palaces of culture and recreation centers, rural community centers, etc.). It is more practical for vendors to rent premises on an hourly basis from municipal institutions rather than from commercial entities. Besides being cheaper, this serves better to attract the attention of the local population. In small settlements, the community center may be the only public place where the local residents get together. Besides, cultural institutions employ many women of a close-to-retirement or post-retirement age who are the largest target group among consumers of health products.

Of course, as a lessor, a cultural center cannot compete with a medical institution. An ideal option would be to present dietary supplements or wellness devices in a clinic. However, this is usually forbidden by the head of the health facility who may be punished for promoting pharmaceutical products within the walls of the clinic. Since recently, this threat has been hanging over their heads like the Sword of Damocles. We recorded only one case when notice of an itinerant trade event was placed in a medical establishment—the municipal clinic in Chusovoy. Another similar option—renting premises in a pharmacy—is more common; it is used to sell hearing aids, healing oils and balms, as well as physiotherapy devices for home use. However, due to higher rent costs, even this option is rare as compared to selling events held at the premises of cultural institutions.

Do cultural institutions benefit from such arrangements? On the one hand, leasing out premises to third parties is an established way for municipal institutions to raise additional income. Leasing is the easiest way to increase the budget, especially if it is not a question of long-term lease. For this purpose, dietary supplements, balms, hearing aids, and physiotherapy devices are no different from other consumer goods offered at visiting fairs: fur coats, pots, and bedlinen from the manufacturer or from a customs warehouse. By volume, health products may even fall behind the other categories.

On the other hand, rental fees are low, and do not bring the administration of the cultural institution big profits. Thus, municipal palaces of culture in the surveyed towns charged RUB 400–500 ($12–$16) per hour. Generally, for this amount they provided a table in the lobby rather than a separate room. At the editorial office of the municipal newspaper in a district center the rate was even lower—RUB 150 ($5). A rural community center or a library may charge as little as RUB 100 ($3) or even RUB 50 ($1.5). One of our informants—an administrator at a palace of culture—pointed out, "All rates are approved by the finance department; we may neither raise, nor reduce the rental fees."

Local residents are perplexed that cultural institutions should be used to distribute wellness products and sell consumer goods. The founders of such institutions and the supervisory bodies are also annoyed, since they would like municipal leisure facilities to serve their intended purpose rather than turn into shopping centers. We heard that the administration of some cultural institutions refused to lease premises to visiting vendors. There were cases when the interviewers were told that the premises were not for rent, although newspaper ads and on-site observations indicated otherwise. Non-municipal cultural centers demonstrated more freedom in disposing of their premises.

The administration of the leisure facilities may or may not believe in the efficacy of the wellness products and services distributed on the premises they rent out. In any case, the impression from interviewing them is that they do not care what the visiting peddlers sell; whether such sales violate any legal provisions; whether the products are safe; whether advertising reflects the actual properties of the goods, and so on. In other words, they are willing to provide their premises for itinerant trade events to honest lessees and apparent swindlers alike.

In general, the described itinerant trade practice is a grey area for state control and accounting, as it develops in the absence of distinctly defined regulations and bans. However, there is another—related—type of peddling, which is clearly associated with fraud.

This concerns door-to-door and street vending of health appliances (primarily portable physiotherapy devices and massagers) based on a deliberate deception of the buyer. In contrast to itinerant vendors, such traveling salespeople incur no advertising or rental expenses. Unlike network marketers, who strive to win the confidence of the buyers and increase the number of loyal clients in their own locality, they work in any place only once. Their visit is afterwards remembered as an attempt to cheat the local residents.

Judging by the records of our field research in the Kama area, in 2010–2013, such street vendors coming from other places operated throughout the area. We heard stories about them in towns and villages. With minor deviations, the operating pattern is typical. The visiting vendors offer elderly people to buy physiotherapy and/or massage devices for home use, presenting them as a remedy against all diseases. Such devices are obviously overpriced, but the vendors insist they are selling them at a preferential price. They declare that the buyer is a participant of some state program (beneficiary of a charity fund, etc.) and is therefore entitled to purchase the goods at a big discount. They work with the target audience using the social services database (somehow obtained), or make a round of the households (in a village) inviting the people to come and listen to important information about the social policy of the state.

The local authorities and law enforcement bodies clearly define such activities as fraudulent and warn the population thereof through respective notices on noticeboards and in the local press. Despite this, it is very difficult to hold a vendor liable or compensate a buyer for damage, because selling at an inflated price is not an offense as such,[61] and the vendors are usually hard to find.

Russian law enforcement practice shows that frustrated buyers managed to return the purchased devices and retrieve their money if they appealed for help to a consumer protection association, and that organization represented their interests in civil litigation. Criminal fraud cases against such merchants are opened only when the police link their activities to the operations of a large organized criminal group. In Perm, such a high-profile case was filed in 2013.[62] According to police information, the Permskiy Krai Publishing House recruited staff vendors and trained them to apply respective selling techniques. Then, posing as employees of a certain government agency, the vendors approached veterans and told them about a special federal program for supplying such devices. The money they charged was supposed to be collateral for using the device rather than payment for it. In 2013, a court in Khakassia considered a similar case on distributing Home Doctor devices. The organizer of the trade chain received a minor suspended sentence. This sentence demonstrates that law enforcers consider deliberately misleading customers as to the therapeutic effects of the sold devices to be a major threat only when the enterprising merchants pose as government employees simulating the social policy of the state.

In general, the work of contemporary peddlers selling health products in the lobbies of cultural centers, from small trucks in the street, or from door to door may be perceived as a certain relic of the past amid the existing widespread forms of retail trade (shopping centers, supermarkets, online shops). However, when it comes to certain types of products, such practices are sustainable, pervasive, and reproducible. Due to this, we cannot consider them yet another rudiment of "the turbulent 1990s"

---

61   We are talking about the situation prior to 2015. Subsequently, peddling medical devices was prohibited and, consequently, door-to-door sales of physiotherapy appliances became illegal.

62   According to the Interior Ministry's Main Directorate for the Perm Territory, "since 2010, the wrongdoers have been selling physiotherapy devices in the region under the guise of entrepreneurs. <...> The police have identified over two and a half thousand victims. Total damage amounts to about RUB 20 million. Twenty-two people have been found guilty". *See* Interior Ministry's Main Directorate for the Perm Territory (website).
URL: https://59.mvd.ru/news/item/2140097/.

along with shuttle trade and peddling products paid out by employers instead of wages. Such activity is the principal vending pattern for goods that cannot be sold through pharmacies or other authorized trade outlets because of difficulties or bans.

\* \* \*

Itinerant trade, alternative health maintenance systems offered by MLM companies, and the pharmacies' latent social functions—these three cases of the activities of "informal healthcare" agents engaged in the retail trade of health products in present-day Russia are very different. What unites them is their invisibility. They do not fit into the government's picture of providing medical products to the population, which is formed by regulations and official statistics. They appear in the media and on the administrative agenda only when regarded as outrageous problems requiring administrative decisions and tighter control. However, we are dealing with established socio-economic practices apparent to ordinary people, because they regularly encounter them in everyday life and even use them from time to time. In the following chapters, we will show that such invisibility is also typical of other "informal healthcare" agents.

# 3 Health from the garden, forest, and market: Procuring and selling gifts of nature

We are interested in those cases when people intentionally gather, cultivate, buy, and sell gifts of nature to address specific health problems. Natural remedies form the basis of treatment methods generally attributed to folk medicine. The word "folk" in this context refers to something natural—something that is not of an artificial (industrial) origin.

The chapter focuses on two areas of activity: production of health products based on private subsidiary farming (cultivation of medicinal plants, beekeeping, etc.); and hunting and gathering, i.e., the collection and harvesting of natural resources. Lawful cultivation and harvesting of natural remedies on a commercial scale for processing and further marketing as dietary supplements or medicinal herbs or for the production of medicines sold in pharmacies remain beyond the scope of the discussion, because such activity focuses on serving formal healthcare.

Since this sphere is heavily dependent on the climate, location, and other natural factors, drawing a nationwide picture based on field data collected in one region would be inappropriate. Therefore, the text focuses on the Perm Territory, and I tried to avoid involuntarily extrapolating the findings to other regions or Russia as a whole.

*Natural remedies: harvesting range and scale*
We shall start with bee products (honey, bee pollen, propolis, royal jelly, and bee venom). They are often used in basic self-medication for colds and in the more "advanced" folk medicine (including, for example, alcohol tinctures on dead bees). Markets for dietary supplements, certain drugs, as well as specific therapies (bee sting therapy) have developed on the basis of bee products. Official medicine recognizes bee products and considers them useful when applied for authorized self-medication approved by doctors. Medical science substantiates the efficacy of their active ingredients: scientists conduct pre-clinical and clinical research, and defend dissertations on bee products.

Beekeeping in Russia exists predominantly on the level of private households.[63] In the surveyed parts of the Perm Territory beekeeping is a widespread occupation in the agricultural areas around Kungur. According to Permstat, 5,391 bee colonies were registered in the Kungur district in 2012, whereas Chusovoy district had only 902. Most beekeepers are private individuals. Beekeeping for them is not the only and often not the main activity. An average apiary contains thirty honey bee colonies. Many informants noted that beekeeping had "shrunk in size" (in the Soviet Union, collective farm work standards provided for one beekeeper to take care of sixty bee colonies; the average size of an apiary was from sixty to one hundred beehives). Urban residents often keep beehives in the countryside—at the dacha or in a village. Small villages can have up to a dozen apiarists. For many of the beekeepers we interviewed, apiculture is a family tradition. Few of them register this as a business activity. For example, only six apiarists in the Suksun district are registered as sole proprietors (the number of honey bee colonies exceeds two thousand). It happens that a person is employed at an apiary of a local entrepreneur and also keeps his own bees.

There is an enormous gap between official figures for honey production and sales. According to Permstat, a total of 2,851 tonnes of honey was produced in the Perm Territory in 2012, but sales reached only 497.3 tonnes. Similar figures for the Kishert district amounted to 112 tonnes and 20.1 tonnes, respectively. This shows that sales of honey from private farming is a grey market segment uncontrolled by the state.[64] Official statistics does not capture any other bee products.

As for the medicinal resources of plants, we should always keep in mind the difference between the positions of orthodox medicine (for which plants are starting materials of herbal origin) and folk medicine. According to the website of the Russian Environmental Federal Information Agency,

---

[63] As at 1 July 2006, the total number of honey bee colonies in Russia was 3,727,800. Of them, 3,490,800 (93.6%) belonged to private households; 180,000 (4.8%)—to agricultural entities; and 57,000 (1.5%)—to farmers and sole proprietors (*Results of the 2006 All-Russian Agricultural Census*, V.5, 2008).

[64] Moreover, there is a significant difference between the figures of the federal statistics service (Rosstat) and its regional branch (Permstat). Rosstat reported that in 2012 the commercial production of honey in the Perm Territory was 1,404 tonnes. Upon request, Permstat, in turn, provided the figure of 2,851 tonnes.

about 2,500 higher plants on the territory of the former USSR have medicinal value, but pharmacological authorities allow using only about 200 of them.[65] General information about the number of species of medicinal plants in the Perm Territory varies depending on whether we are considering only wild plants and only those plants the effect of which has been recognized by official medicine. The popular *Atlas of Medicinal Plants of the Perm Territory* includes 350 species that "grow and can be cultivated" in the region (Shchelokova, Glumov, 2009), whereas the *Russian State Register of Medicines for 2008* contained only 93 plant species growing in this area (Belonogova, 2009).

Cultivation of medicinal plants in the Perm Territory is virtually nonexistent. According to the 2006 Agricultural Census, only 5.3 hectares of land were allocated for these purposes in the area—this is approximately 100 times less than in the Novosibirsk or Ivanovo Regions. For comparison, the overall figure for Russia is 4,558.7 hectares (*Results of the 2006 All-Russian Agricultural Census*, V.4, 2008). In 2013, Permstat informed that such statistics was not collected because medicinal plants were not cultivated in the area. According to expert assessments, commercial harvesting of medicinal plants here is also undeveloped (Belonogova, 2009). In short, the Perm Territory has no robust herbal medicine industry.

However, medicinal plants are widely used in everyday life. As expected, gathering wild plants and using plants from one's own garden is common practice in the surveyed rural communities of the area. The usual winter stock includes from three to five, rarely up to ten plants (interviewees often named oregano, St. John's wort, mint, marigold, lime blossom, coltsfoot, rose hip, cranberry, and cowberry).

Among houseplants, Basket plant (Callisia fragrans) is worth separately mentioning. It is popular with people keen on folk medicine, but it is not a formally acknowledged medicine. Although Basket plant is grown on the windowsill, it is also cultivated for sale. We believe its popularity is purely of a media nature and is due to a certain fashion, like the one for kombucha among Soviet people.

Besides higher plants (herbs, fruit, bark, buds, etc.), folk medicine uses other harvested products: mushrooms (Chaga mushrooms, fly aga-

---

65   *Terrestrial Biological Resources*. The Russian Environmental Federal Information Agency (website). URL: http://www.refia.ru/index.php?13+2#lekarst.

rics), shilajit, and rock oil. In the surveyed localities, the fly agaric (Amanita muscaria) occupies a special place in the list of healing gifts of nature. People apply its alcohol tincture externally against low back and joint pain, and take it as a remedy which "kills off cancer". In informal conversation, a female mushroom picker (about 50 years old) selling fly agarics on the street gave us the following recipe of this folk remedy: "For cancer, place the mushrooms in a glass jar and bury the jar for forty days; take the resulting mushroom juice in drops". We heard several stories of miracle recoveries thanks to fly agaric.

Of the animal derivatives used in Russia for medicinal purposes, the best known and most popular remedies are badger fat, bear grease, bear bile, castoreum, and antlers. The last three (along with deer musk) are an integral part of traditional Chinese medicine; however, Russia has its own national traditions of using these remedies.

Products of hunting which are attributed medicinal properties are processed and widely sold as dietary supplements. They are traditionally included in the product mix of online stores and networks distributing natural remedies and are sold in the form of tinctures, exudates, elixirs, capsules or simply poured into jars. The scale of sales suggests that a large portion of such products are either counterfeit or made from poached derivatives.

Often such derivatives are advertised as universal remedies for many diseases, although specialization also exists (e.g., badger fat—for treating respiratory diseases). From the standpoint of orthodox medicine not all of them possess adequate evidence of efficacy.[66] Demand for such products depends not only on tradition, but also on fashion and media promotion. Sometimes medicinal properties are attributed to certain animal derivatives not only due to the popularity of Eastern medicine, but also because of the passion for occult practices or simply for marketing purposes.

Bears, badgers, and beavers can be found in the geographical area of the Perm Territory. However, obtaining a permit for hunting wildlife

---

66 Synthesized ursodeoxycholic acid, found in large quantities in bear bile, serves to produce hepatoprotectors. The therapeutic effect of antlers and deer blood is a subject of scientific research; they are ingredients in some tonics. Physicians believe badger fat to have a certain therapeutic effect when applied externally (warming effect). And castoreum is formally used only in the perfume industry. Only folk medicine recognizes its numerous healing properties.

is a very costly affair. Hunters say that "only the rich can nowadays afford hunting". A hunter must buy a one-time personalized license indicating the bag limit and a voucher to a hunting farm.[67] For an ordinary villager the total cost of the permits is quite high.[68]

The administration of the hunting farms is currently the main regulator determining the scope of the legal market for medicinal animal derivatives. It sets the price of the voucher, and based on the number of game animals on the farm grounds determines the share that may be harvested (the general standard is ten percent from the official number of animals registered with the farm). Although the prices vary from farm to farm, the difference is insignificant. Further we will show that hunting farm managers also act as information mediators and market moderators, since they possess information about the allocation of resources and have the contact names and numbers of the local hunters.

The scale of legal harvesting is very small. For example, in 2013, Suksun Hunting Farm with an area of 52,000 hectares had 44 registered bears, of which four animals were designated for hunting (in practice, fewer animals may be harvested); and 45 registered badgers, with also four of them designated for hunting. In the Kishert district we were told that hunters do not purchase vouchers for bears at all due to their extremely high price. In 2012, four badgers and three bears were legally harvested in the grounds of the Sylva Hunting Farm (which include the area around Kungur and Uinskoye village).

The official harvesting figures seem negligible when compared with the number of hunters. According to the hunters themselves, not all of them have the skills required to harvest a badger or a bear. All-in-all, a district may have only several professionals who can be contacted for medicinal derivatives.

Along with legal harvesting, there is a shadow market for animal derivatives, which according to an informant, is largely driven by the "anti-popular law" on hunting. The ill-conceived policy of the state forces people to hunt illegally.

---

67　In the Russian Federation, a hunting farm is a public or business entity authorized to use game animals in a particular area.

68　Annual hunting licenses for a bear cost RUB 3,000 ($95), for a beaver or badger—RUB 60 ($2). In the surveyed rural areas, a voucher to harvest one bear cost from RUB 30,000 to RUB 50,000 ($942–$1570); one beaver—RUB 800–RUB 1000 ($25–$32); and one badger—RUB 600–RUB 2000 ($27–$63).

The situation with the beaver has markedly changed in the past decade. Beavers used to be rare animals in this geographical area, and their harvesting was strictly rationed. The exudate from a beaver's castor sacs (castoreum), which according to rumors was a "natural Viagra", was a scarce commodity and highly valued on the black market. However, the beaver population has significantly grown in recent years, and beavers have spread virtually across the whole territory. At the same time, they are no longer perceived as such a valuable source of medicinal components. According to interviewed hunters, people are now very reluctant to obtain hunting permits for this animal.

In general, the Perm Territory is not an outstanding region in terms of using gifts of nature for medicinal purposes. Unlike the Far East, for example, it has no particularly valuable natural resources that could serve as a basis for international black markets or large-scale industrial processing. The emerging supply is aimed primarily at satisfying the self-medication needs of the local population.

*Folk medicine amateurs and professionals*
Procuring (gathering, producing, cultivating) healing gifts of nature is part of the household economy aimed at ensuring the self-sufficiency of households, especially in rural areas.

Gathering well-known medicinal plants is the most widespread practice ("we are all herbalists ourselves", one of our interviewees said). However, few people possess in-depth knowledge of the subject. It implies, on the one hand, using rare plants, the collection of which requires special efforts, like traveling to remote places; and on the other hand, the habit of seeing healing properties in garden plants and weeds, which are always at hand.

Cultivating medicinal plants in one's own garden for wellness purposes is another specialized practice. The simplest options are to plant chamomile, peppermint, marigold, etc. Cultivating also means growing Basket plants or Aloe vera on the windowsill and sometimes nipping off parts of the plant to fight a cold or reduce inflammation.

However, rather than among villagers, we encountered a comprehensive approach to maintaining "a medicinal garden" among urban dwellers with summer cottages in the countryside or living in private houses with an adjacent land plot. Medicinal gardening is primarily intended for private consumption; even that is rather symbolic, because it is impossible to cultivate herbs on a vegetable patch in amounts sufficient for long-term use. A real apothecary garden is a very rare phenomenon, although gardening websites abound with respective recommendations.

A passion for cultivating medicinal herbs is a rather rare occupation, but it implies a circle of like-minded people to exchange plants and recommendations. Among our informants those were women in their post-retirement or close-to-retirement age that advocate alternative medicine, participate in network marketing, and live in urban rather than rural areas.

Interviews with healthcare professionals give the impression that along with harvesting, people in rural areas readily buy medicinal herbs in pharmacies. However, despite the mediation of pharmacists, medical experts consider such self-medication chaotic and unprofessional.

Our observations show that there is no developed market for medicinal herbs even in rural areas. There are very few professionals with good knowledge of medicinal plants who can prepare herbal combinations. Customers say about them: "The sellers are normal people—herbalists, not vendors". Informants often refer to professional herbalism as an old-time folk tradition. Even people who actively use original techniques and alternative therapies (urine therapy and others) to maintain their health, are sometimes skeptical about being involved in phytotherapy.

Folk herbalists are gradually replaced by people relying on book knowledge. In rare cases, they are professionals, physicians or biologists, who convert their scientific expertise into services for proponents of herbalism. We encountered one such professional in Perm at the regional expo *Health and Medicine—2013*. An elderly female biologist had turned into phytotherapist—she collected herbs and prepared herbal combinations customized to the individual requirements of her clients. Her prices were quite at the market level.[69] In addition, she promoted her services and raised the awareness of the population by taking part in local TV broadcasts, lecturing at health resorts, publishing books, and participating in various health fairs. She emphasized the scientific basis of her services, thus opposing herself to "quack" folk healers.

However, most herbalists engaged in street vending gain knowledge about the effect of plants from periodicals and pamphlets. Our informants named such sources as "a book on plants" bought at a village

---

[69] A consultation cost RUB 500 ($15), and the herbal combination intended for a two-month treatment—RUB 2,000 ($63).

market; a selection of "small pamphlets" with "old recipes" that used to belong to the vendor's mother; the magazine *Apiarist*; books by Valentina Travinka; a collection of folk recipes from Siberian healer Natalia Stepanova; and, naturally, the *HLS Bulletin*. The latter, in particular, encouraged an herbalist from a surveyed Orthodox convent to start making medicinal herbal tinctures and oils for sale.

It is noteworthy that street vendors use such pamphlets and periodicals as evidence of their competence in the eyes of customers. Thus, a woman selling medicinal herbs near the Klyuchi resort in the Suksun district always brought along newspaper clippings to demonstrate that her information came from reliable sources. Another vendor claimed relying on books "where everything is written" and carried around photocopied pages from them.

Notably, even where there is a developed market for gifts of nature, the gatherers remain quite ignorant about the properties of the plants. We encountered this in 2011 in the Charysh district of the Altai Territory.[70] Local poachers selling bagfuls of rare medicinal herbs to tourists and dealers had only the vaguest idea of the actual effect those plants produced. For example, when we asked about the application of the red root (Hedysarum neglectum), we were told at best that it "was very good for men". To locate the required herbs, gatherers relied on old Soviet atlases of plants listed in the Red Data Book of endangered species.

So, we do not find any clear correlation between the gatherers' occupation associated with supplying medicinal herbs and their involvement in folk medicine. Probably, the situation is different with beekeepers? When communicating with apiarists in the Perm Territory (altogether eleven people), we always asked about their attitude to treatment with bee products and awareness of their medicinal properties. Opinions varied from active commitment to indifference and ignorance. Only two or three people knew in detail the medicinal properties of bee products and used them regularly to treat their friends and family. Some sold only honey and from time to time used propolis and bee pollen to treat their family members and other relatives. The products that beekeepers offer for sale are rarely "loaded" with those super healing properties that dealers usually attribute to them.

---

70  Fieldwork in the Altai Territory was conducted in July 2011 under *The Health Maintenance System* project funded by the Khamovniki Foundation for Social Research.

The attitude has nothing to do with whether or not the beekeeper is a health professional. Thus, one of the informants extensively relied on the medicinal properties of bee products and utilized everything possible for health purposes. She said, "My father used only honey and propolis; and I, as a former feldsher, use other products as well." Another female beekeeper—also a rural feldsher—did not use bee products for medicinal purposes preferring to rely on conventional medicine: "Well, I believe if I take pills, the effect will be better." Yet another informant criticized folk medicine referring to the opinion of his wife—a physician:

> I do not believe in folk medicine and go to hospital for treatment. You must consume bee products permanently for them to be of any benefit. It's not as if you can get cured by just eating a jar of honey.[71]

*Markets for natural health products*
In order to understand how such markets function at the local level, we first of all inspected marketplaces and the popular locations of unauthorized street trade. Then, when speaking to experts and ordinary residents, we enquired about the people to whom one turns in need of healing gifts of nature, and contacted the beekeepers, hunters, and herbalists ourselves.

Theoretically, there are several ways to dispose of the medicinal products obtained by gathering and hunting or privately cultivated:
- Consume personally and offer as gifts
- Sell through acquaintances
- Sell at home, but to order or through local media and outdoor advertising
- Sell through retail trade outlets or by peddling
- Sell to dealers or to procurers for processing

Observations in the Perm Territory show that the first two forms prevail. We rarely came across announcements in the local district newspapers (one or two cases per year) or saw any evidence of outdoor advertising (there were a lot more advertisements in the cities).

As for street trade, the areas designated for authorized sale of agricultural products from private plots, including farm markets and street stalls allocated by the local administration, are not the principal outlets for natural health products. Authorized marketplaces are trade platforms for

---

71  Informant: male, about 60 years old, beekeeper, village.

imported consumer goods—food, clothing, and footwear, which are usually referred to as "Chinese stuff". Local gifts of nature can be found most often at unauthorized sales points which spontaneously emerge in crowded spots and where there is no need to pay for retail space: around major public transport stops, at busy intersections, on the central street sidewalk or next to the fence of an official market.

Of the ten authorized markets surveyed in Perm in the autumn of 2013, only three offered healing gifts of nature. The Central Market had the largest number of sellers; however, the wide range of goods (different kinds of honey, several dozen species of medicinal herbs, badger fat, and shilajit) and high prices allow to assume that the vendors were professional dealers. At the same time business was flourishing in spontaneous "spots" of unauthorized trade.

Street vending of healing gifts of nature has certain features that indicate the absence of large-scale developed markets in this field; moreover, such markets are unlikely to emerge, at least in the Perm Territory.

First, street trade is characterized by seasonality. We conducted fieldwork from May to November, and the situation varied depending on the month. Natural remedies were available in the market only during limited periods: the most popular medicinal herbs (St. John's wort, oregano, motherwort, lime blossom, and others)—in midsummer; fly agarics—in autumn; bee products—in late summer and autumn; badger fat—in late autumn and winter. In autumn and winter, one can also buy cranberries, medicinal alcohol tinctures and dried rowan berries, viburnum berries, rose hips, and hawthorn berries.

Second, in most places (except for tourist ones), the individual vendors neither harvest nor cultivate health products specifically for sale. Generally, they offer passers-by what remains from their personal consumption and what has not been sold through acquaintances. "They gather herbs mainly for their own needs and sell only the surplus", clarified an interviewed expert representing Kungur's municipal administration.

We can assume that the demand for such goods is low, since street vendors often gather and bring healing gifts of nature only "to order", if somebody requests them. For example, due to unstable demand mushroom pickers do not offer fly agarics for sale every day, "because they don't keep long—their caps open out".

For rural beekeepers, street vending in the cities is often only a way to find new regular customers. Here is how a hereditary 60-year-old beekeeper, who came to trade in Chusovoy from neighboring Beryozovka district, described his strategy: "We use the marketplace to establish contacts, and then people buy from us year after year. Some clients have been purchasing only our honey for ten years in a row." By the marketplace he meant unauthorized sales spots near major stores.

Finally, street vendors have minimum knowledge of the medicinal properties of the gifts of nature they are selling. As mentioned above, they mainly gain such knowledge from popular literature. However, they often readily consult the buyer as to the best treatment methods. For example, one female informant inserted a kind of instruction for use in the bags with herbs—a handwritten A4 sheet of paper recommending in what forms to take the herbs (as alcohol tincture, tisane or lotion). The vendor also indicated her mobile phone number on the sheet.

Street trade is somewhat different in tourist places. Here sales outlets for natural remedies develop with a focus on urban clients. Sellers compete, often accusing each other of incompetence or poor quality of the goods. The products are harvested specifically for sale, the prices are generally higher than in other locations, and the therapeutic effect of the goods is more aggressively advertised. In Kungur district, for example, such a spontaneous marketplace is located at the entrance to the Belogorsky St. Nicolas Monastery. In July, several elderly women from the neighboring village sold herbs (St. John's wort, oregano) there, which they had gathered in the vicinity. The monastery also buys medicinal plants from the locals. It dries, packages, consecrates them, and sells in the church shop.

Street vending of medicinal animal derivatives is rarer; it involves the most relevant products—badger fat and bear grease. In the countryside, such trade takes place along intercity roads; in the towns—in marketplaces. However, villagers are unanimous in their opinion that such purchases are risky. First, the product may be counterfeit (according to the hunters, "it may contain only margarine" instead of grease). Second, one can very likely run into a product obtained from an animal that is sick or infected with parasites. Since predominantly poachers trade "on the road", their prey obviously does not pass any sanitary-epidemiological control.

How do herbalists engaged in street trade operate? Many of them sell medicinal herbs in addition to other products they gather or cultivate: honey, berries, mushrooms, saplings, vegetables, jam, etc. We were more interested in those who harvest and sell medicinal herbs regularly and offer customers homemade preparations from them, thus demonstrating a more or less in-depth knowledge of the subject. Following are two examples showing the different approach to this occupation.

The first informant was an elderly woman, long retired, a city-dweller. It was her first year in street vending ("earlier I had neither time nor need for this"), but she had been processing natural raw materials for her friends and family for quite some time using folk medicine recipes. For her, this was actually a hobby, a certain way of making her old dream of becoming a doctor come true. Her knowledge came from popular health periodicals (she was subscribed up to four newspapers at a time) and books, and she readily shared it with others. A resident of Perm, she spent six months at her dacha in the village. The geography of her harvesting was very wide—she gathered some plants in the vicinity of her relatives' village in the Perm Territory, cultivated others on her own land plot in the far away Kursk Region, and even grew something at home on the windowsill. On top of that she bought some missing ingredients in the Central Market in Perm. She did not regard pharmacies as a source of starting materials for her preparations: "I do not trust them. Who knows, whether their herbs are not expired." She prepared Basket plant and fly agaric alcohol tinctures, as well as dandelion root tincture with oil; sold "roots" (comfrey), hawthorn berries, rose hips, and four-five various herb species. Upon request, she also prepared herbal combinations. Her prices were arbitrary, cost-based, and in general substantially (sometimes twice) lower than in the Central Market.

The second informant was a middle-aged woman living in a village near a resort. Like her fellow villagers, she tried to benefit from the proximity of the wellness facility to earn some money—in the evenings she came to the entrance to sell herbs, roots, and blue clay. She was a former nurse; so, in presenting and advertising her goods, she used expressions which gave folk remedies the appearance of medicinal products. And that, despite the fact that like the first informant she gained knowledge about them primarily from popular books and newspapers on folk medicine. Her product range was quite extensive (about ten items), but included only locally growing herbs. The prices varied depending on the customer and were established arbitrarily in the process of communication. She did not follow any particular attendance schedule and spent her "work shifts" near the resort not only trading but also establishing contacts. She had built a client base from some former and present guests of the resort who placed orders with her. Upon request, she sent them goods by post, sold large quantities of clay and medicinal herbs at home, and also acted as guide—accompanied those interested to places where the herbs grow. She used hired labor to procure the raw materials: "Clay is very hard to get; it is deep down in the river. I don't dig myself—I hire people to do it." Unlike the first case, where herbalism was nothing but a hobby, here the gatherer planned to make a living from selling wild plants. She was even considering wholesale business—she had a one-time experience of selling several sacks of herbs to a dealer from Perm, and was negotiating regular supplies of plants to local entrepreneurs running a tourist camp.

If medicinal herbs can be harvested and cultivated for personal needs only, in beekeeping output usually exceeds such needs, and beekeepers must find ways to sell the honey. For lots of them this becomes a real headache, especially in the villages, where many people have their own honey, but business skills are lacking. Most of the beekeepers we interviewed complained about low demand and the absence of an established market for their products.

They try to sell honey through acquaintances or at home (to anyone "who looks in"). Customers also benefit from such informal purchasing, because it is cheaper and the risk of buying counterfeit or poor-quality goods is lower. Beekeepers establish their own client networks of friends and acquaintances, colleagues, and regular customers from big cities. They told us in interviews that they were sending honey to neighboring big cities (Perm, Ekaterinburg, and Pervouralsk) for further marketing through acquaintances.

However, this turns out to be insufficient. Competition forces people to find ways out, and they resort to unregulated market techniques, which were widespread in Russia in the early 1990s, but became illegal due to increasing legislative pressure. Such techniques include trading in the immediate proximity of farm markets, in other public places, and along highways; pasting private ads in the street; and making door-to-door rounds of offices. Although sales of products from private subsidiary farming are not taxed, beekeepers tend to avoid authorized retail trade outlets because of additional charges—the need to obtain a certificate for the goods and pass veterinary control.

The amount of honey harvested from an apiary varies depending on the weather and the intensity of flowering. On average, a bee colony produces from twenty to thirty kilos of honey per season. When setting sales prices, private beekeepers take into account prior-year prices, the honey yield in the current season, and average local prices. They are also guided by the prices set by market dealers. Generally, as the purchase volume increases, the price of a liter goes down. In the summer and autumn of 2013, a three-liter jar (about 4.5 kg) of honey cost in the surveyed localities from RUB 900 to RUB 1,500 ($28–$47). Thus, from thirty beehives, a beekeeper earns on average RUB 200,000–RUB 300,000 ($6,300–$9,400) per season.[72] Given that beekeeping is physically demanding and time-consuming, it can hardly be considered a highly lucrative business.

As in the case of herbalism and beekeeping, rather than search for a product in shops or on the market, local residents prefer to address hunters directly when they need medicinal derivatives of wild animals. Negotiations between the customer and the hunter may be mediated by the manager of the local hunting farm.

Note that under legitimate allocation of hunting resources a badger is harvested only when there is a specific customer—consumer of medicinal fat. However, the requirements of a particular patient are always less than the amount of fat (two-three liters) a hunter obtains from one animal, so he needs to dispose of the surplus. This is usually done through friends and family. In the surveyed rural areas, a standard portion of badger fat (in a 250 ml "mayonnaise" jar) costs anywhere from RUB 600 to RUB 1,000 ($18–$32). In emergency situations (for example, when a child is sick), a hunter can give away some product for free. A hunter makes approximately RUB 5,000–RUB 8,000 ($155–$250) from one animal. This covers the overall hunting costs and leaves "just enough to buy a bottle of vodka". Bear derivatives (bile and grease) are rare and expensive even when compared to badger fat. Hunters sell them (if at all) only through acquaintances and only "for insiders".

---

72  For comparison: according to locals, villagers specializing in picking mushrooms and berries for sale (on the market, through acquaintances, or along highways), during the summer season earn up to RUB 100,000 (about $3,200).

As for selling natural remedies to dealers and processors, this option is the least common in the surveyed rural communities. The Soviet system of consumer cooperatives on which all harvesting activities were focused (Kuznetsova, 2012) is no longer in place, and selling products obtained through hard labor to dealers is unprofitable. Pharmacies currently do not purchase medicinal raw materials either. Monasteries are a rare exception—they buy wild plants and agricultural products from residents of the neighboring villages, process them for their own needs, and sell to pilgrims.

Besides, dealers are not active in the area, which means that extra efforts are needed (like going to a major city, etc.) to deliver a large quantity of goods. Thus, an informant who used to harvest castoreum for wholesalers cannot sell the remaining amount of three kilograms after having lost contact with the intermediaries.

We observed the activity of dealers only at the stage of retail trade in products of private subsidiary farming and hunting. It is, however, difficult to determine the share of the authentic local product in the end goods, which may also contain various supplements or even be imported. Dealers most often sell certified bee products attractively packed and "loaded" with additional advertised healing properties. They invent the healing effect according to the medicinal properties of particular plants, thus offering a variety of honeys ("acacia", "chestnut", etc.), which a beekeeper, familiar with how bees collect and produce honey, cannot understand and accept. Their prices can be both higher and lower than the average market ones, thus allowing them to compete with private producers.

Entrepreneurs who have their own apiaries and also buy up honey operate through specialized sales outlets in cities or tourist locations. They have several options: engage in itinerant trade at premises leased for an hour or a day in cultural centers or other facilities; participate in specialized trade fairs paying for a place/stall; distribute through retail chains; and, finally, open their own stationary shops. In the surveyed localities, visiting entrepreneurs serving several regions engage in such retail trade rather than the local business people.

***

Summarizing the observations set forth in this chapter, we can say that no developed markets for natural health products emerge in areas where there are no particularly valuable natural resources that could serve as a basis for international shadow trade or large-scale industrial processing (as in Eastern Siberia and the Far East).

Gathering wild plants, cultivating medicinal herbs, beekeeping and hunting—these rural occupations serve primarily to satisfy the personal requirements of the local population in self-medication and help their friends and relatives. Lots of efforts are needed to sell large amounts of products that would generate some income from harvesting. Especially if we are talking about legal activities. Considering the details of how natural remedies are procured and sold in rural areas, one inevitably starts doubting the authenticity of the health products that in processed form are widespread in the market for dietary supplements.

The image of folk medicine as a field of expertise and skills drawing on the Russian people's in-depth knowledge of the nuances of harvesting and using healing gifts of nature—a knowledge passed down from generation to generation—tarnishes. The relationship between passion for folk medicine, practicing it as a profession, and providing customers with products obtained from private subsidiary farming, hunting, and gathering is far from linear. Where it exists, traditional knowledge is replaced by a compilation of ideas picked up from the media.

# 4 Shadow and respectable alternative medicine: From healers to "complementary" specialists

The main heroes of this chapter are healers, which constitute the most obvious opposition to classic doctors. In everyday language, they are usually associated with alternative medicine, although, as can be seen from the previous sections hereof, they are not the most popular and mass agents of "informal healthcare". In contrast to suppliers of goods and ideas for self-medication, representatives of this segment provide therapeutic and diagnostic services themselves. Orthodox medicine treats their various methods differently.

It rejects some services completely, since they are based on supernatural phenomena that modern science cannot explain. The state classifies them into two categories. *Occult and magical services* have nothing to do with medicine at all. A medical background is required to practice *traditional medicine*, but such services are not automatically permitted in regular healthcare facilities. In the early 1990s they were widely integrated into formal medical practice in the wake of increased interest in alternative therapies in Russia. These circumstances still determine the tactics of professionalizing and promoting the services of healers.

Other services are permitted in medical institutions, and the state grants health professionals the exclusive right to practice them. They are often designated by the fixed expression "complementary and alternative medicine" (CAM). Some CAM practices become part of the treatment process; they are admitted into the public health system and monopolized by the professional medical community. However, even in this case, they are "stepdaughters" among the modern medical specialties. On the one hand, evidence-based medicine challenges their right to be a decent medical occupation. On the other hand, CAM specialists promote their services by contrasting them with the basic approaches of orthodox medicine.

Hence, our description of "informal healthcare" services includes two large sections focusing on healers and CAM physicians, respectively. The last—third—section addresses mental health specialists that replace other medical professionals. Despite being the shortest, it concerns an extensive and popular segment of services in Russia. This segment is generally not regarded as part of traditional or folk medicine, and I believe it is worth a separate discussion.

## 4.1. "People remember a certain Baba Vanga, so they will also remember me": Healers

This group includes people who according to their patients provide health services due to paranormal abilities, skills, and hidden (esoteric) knowledge.[73] Such healers can have different designations: witch doctors, psychics, magicians, sorcerers, shamans, babushkas, bonesetters, traditional healers and so on.[74] The term "healers" in this case is used as a universal reference.

This mixed group of "informal healthcare" agents currently operating in Russia resorts to a vast arsenal of methods, including:
- Treatment by a special type of energy, the knowledge of which has been drawn from esoteric teachings and pseudoscientific concepts (psychics, Reiki masters, cosmoenergy- and bioenergy therapists, and others)
- Traditional magical practices: charms, prayers, and rituals using particular items
- Manual skills unrecognized by conventional medicine (bonesetters, Philippine healers), etc.

The variety of these diagnostic and treatment methods includes practices adopted from Russian traditions, imported from other traditional cultures, and relatively recent ones that are associated with occult knowledge and new spiritual teachings. Accordingly, many of them do not fall under the definition of "folk medicine"—you cannot say about them that they are entrenched in folk traditions and are passed down from generation to generation.

---

[73] At the same time, they are not controlled by religious organizations whose representatives can also engage in treatment with the help of God, i.e. the supernatural.

[74] For example, the catalogue of healers on the Russian esoteric website *Psychic Universe (Mir Extrasensov)* identifies, among others, the following categories, or specialties: numerologist, cosmoenergist, witch doctor, wizard, enchantress, fortune-teller, prophet, eniologist, medium, sorcerer, healer, witch, astrologer, seer, psychic, magician, soothsayer, shaman, bioenergy therapist, bioenergist, clairvoyant, and palmist. URL: http://www.extra-mir.ru/celiteli.

Amendments to the legal definition of "folk medicine" introduced by the law *On the Fundamentals of Public Healthcare in the Russian Federation* can be interpreted as the state's intention to distinguish this activity from esoteric practices. By contrast, people applying such methods follow the strategy and tactics of integrating occult practices with medicine.

In addition to those who specialize primarily in treating physical diseases, there are also general consultants who address people's problems (including health problems) using skills and abilities that science cannot explain. These are predictors of the future (fortune-tellers, astrologers, clairvoyants, and palmists) and magicians/sorcerers/psychics who undertake to neutralize the negative effects suffered by humans from supernatural forces (jinxes, evil eye, negative karma, and black magic). Since such occupations are all based on a holistic approach to human nature, the practitioners fight the disease by eradicating its cause, which allows enhancing all aspects of the client's life—brings him health, wealth, and family happiness. Consequently, such specialists also participate in "informal healthcare" and are relevant to our description, although at first glance they do not fall into the category of healers.

It is also necessary to consider the difference in positioning the activities. Thus, anthropologist Galina Lindquist identified two independent social roles when describing Russian magicians and healers in the early 2000s. People seek the help of magicians mainly to address social and personal problems. Difficulties in romantic relationships top the list, followed by the need to bring adult children that had gone astray to their senses. Domestic alcohol abuse and problems in business and finances rank third and fourth, respectively. Healers, in turn, promise to deal primarily with health problems and define their activities in the biomedical paradigm. Although it is sometimes difficult to notice any difference in the ways magicians and healers work (for example, both make similar passes with their hands), the latter extensively use medical symbols and attributes when presenting themselves (Lindquist, 2001).

It is difficult to determine the scope of healing in contemporary Russia, as this sphere is mystified and largely in the shadow. It seems that estimates of this phenomenon that appear from time to time in the media are mostly arbitrary and depend on the imagination of the author. Thus, in March 2013, the media widely publicized the statement of Moscow's chief cardiologist that Russians annually spend over $30 billion on psychics, sorcerers, etc.[75] An earlier declaration by State Duma deputy Tatiana Yakovleva that 800,000 psychics are operating in Russia also seems taken "out of thin air".[76] In 1995, experts spoke about 300,000 healers that were using methods and techniques based on energy-informational approaches, whereas representatives of the Russian Orthodox Church estimated the number of healers at the beginning of the 2000s at about 250,000 (*Traditional Medicine,* 2011).

We can be certain only of one thing: there is a stable demand in the country for treatment by paranormal methods, this being associated with a widespread belief in the supernatural. Notions about the ability to cause harm by magical techniques—jinx, evil eye—are common. They are a familiar way for members of the traditional (rural) society to interpret social relations and explain the emerging problems; therefore, they are quite persistent. As anthropologist Olga Khristoforova notes, it is a flexible but very sustainable mental and emotional framework where the real and the imaginary intertwine (Khristoforova, 2010).

The facts about healing that our team gathered in the Kama area in 2013 come from two principal sources: stories told by local residents about the living and deceased healers in their localities, and direct contacts with such specialists (seven interviews and two informal conversations). The resulting picture is a far cry from widespread media representations of healing.

The media landscape is largely shaped by institutions whose main function is to streamline the market of occult-magical or esoteric services and professionalize healing as its integral part (professional associations, educational organizations, specialized websites, etc.). For such institutions, establishing a professional community and an integrated organizational field is not just a mission, but also a kind of business, i.e. an income-generating activity. Healers involved in their work regard their occupation as entrepreneurship; they resort to advertising and seek—if only formally—to comply with the requirements imposed on them by the state. It is important for them to be recognized by the society and their colleagues-competitors. The strategy for winning recognition includes simulating

---

75 *Russians Spend $30 Billion on Sorcerers and Psychics.* Interfax.ru. 20.03.2013. URL: http://www.interfax.ru/russia/296568.
76 Pleshakova S. *Russia Launches a Witch Hunt.* Moskovsky Komsomolets. 05.04.2011. URL: http://www.mk.ru/politics/russia/article/2011/04/04/578224-v-rossii-obyavlena-ohota-na-vedm.html.

a scientific infrastructure and integrating into complementary medicine. For example, the ENIOM All-Russian Research Center for Traditional Folk Medicine promotes the idea of eniomedicine which "includes homeopathy, phytotherapy, bioenergy therapy, psychic studies and practice, and many other branches".[77]

By contrast, field data presents healing as an individual non-professional activity targeting friends and relatives—non-public and quite ordinary, not conspicuous (in particular, neither the dwellings of the healers, nor their appearance stand out in any way). Apart from Perm, this was the main category of healers, either located personally or mentioned in conversations with the local residents in the surveyed towns and villages.

Informants presented healing as a common miracle. When asked whether there were any healers in the settlement, they often related stories of their personal experiences of being treated by such healers, or about relatives that were providing such services. Even people with a medical background told us about healers in their families. Thus, a retired doctor said that her father in an inexplicable manner "charmed away hernia by drawing something"; a former feldsher revealed that her aunt had been a witch doctor who could cast spells over water, remove jinxes, and do other things.

Many informants expressed the view that healing was a tradition rooted in the past, which was dying out together with the villages. We frequently heard the following answers to our enquiries about local witch doctors: "She used to live here, but she has died"; "I haven't heard anything about her for ages"; "She has gone and taken the gift of healing with her". Nevertheless, evidence suggests that such activity is continuing, although its external features are somewhat changing.

Not every village or settlement can "boast of" people with supernatural healing powers, but local residents concerned about their health are able to indicate the whereabouts of such healers in the immediate vicinity. In the surveyed district centers and small towns, we recorded from two to seven healers whose names were well-known. As was to be expected, most of the information came from people involved in socio-economic relations of "informal healthcare" as agents or clients, while representatives of official bodies (local officials, physicians) were convinced

---

77   ENIOM All-Russian Research Center for Traditional Folk Medicine (website). URL: http://www.eniom.ru/centr/history.

that there were no traditional healers in the area under their competence. Perm's online forum *teron.ru* contains reference to over a dozen well-known local babushkas specializing in children's ailments (treating umbilical hernias in infants with bites and spells, curing stuttering, etc.) and in general diseases. They usually live in private houses on the city outskirts or in the suburbs and do not publicize their occupation. There are also those who openly advertise their services in this field ("experienced magicians", fortune-tellers, psychics, cosmoenergy therapists, etc.). We identified over thirty of them based on newspaper and other ads, although such data must be treated with caution. There are also at least a dozen Reiki masters in Perm engaged in treatment and training.

The shadow nature of healing activity in Russia is worth mentioning. Although legislatively not prohibited, it is illegal in the vast majority of cases. There are no regulations governing occult-magical services, but in order to treat people openly, a healer must obtain a permit to practice folk medicine. The permit is valid only in the issuing region. A recommendation from a professional medical association, which tests the skills and abilities of the healer, is needed to obtain it.

Very few permits are issued. According to media reports, only several hundred healers were registered in Russia in 2012.[78] It took long for the required regulatory framework to take shape on the regional level. When the regional authorities finally established the requirements for applicants for a diploma in healing, it turned out that most traditional healers, especially in rural areas, could not comply with them. Thus, pursuant to Order No. 3 of the Ministry of Health of the Perm Territory of 12 January 2009, only individuals with a higher or secondary medical education, possessing a diploma and special title, and registered as legal entities or sole proprietors are entitled to practice folk medicine within the region. According to the authorities, practicing folk medicine at home is also inadmissible—the premises where healing sessions are held must meet sanitary standards established for public buildings.

In short, the requirements of the state are such that the vast majority of practicing healers do not fit into the specified framework. Therefore, the number of people legally treating others by means of psychic powers, esoteric knowledge or magic is negligible in Russia. In June 2013, the

---

78    Reznik I. *Moscow Insists on Herbs with a Diploma. Metropolitan Authorities Intend to Establish Control Over the Activities of Local Traditional Healers.* Gazeta.ru, 08.10.2012. URL: http://www.gazeta.ru/social/2012/10/08/4805193.shtml.

Department for Licensing Certain Types of Activity of the Ministry of Health of the Perm Territory informed that it had issued only five diplomas over the entire period of keeping a register of healers (2010–2011). It is noteworthy that four of the five healers were registered as sole proprietors, lived in the Kirov Region, and worked in the same organization.

The activity of healers can be classified by various parameters. The easiest would be to do it based on the applied diagnostic and treatment methods. However, this approach does not provide a socio-economic characteristic of contemporary Russian healing practice. Classification options by the economic nature of the service, by ways of being drawn into such activity and level of professionalization, and by the client base would be more appropriate. We shall examine each of these criteria separately.

*The price tag. Commercial and nominally free of charge healing*
If we present the variety of healing practices as a single spectrum, nominally free of charge services will be at one end of it. They are generally provided by the so-called *babushkas (old ladies),* who can also be relatively young women. Such healers help people out of compassion, enthusiasm or because "they cannot do otherwise" ("God commands" and so on) accepting gratitude in the form of food or money, according to the principle "whatever people choose to give". Their work can be called nominally free of charge because gratitude is after all common.

Such healers do not advertise their services—information about them spreads "by word of mouth". Their clientele consists of friends and relatives, the friends of friends, neighbors, and local residents. Moreover, they do not always perceive their activity as a professional occupation, saying that they are "just helping". Anyway, they do not regard this work as the main source of income. "One will give a loaf of bread, another— 50 rubles. Indeed, not everyone in the village is rich,"—this is how an informant—a 70-year old village healer—described her income.

Shadow services of unregistered healers, unaccounted for by the state, are in the middle of the spectrum. The price for such services, however, is usually clearly established, even if it is called "gratitude" or "reimbursement". In other words, there is an understanding of how much such services may cost. Rather than pricing services based on the work input, the healers we talked to set their fees by reference to those charged by conventional and alternative medicine professionals to whom people turn with similar health problems, but at a lower level.

According to the information we managed to obtain in the Kama area, the fees of such healers range from RUB 200 ($6) per session charged by a bonesetter (plus a mandatory additional symbolic payment in small change—three coins with a par value of 10 kopecks each) to RUB 2,500 ($78) charged by a healer working with alcoholics.

The client flow varies. Most informants noted a decrease in the number of patients in recent years, also because they themselves had shortened the visiting hours due to poor health. Usually, they claimed consulting several people a day; however, this did not happen on a daily basis (the average number was rather several patients a month). The most well-known and popular healer from among our informants, who according to the local residents used to consult about a dozen people daily, at the time of the interview had only three patients a day (a consultation cost RUB 500 ($16); previously, she used to work under the principle "whatever people choose to give").

Thus, in the best-case scenario such activity can generate annually approximately RUB 300,000–RUB 400,000 ($9,500–$12,500), which is a substantial amount for a village, but comparable with average wages in Russia. None of the surveyed healers stood out from the local residents by a more luxurious house or higher standard of living (in contrast to entrepreneurs or local officials). In most cases their houses looked very modest and even shabby; if a homestead was prosperous, this was due to the diligence of the owners.

None of them purposefully advertised their services. However, there are also other healers—those who attempt to win clients by placing classified ads in newspapers and promoting their services in public places frequented by people interested in esoteric knowledge. Usually they practice modern healing techniques (Reiki, cosmoenergetics) or provide general magical services that do not focus on addressing health problems (predict the future, remove jinxes, break the evil eye, etc.). Most advertisements contain no reference to prices, but there are exceptions. Thus, a séance with a "powerful psychic, parapsychologist, and magician" from Perm cost RUB 1,000 ($32). Another advertisement offered to remove a jinx for only RUB 200 ($6). Note that classified ads about such services are common for cities; in rural areas, they are rather an exotic rarity.

In the opinion of potential clients, real healers are selfless, work free of charge, and accept only gifts. It is widely believed that a fixed fee means the healer is "just making money", so he or she is either a quack or a black magician. Thus, the non-profit nature of healing becomes a criterion of the quality of services and enhances the credibility of the healer. For example:

> I like such babushkas that don't take any money at all. < .... > Then the chances are higher that she will help < .... > If a person has the gift, it is God-given. And the treatment must also come from God.[79]

The other end of the spectrum is represented by legalized or partially legalized business-focused healers with the status of sole proprietors or LLC. They tend to promote their services openly on their own websites, through advertising, membership in associations of healers, and if lucky— by participating in TV shows. They work under tariffs that may be determined absolutely arbitrarily. As St. Petersburg sociologist Oleg Pachenkov (Pachenkov, 2001) noted, when it comes to well-known widely promoted healers, we can speak about the "entrepreneurial strategies" of their operations and entire business teams organizing the work of a person with paranormal abilities.

Healing as a business is often combined with other, related activities. In this case it serves primarily to enhance the image of the "informal healthcare" agent and promote its core businesses—sale of ideas or goods. Such businesses include spiritual teachings and "health promotion systems" with associated training centers; trade in esoteric literature and occult goods; astrology schools; psychology and personal development centers; direct selling of therapeutic devices, etc.

Speaking about healing as a business, we should also mention the associated fraud. According to media reports, up to ninety percent of newspaper classifieds advertising magical services, including healing, come from fictitious, "not real" psychics and magicians (i.e., those who are not engaged in healing).[80] Their main goal is to collect information on

---

79   Informant: male, about 50 years old, local resident, medium-sized town.
80   Rakshenko L. *Magic Business: Wholesale and Retail Miracles.* Harvard Business Review—Russia. 2012. Nos. 6–7.

those who respond to the ads and create a database of client phone numbers. The database is then used in phone and sms fraud, for blackmailing, and consulting by telephone in the name of popular psychics.

Court practice shows that the most common type of criminal cases associated with healing, which fall under Article 159 of the *Criminal Code of the Russian Federation* (fraud), involves trivial "Gypsy-style" cheating. The swindler, being well aware of having no special abilities, *poses as* healer and convinces people that a curse has been put on them, which can be broken by magic procedures of "purifying" money, jewelry, and other valuables. Contact with the victim usually takes place in the street or at the victim's home. That is, there is no question of regular healing practices.

According to the Public Computerized Database *Justice*,[81] there are very few charges in this sphere: in 2010–2014, courts of the first instance heard only about forty criminal cases. This means that very few incidents of this kind are taken to court. Civil cases where clients try to claim compensation from the healers for an undesirable effect of their services or lack thereof generally end in a ruling against the plaintiff.

*Customer base and status of healers in the local community*
Where does a healer's clientele come from? If a healer uses traditional business tools to gain clients, the customer base is limited to the area covered by advertising. As besides treating people professional healers are often engaged in related activities and businesses, patients learn about them primarily at specialized locations: centers of alternative medicine, massage parlors, esoteric goods shops, schools of healing or spiritual associations. Accordingly, they serve an audience already involved in "informal healthcare"—well-prepared and anticipating a therapeutic effect.

It is a different case with healers who do not seek publicity. Attempts to find out from local residents the whereabouts of familiar healers brought unexpected results. As information about the babushkas and bonesetters that do not advertise themselves in the media spreads "by word of mouth", from acquaintance to acquaintance, the path that leads customers to them is sometimes long and winding. The general trend is such: rather than turning to healers who live nearby, patients prefer those

---

[81] URL: bsr.sudrf.ru.

with good references. For example, in interviews, Orda residents mentioned going to the neighboring Suksun district for treatment of alcoholism, while some Suksun residents went with the same problems to the Oktyabrsky district. Contrary to widespread belief that healers live mainly in remote villages, some informants from Lysva and Kungur traveled to Perm to see people with healing abilities. So, the geography of services develops spontaneously, especially in the era of Internet technologies.

In conversations, healers love to show off their extensive clientele, "collecting" visitors from afar:

> Only Putin and Medvedev haven't visited me yet; yes, those two I haven't seen. Otherwise, people are coming from everywhere. How did you find me, I ask them? They say, "Through the Internet." They are all coming to me. Let them come while I am still alive. People remember a certain Baba Vanga, so they will also remember me, yes.[82]

Healers who are not widely known serve mainly relatives, friends, and neighbors. They actually partially compensate for the lacking healthcare resources in rural areas, and therefore enjoy the respect of the local residents.

However, in the Perm Territory we also witnessed the opposite occurrence. Some healers served primarily visiting patients, but the locals did not trust them, often substantiating their skepticism by the lack of medical background. However, in other cases the absence of a medical diploma was no obstacle to contacting the healer, because he or she "helped". Apparently, relationships within the local community are more important than education: the healer's reputation is largely due to his or her personality and ability to communicate with neighbors.

*Gift and diploma. The industry of professionalizing healing practices*
For some, healing is an innate and inherited gift ("hereditary healers"), for others—skills acquired through special training or initiation (as in the case of Reiki), self-study of esoteric literature, experienced religious revelation or grave illness. The two ways of becoming a healer can be combined: people discover in themselves unaccountable abilities to treat others following contacts with the community of experts on paranormal phenomena. I believe that like in the case of herbalism, healing in Russia has long been characterized by the process of replacing the traditional transfer of

---

82   Informant: female, healer, about 90 years old, village.

knowledge and skills with generally available self-studies relying on the media and fee-based training.

There is no generally accepted notion of "gift" and of how the innate talent for healing appears. For example, newspaper advertisements for such services often emphasize the transfer of unique powers from ancestors referring to *generations of healers*. However, in interviews we heard different versions of what option of acquiring the gift was considered legitimate. In one case a healer assured that her powers were God-given; in another—that the gift may not be transferred to anyone (i.e., it cannot be a willful act of the healer); in the third—that it may be transferred to strangers, but not to relatives, etc. Apprenticeship exists, even among our informants. However, it is not common, and both experts and local residents believe this to be the reason why folk healing is fading into the past.

The healers from among our informants had mainly acquired their treatment skills at relevant courses (workshops) widespread in the 1990s, as well as from specialist and popular literature on health and esoteric knowledge. Virtually none of our interlocutors had any professional medical background; however, some of them were trained veterinarians with hands-on working experience, which they believed gave them all the required knowledge about the human body. With luck, after assimilating and creatively elaborating miscellaneous ideas they developed their own techniques, which gained the clients' confidence.

For example, a female informant (about 70 years old) has been practicing healing since 1994. Prior to that she had worked as educator and member of a trade union committee at an industrial enterprise. Like many others, in the 1990s she tried to learn some new skills to earn a living, and became fascinated by the esoteric. During that period of spiritual and professional pursuit she attended massage courses ("manual and under Djuna's [famous faith healer] technique"), participated in "American-style autogenic trainings", went to a hypnotist, and practiced "immersion in the underworld". She said that at some point the gift of healing inherited from the ancestors was awakened in her. She provided the following proof of the inherited nature of the gift: her grandmother from one branch of the family had been an herbalist, a great-grandmother from another branch—a sorceress. "Of all our big family, the gift was transferred to two people only—my sister and myself." Having discovered her healing powers, she went to a health center and enrolled for a training course on applying hypnotherapy for smoking cessation "using Dovzhenko's method" (generally "only medical workers were admitted" but for her an exception was made). After completing the course, the healer enhanced the technique and started using its adapted version to treat alcohol abuse.

Training healers is a specific business in Russia. It is characterized by an exaggerated imitation of the external features of scientific hierarchy and public education, although naturally without any licenses for educational activity.

The main players in this field are industry associations and "academies", such as the Academy of Traditional Folk Medicine; Professional Visceral Therapy Association; ENIOM All-Russian Research Center for Traditional Folk Medicine; Guild of Traditional Medicine Practitioners, Healers, and Applied Psychologists; Moscow School of Parapsychology; International Academy of Clairvoyance and Energy Therapy with an in-house "theosophical-parapsychological university", and many others. Every region has training facilities. Well-known healing centers and popular magicians that widely promote themselves are also engaged in teaching. For example, several followers of Marina Krymova—a popular esoteric psychologist with a focus on pre-Christian Slavic culture—provide healing and esoteric services (clairvoyance and magic, rehabilitation massage, "Russian stretching", and other) in Perm.

Such schools simulate and reproduce formats of modern vocational training with its lectures and examinations and traditional apprenticeship with its magic rituals of initiation and transfer of supernatural powers. Offers vary: one can choose between full-time, correspondence, and distance (by Skype) learning; enroll for comprehensive or specialty programs, select multi-level long-term or express courses. Training healers may be combined with teaching fortune-telling, clairvoyance, magic techniques or astrology. The cost of such educational services is rarely published; however, the available information indicates a wide price range. Apparently, fraud is also thriving in this sphere—a widespread option is to charge money for some "distance training course" without actually providing any educational services. Online sales of all kinds of healing manuals—DVD video course and others—are also common.

A review of publicly available sources shows that the market of educational services for healers is so mature and accessible that it seems self-sufficient. In other words, it is much easier to make money on training people who wish to become healers and magicians than on providing the actual healing services. It appears that few of those students who had obtained "diplomas" and "certificates" succeeded in turning healing into an occupation generating enough income to make a living. A similarity with network marketing is traceable—there, rank-and-file distributors attracted by potential earnings are the main consumers of goods and services provided by their MLM companies.

The training business is an element of the infrastructure for professionalizing healing practices in Russia, which, as mentioned earlier, is dominant in the media and shapes the public perception of this occupation. The infrastructure also includes professional unions (associations, societies), competitions and titles, certification, and specialist periodicals. It started developing in Russia in the early 1990s as part of the general normalization of supernatural studies. Pavel Romanov and Elena Iarskaia-Smirnova noted that this normalization was an integral part of the public discussions focusing on esoteric issues (Romanov, Iarskaia-Smirnova, 2007).

The most distinguished and respectable professional union in this field is the Russian Association of Folk Medicine (RANM[83]). It was established in 1990 when the First Congress of Russian Healers took place. Regional health authorities consider the recommendations of RANM's Central Expert Qualification Commission when issuing permits to practice folk medicine (formerly—diplomas in healing). Delivering such documents is a source of income for the Association. According to an informant, an expert review costs about RUB 50,000 ($1,600).

The Global Association of Physicians, Psychologists, Traditional and Faith Healers;[84] the Guild of Traditional Medicine Practitioners, Healers, and Applied Psychologists; the International Professional Medical Association of Complementary and Folk Medicine Practitioners, Psycholo-

---

[83] The full name is the Russian Professional Medical Association of Traditional and Folk Medicine Practitioners. Former names: Association of Folk Healers of Russia, Professional Medical Association of Folk Healers of Russia, All-Russian Professional Medical Association of Traditional and Folk Medicine Practitioners and Healers.

[84] Sociologist Elena Salo believes that the Global Association of Physicians, Psychologists, Traditional and Faith Healers is the only organization of this kind in Russia, "which is somewhat closer to the Western model of a professional association" (Salo, 2009, p.26).

gists and Healers, and other organizations claiming to represent the interests of the professional community are less conspicuous in the public sphere.

The diversity of professional titles and awards on the websites of some widely promoted healers is astonishing. They may include medals: *For Achievements in Folk Medicine, Master's Star, First Degree Honored Healer, For Educational Activity, For Healing Activity, Magic Touch,* and *Healing Elite*; titles of award winners in competitions *Best Healer, Best Russian Healer of 1999, the Last Decade of the Twentieth Century, Best Russian Healer of 2000–2002, Best Healer of the Last Decade of the Twentieth Century, Best Healer of the Third Millennium,* etc. As an overview of the media revealed no information on the procedure for selecting competitors and holding competitions, we can assume that such titles and awards are attributed against payment and are a source of income for professional associations.

Basically, institutions for the professionalization of healing are first of all business projects aimed at making money on people wishing to become professionals. Therefore, their scope of work is typical: training, certifying educational programs, holding forums and congresses, organizing excellence competitions and granting awards, issuing publications like *The Best Healers of Russia*.

Legal professional institutions in Russia unite a negligible minority of all the people who provide treatment relying on supernatural powers and skills. This is evidenced by data from the registers of associations and unions. Thus, the catalogue of the leading Russian-language esoteric website *Psychic Universe (Mir Extrasensov)* contains about 1,700 registered specialists, of them only twelve—in the Perm Territory.[85] The Russian Association of Folk Medicine had about 350 members at the end of 2014.[86] ENIOM's International Register (Directory) of Psychics, Parapsychologists, Bioenergists, Healers, and Clairvoyants contains about 330 people, of whom at least a quarter live abroad.[87]

---

85  Data from the *Mir Extrasensov* (website) as at May 2015.
    URL: http://www.extra-mir.ru/celiteli.
86  Data from RANM (website) as at November 2014.
    URL: http://www.ranm.org/roll/index.phtml.
87  Data from ENIOM (website) as at May 2015.
    URL: http://www.eniom.ru/rossiyskiy-registr-celiteley).

Finally, all attempts to introduce certification of healers in Russia that would protect consumers from fraud and indicate the existence of a civilized market of services in this field have so far failed.

In January 2006, Roszdravnadzor of Russia issued a special order (No.154-pr/06) announcing the introduction of the *Register of Healers*—a system of voluntary certification of folk medicine services. FCTRC TDTM was charged with issuing the certificates. In a separate information letter No. 01i-363/06 of 27 April 2006—*On the Activity of Folk Healers*—the Head of Roszdravnadzor clarified that it's regional branches would consider the certification results when inspecting the work of legal entities and sole proprietors "engaged in folk medicine".

According to the media, very few healers expressed the desire to be entered in the Register, and only twenty percent of the applicants succeeded in proving the efficacy of their methods.[88] In 2008, a representative of Roszdravnadzor informed that over two years the agency had carried out only forty-five certification inspections, issued thirty-three certificates of compliance, and turned down twelve applications (Kazakov, 2008). In 2015, access to this register was no longer publicly available. By then, the organization in charge of issuing the certificates had been liquidated. We can therefore assume that the certification system is not operational. Meanwhile, the idea is in the air, because it gives the operator of the certification system wide opportunities to control the access of professionals to the market and has an obvious business potential. RANM, for example, is advancing this initiative.

Although visible in the media, the institutions for the professionalization of healing practices are not very popular with their target audience. The reasons may be their focus on profit-making, and no real need for the healers to have their professional interests represented or their activity legalized. Therefore, we believe they cannot serve as an indicator of the actual situation in this sector and may not be used to evaluate the level of professionalization of healing practices in Russia.

Another aspect of their activity is more important. Such associations unite under their roof phytotherapists, homeopaths, professionals in

---

[88] Reznik I. *Moscow Insists on Herbs with a Diploma. Metropolitan Authorities Intend to Establish Control Over the Activities of Local Traditional Healers.* Gazeta.ru, 08.10.2012.
URL: http://www.gazeta.ru/social/2012/10/08/4805193.shtml.

Ayurveda, or Tibetan medicine, Reiki, as well as those who heal with prayers and bioenergy effects. Specialists in complementary medicine and professionals in occult-magical services sit side by side at their forums and congresses. Members of the associations often demonstrate proficiency in different techniques, both permitted and banned for use in medical institutions. In other words, the institutions for the professionalization of healing practices work to unite "informal healthcare" services as such, whether recognized by the state or not.

\*\*\*

Let us summarize the overview of current treatment practices in Russia that rely on paranormal abilities and phenomena. In depicting them we focused on the socioeconomic aspect of such occupations and deliberately omitted reviewing the applied techniques, which vary considerably. A comparison of methods would have shown us a string of different social roles/types varying by entourage and the ideological roots of their activity. By contrast, comparison by type of income, customer base, and level of professionalization allows presenting healing practices in the form of an iceberg.

The top of the iceberg is formed by institutions for professionalizing such practices as "folk medicine" (schools, associations, register, ratings, media resources). They serve the interests of a narrow stratum of star healers and business-focused healers, and make money on the desire of people fascinated by the supernatural to be admitted to this circle.

The hidden part of the iceberg is the daily activity of semi-professional and amateur healers who work informally and sometimes do not regard their occupation as a service. Patients, for their part, do not identify them with the media image of magicians/psychics and willingly resort to their help in certain cases (curing sprains, bruises and concussions; "biting" umbilical hernia in infants; treating alcohol abuse; removing jinxes, etc.). Some healers serve a wide range of clients and charge a fixed fee. Their names sound familiar, so it is possible to determine their number in a given locality. But there are also others: they are invisible to the outside observer; they help only friends and relatives, either for a symbolic fee or out of mutual assistance; and they do not position themselves as healers. Their interaction with the patient is based only on the shared belief of both parties that health problems can be addressed by means of the supernatural.

## 4.2. Frontier zone: Ambivalent status, recognition problems and shadow practices of complementary and alternative medicine specialists

While professional medicine decisively dissociates itself from paranormal healing practices, some non-conventional methods are privatized by it and included in the arsenal of healthcare institutions. The process of recognition is accompanied by heated professional discussions about the efficacy and evidence base of one or another diagnostic or treatment method.[89] A sociological approach allows to distance oneself from these discussions and focus on the frontier status of complementary and alternative medicine specialists.

However, even here many questions arise. The academic discussion of our findings was a perfect illustration. There was always someone in the audience who objected to using the words "informal" or "alternative" with regard to homeopathy or reflexology, for example, and referred to laws, regulations, and public opinion to substantiate this position. For instance, if a method is taught at a medical school, can it be classified as CAM? Does the official admission of a treatment method to medical practice make it an integral part of conventional medicine? In order to find the answers, it is necessary to review in detail the regulatory framework, and, what is more important, forgo the straightforward approach to healthcare as a sector with clear boundaries determined by the mere reference to them in the documents regulating medical activity.

The market for services of CAM professionals is a frontier zone of "informal healthcare", so we cannot depict it without examining how the state and official medicine recognize their activities. The first part of this section focuses on these processes and shows how the scope and prerequisites for integrating CAM practices into Russian healthcare affect the

---

[89] The article of V.V. Vlassov, President of the Russian Society for Evidence Based Medicine, titled *Bar Homeopathy from Medicine* published in the *Medical Newspaper (Meditsinskaya Gazeta)* (No. 55 of 23 July 2010) and the reaction of A.A. Karpeev, Chairman of the National Council for Homeopathy could serve as an example of such public debate. *See* National Council for Homeopathy (website). URL: http://homeosovet.ru/articles.php?article_id=3.

provision of services in this sphere. The second part deals with Russia's most prominent shadow markets of CAM diagnostic and treatment services, where other agents (sometimes winning the competition for the customer) participate along with physicians.

*Recognition institutions and the boundaries for legal activities of CAM physicians*
As mentioned in the first chapter, in view of the corporate nature of Russia's medical community, recognition of alternative treatment methods by the state and by official medicine is possible only in one way—in the form of a take-over. Medical professionals monopolize the right to use such methods, and from then on, the physicians practicing them must comply with the principles of the national health system. Integration results in the emergence of a medical specialist built into the work of an appropriate institution which has all the legitimate grounds to claim part of the system's resources. Only this specialist is from then authorized to provide certain services to patients.

However, state regulation of a medical activity implies that besides the permission to practice it according to the specialty, this activity must also be included in the respective supporting (educational, HR, scientific, informational and statistical, organizational and managerial, etc.) infrastructure of the Russian health system. Thus, for a gastroenterologist to provide services, the system must have: the ability to obtain a license to provide medical care in gastroenterology; a diploma of higher education and a respective professional certificate; a position in the staffing schedule of a medical institution; approved standards regarding the number of gastroenterologists in the healthcare facility, the number of specialized wards in hospitals and the equipment of their consulting rooms; reference to gastroenterologists in statistical reporting forms, as further allocation of budgetary resources is based on official statistical data; research specialization enabling to establish a dissertation council, conduct research, and develop medical science in this field, etc.

This supporting healthcare infrastructure is established and regulated by separate laws and regulations. Let us see what role is accorded to CAM practices, or, according to the terminology accepted in Russia, traditional medicine practices.

The first step towards integrating an alternative medicine field into Russian healthcare is obtaining an authorization to use certain therapies in clinical practice. CAM professionals often refer to orders of the USSR Ministry of Health that were issued expressly to introduce their methods into healthcare practice, and to methodology guides (*metodicheskie rekomendatsii*) written by groups of authors (mainly from FCTRC TDTM) in the late 1990s—early 2000s and approved by the Russian Ministry of Health. For some alternative techniques, the once developed methodology guides still remain the only document proving their involvement in formal healthcare, which they would like to emphasize.

The methodology guides were an element of the system, which existed in Russia in the 1990s–2000s for the purpose of admitting medical methods to practice and keeping track of them.[90] Under its general logic, a new method could appear in medical practice only following research by a specialized institute subordinated to the Ministry of Health—the academic institution invented the method (technique), performed its clinical trials, substantiated it, and introduced into healthcare practice. The recognition of CAM methods also followed this procedure.

For example, the third edition of the *State Register of New Medical Technologies* contained 1218 "prevention, diagnostic and treatment technologies and organizational methods of work" approved for use in medical practice; of them, the traditional medicine section contained 15 medical technologies, such as, "variational thermo-algometry in traditional diagnostics" or "combined homeopathic and manual therapy of patients with pain syndromes associated with spinal osteochondrosis" (*The State Register*, 2002). By comparison, the 2009 list comprised also medical technologies developed by business entities, which thus introduced their products into widespread healthcare practice. Thus, along with prosthetic replacement surgery and coronary stenting, new technologies included such methods as "the *Oculist* dietary supplement for the correction of

---

90  Pursuant to the *Fundamental Principles of the Legislation of the Russian Federation on National Healthcare* (Article 43), only approved preventive, diagnostic, and treatment methods were allowed in Russia. They were included in the *State Register of New Medical Technologies*, which from 1995 to 2002 was published as an official document of the Russian Ministry of Health. Every method in the Register contained a reference to a methodology guide (*metodicheskie rekomendatsii*) or practical guidance (*metodicheskie ukazania*) developed by the research institution applying for approval of the technique. In the period from 2004 to 2012, Roszdravnadzor of Russia was in charge of registering new medical techniques and keeping their register (list).

functional vision disorders" from JSC DIOD Plant of Environmental Equipment and Organic Food, and "informational radio-wave screening diagnostics and correction of the functional state of the human body" from CJSC Informational Medicine Research Center.

The new system for standardizing medical care stipulated in the law *On the Fundamentals of Public Healthcare in the Russian Federation* (2011), implies that only methods included in the standards of care and the procedures for providing medical care by type of disease (*poryadki okazaniya meditsinskoi pomoshchi*), hereinafter referred to as *poryadki*,[91] may be applied in healthcare practice. An exception is made for innovations undergoing clinical trials. The standards, in turn, are based on the *Nomenclature of Medical Services* approved by the order of the Russian Ministry of Health.

The process of developing the standards of care for every disease and having them approved by the Ministry of Health is far from completed; therefore, it hardly makes sense to analyze the place of CAM methods in them. If we look at the *poryadki* (i.e. documents of a more general nature, which determine the resources that healthcare must allocate to fight diseases), we will see that CAM methods are included in medical rehabilitation. According to Order No. 1705n of the Russian Ministry of Health dated 29 December 2012, medical rehabilitation includes "integrated application of drug and non-drug (physiotherapy techniques, exercise therapy, massage, therapeutic and preventive nutrition, manual therapy, psychotherapy, reflexology, and methods involving natural healing factors) therapies." Besides massage, physiotherapy, and reflexology rooms, the same document also refers to leech therapy, apitherapy, and homeopathy facilities.

The *Nomenclature of Medical Services*[92] does not explicitly distinguish traditional or folk medicine services either. Services there are classified strictly in the spirit of biomedicine. Many services, which used to belong to traditional medicine, are mentioned in the nomenclature, but placed in different categories. Various types of massage, acupuncture, and manual therapy can be found in the section "treatment by simple

---

91   *Poryadki* determine the rules of work, equipment, and staffing of medical facilities for a group of diseases (e.g., tuberculosis), medical specialty (e.g., urology, neurology) or type of medical care (e.g., medical rehabilitation).
92   The nomenclature was approved by Order No. 1664n of the Russian Ministry of Health and Social Development on 27 December 2011.

physical impact on the patient". Phytotherapy, along with other services of wellness institutions (mud therapy, baths, ozonation, mineral waters), have been placed in the category "treatment by exposure to climatic factors (water, air, etc.)". The only reference to bioresonance therapy ("bioresonance therapy in reflexology") appears in the section "electromagnetic therapeutic impact on organs and tissues".

The *Nomenclature of Medical Specialties*[93] is the key regulation for the internal structuring of the Russian professional medical community. It demonstrates which specialties are recognized by the state at a given time and plays an important role in the emergence of medical corporations. The nomenclature's direct, practical purpose is management of human resources and educational policies in healthcare. However, in fact it regulates the access of doctors to professional occupations and allows medical corporations to qualify for budgetary resources. The nomenclature of specialties serves as a basis for developing areas of healthcare, approving staffing schedules for medical institutions, and issuing permits to engage in medical activity. Therefore, in the recent history of Russian healthcare, entering a specialty in the nomenclature has always been a matter of extensive lobbying by its representatives.

A review of the nomenclatures of medical specialties for the past two decades shows that from 1997 to 2015 manual therapy and reflexology were the only areas of traditional medicine included in them. At the end of 2015, osteopathy was also added. Other areas of traditional medicine were not mentioned in the list of medical specialties, although until 2012 a license was also required to practice them, so doctors had to complete special postgraduate training.

---

[93] In my analysis, I used the nomenclature, which was effective at the time the book was written. It was called the *Nomenclature of Specialties of Professionals with Higher and Postgraduate Medical and Pharmaceutical Education in the Healthcare System of the Russian Federation* and was approved by Order of the Russian Ministry of Health and Social Development No. 210n of 23 April 2009 (as amended and supplemented). Later it was replaced by another document—the *Nomenclature of Specialties of Professionals with a Higher Medical and Pharmaceutical Education*, approved by Order of the Russian Ministry of Health No. 700n of 7 October 2015. The new Nomenclature was significantly amended (among other changes, it no longer classified medical specialties into basic specialties and those that required additional training). I do not consider these amendments, except for the situation with osteopathy.

Besides manual therapy, reflexology, and massage,[94] FCTRC TDTM in its practical guidance (*metodicheskie ukazania*) distinguished four more occupations subject to licensing as "works and services involving methods of traditional medicine". These were bioresonance therapy, homeopathy, natural therapy, and traditional diagnosis (implying methods approved by the Russian Ministry of Health—electroacupuncture according to Voll and Nakatani, electroacupuncture vegetative resonance test, and auricular diagnosis). It was stipulated that traditional medicine also included "traditional healing systems", such as "the systems of Ivanov and Malakhov, Chinese and Tibetan medicine, Ayurveda, yoga, and others", but they are not approved for use in healthcare practice and may not be licensed (Karpeev, Kiseleva, 2003).

The introduction of the medical specialty "recreational medicine" may be considered an attempt to find a place for non-conventional practices in the personnel infrastructure of the healthcare system. The specialty existed in the nomenclature several years (2003–2011); subsequently, the scope of its competence was assigned to medical rehabilitation. A doctor with this specialty was supposed to work primarily at health resort facilities. The twists and turns of recreational medicine and the related balneology and medical rehabilitation in the system of medical specialties are a sensitive issue for physicians engaged in this field, since their formal status, as well as education requirements, are constantly changing. Moreover, as the nomenclature of specialties allows building a robust training and research infrastructure, its changes always mean a blow to the educational and scientific resources of the specialty.

The fact that traditional medicine is not included in the list of medical specialties and since 2012 is no longer subject to licensing reduces the opportunities to professionalize CAM practices within formal healthcare. The status of doctors who have chosen one or another non-conventional practice as their main occupation is currently ambivalent, since public clinics have no appropriate jobs for them, relevant positions are not provided for in the staffing schedules, and so on and so forth.

---

94 "Medical massage" exists as a specialty, but it applies to nursing staff. *See* the *Nomenclature of Specialties of Professionals with Secondary Medical and Pharmaceutical Education in the Healthcare System of the Russian Federation*, approved by Order No. 176n of the Russian Ministry of Health and Social Development on 16 April 2008.

There is also a certain downsizing in the public educational infrastructure, which enabled doctors to retrain and develop skills in different areas of traditional medicine. According to some reports, postgraduate medical education in Russia in the mid-2000s included seven departments and courses of traditional medicine, eight departments of reflexology, five—of manual therapy, and three—of natural therapy, phytotherapy, and homeopathy (Gotovskiy, Moskaleva, 2007). In the late 2000s, some well-known educational and scientific institutions were consolidated, liquidated or reorganized. The number of subject and general development courses in certain CAM areas declines; they are increasingly integrated into educational programs in sports medicine and rehabilitation. The opportunities for special training and research needed to integrate CAM methods into orthodox medicine are shrinking. Finally, CAM occupations, even those that have been assigned medical specialties, have no proper place in the list of research specialties; they fall into the broader 14.03.11 section—"Recreational medicine, sports medicine, exercise therapy, balneology, and physiotherapy".[95]

The above mentioned regulatory acts and elements of the infrastructure supporting the work of physicians reflect the unstable, frontier position of CAM professionals in the healthcare system. Moreover, cases differ—the status of an osteopath is different from that of a chiropractor or a leech therapist. Each has his own history of recognition. I will analyze some of them in detail further on.

We shall now turn from the framework established by formal healthcare for the activities of complementary and alternative medicine physicians to their own professionalization resources and service markets.

According to Russian sociologists, the distinctive feature of CAM professionals is their contradictory self-identity—they consider themselves both mainstream physicians and alternative/folk medicine specialists at the same time (Samarskaya, Teper, 2007). This feature is usually regarded as an indicator of their marginal position in the health system. It seems that the inconsistency of the self-identity can either build up or diminish depending on two factors:

---

95  See the *Nomenclature of Scientific Specialties for Which Academic Degrees are Awarded*, approved by Order No. 59 of the Russian Ministry of Education and Science on 25 February 2009.

- Whether CAM doctors are occupied only in these branches of medicine (i.e., they *work* as homeopaths, leech therapists, osteopaths, phytotherapists, etc.), or they have a parallel conventional medical practice of general practitioner, neurologist, pediatrician and so on.
- How they use CAM techniques in their medical practice: as an alternative to the methods of conventional medicine or as a complement (e.g., they prescribe a patient suffering from asthma herbal combinations and yoga exercises in addition to ordinary medication).

In other words, the use of CAM methods in clinical practice per se and a relevant education are not necessarily the basis of professional identity.

If the state establishes the legal framework for CAM services by regulating various aspects of the work of medical professionals, the representatives of these occupations formalize their professional identity primarily through public associations. The purpose of such non-profit organizations (NPOs) consists in facilitating communication within the professional communities and lobbying their interests in the public sphere. As can be seen from the programs and the statutory documents of the Russian associations of CAM physicians, their key concern is to have their occupations formalized as medical specialties and supported by the regulatory framework.

Ideally, such an NPO should unite all professionals of a given occupation and possess self-governance and self-regulation powers. In the sociology of professions, the establishment of such a community is regarded as an integral stage in the emergence of an independent profession in its Anglo-Saxon meaning (Popova, 2013). However, in reality the situation with professional associations of CAM specialists in Russia is different.

First, organizations with familiar names often actually represent the interests of domestic manufacturers of CAM-related products rather than the interests of the physicians: homeopathic remedies (National Council on Homeopathy), medications based on herbal substances and dietary supplements (Professional Association of Naturotherapists), medicinal leeches (Association of Hirudologists of Russia and the CIS), imported products of traditional Chinese medicine (Professional Association of Reflexologists), etc.

Second, the associations are often established on the basis of prominent medical and educational centers, i.e. they actually represent a school consisting of a leader (founder, author of a patented technique, etc.) and his followers. Such NPOs divide CAM practitioners instead of uniting them on professional grounds, which would be best for the public promotion of their interests and the development of the evidence base of their methods.

Third, CAM associations tend more to integrate with other types of alternative medicine rather than protect their own identity and monopoly to their occupation. This is evident from the programs of conferences and training courses held by such associations.[96]

Where do CAM physicians work? If we list the data obtained in the Perm Territory from the more to the less common options, the following picture emerges.

Private alternative medicine centers and wellness facilities where consultations of CAM professionals complement the range of spa procedures and practices (yoga, herbal steam bath, etc.) top the list. This sphere of activity is fully or partially in the shadow: without a license or with an incomplete list of services in it and so on. Alternative medicine clinics are predominantly a personal or family business registered as a sole proprietorship. The founder acts as a multidisciplinary specialist. For example, he consults patients as psychologist, bioresonance therapist, homeopath, and phytotherapist; combines reflexology and leech therapy; and works with different techniques of manual therapy. Invited sub-lessees, who may be employed as neurologists, general practitioners, pediatricians, etc. in a conventional public clinic, provide the few other services. As noted in the second chapter, MLM distributors sometimes come up with the initiative of establishing an alternative medicine center. However, even if that is not the case, promotion of dietary supplements or health devices for external application becomes common practice in such clinics.

Health resorts of various forms of ownership rank second. They are medical organizations, but their purpose is to improve health rather than cure; they work with patients who have no acute diseases. Therefore,

---

[96] In the Kama area, for example, the Perm Association of Reflexologists serves as a venue for discussing bioresonance therapy and homeopathy, whereas the Professional Visceral Therapy Association organizes meetings with cosmoenergy therapists and healers.

therapies that can cause no harm to the health, especially under the supervision of medical professionals, are more common here than in regular clinics and hospitals; however, according to evidence-based medicine, their effect on the body is that of a placebo. Key spa services generally included in the price of the voucher (exposure to natural healing factors, physiotherapy, massage, and exercise therapy) have long been adopted by conventional medicine. In addition, guests can purchase fee-based CAM services. Judging by the offers of the health and recreation resorts in the Kama area, reflexology and leech therapy are the most widespread services; however, they are provided not everywhere, but mostly at the wellness facilities in and around Perm.[97] At the surveyed health resorts, we saw that it was common practice for third-party lessees (rather than staff employees) to provide CAM services by appointment under a predetermined schedule. Health resorts also practice treatment using devices widely represented in direct selling and unauthorized itinerant trade (Almag, DENAS, Nuga Best, and other). Another common practice is positioning non-medical services—cosmetic, psychological or sports and recreational ones—as therapies bringing relief from different ailments.

CAM services are also provided in private medical centers specializing primarily in conventional medicine. The general list of medical areas in such clinics is determined exclusively by their business potential. The standard package is ultrasound diagnosis, gynecology, urology, dermatology, cosmetology, issuing certificates and opinions. Profit-focused private clinics are responsive to consumer demand, so their price list is a good indicator of the popularity of one or another medical professional. Manual therapy, acupuncture or bioresonance therapy are included in the offer, because such services are fee-based and usually not covered by the package of free medical care under the program of state guarantees. However, the share of CAM services in such clinics is small, which may indicate low demand for them, at least in Perm.

Finally, public health facilities are the least common place of work for CAM physicians (meaning legal licensed employment with a relevant

---

[97] There are altogether slightly over forty health resorts in the Perm Territory. Of them, fourteen offer reflexology (acupuncture); ten—leech therapy; six—various options of bioresonance therapy; four—manual therapy; three—apitherapy; two—visceral massage of internal organs; and one—homeopathy. One health resort offered an original technique for getting rid of parasites.

position in the staffing schedule). This is a logical outcome of the unfavorable environment prevailing at conventional health facilities because of the legal framework governing the activity of CAM professionals and non-inclusion of their services in the program of state guarantees.

Such is the snapshot of the market for CAM services at different medical facilities. What is the development trend? In general, two key factors determine the legal market dynamics (and, respectively, integration of these occupations into conventional medicine and further professionalization of specialists in this sphere): changes in the government regulation of these activities and consumer demand. As mentioned earlier, the second, market, factor is important, since in most cases such services are not covered by the state, and thus the well-being of CAM professionals directly depends on the willingness of the patients to pay for them out of their pockets.

Over the past 10–15 years, these factors have not been promoting the development of complementary and alternative medicine in Russia. On the contrary, both medical professionals and their audience demonstrate a diminishing interest in these occupations. During fieldwork, we often heard that local out-patient clinics used to have reflexology, leech therapy, and other consultations, but such services were no longer available. This was triggered by changes in the regulation of medical practice: increasingly stringent requirements for specialty medical education, cancelled licensing of work (services) based on methods of traditional medicine, and reduced training opportunities.

Besides, many CAM practices accepted by formal healthcare initially have a limited clientele. Although such treatment is usually advertised by contrast to unsafe drug therapy with an emphasis on its versatility, it can have numerous contraindications, adverse side effects, and be simply unpleasant for the patient, as is the case with acupuncture, leech therapy and apitherapy. It also tends to be quite expensive, as it involves a treatment course. For example, a course of ten acupuncture sessions in the surveyed localities cost on average RUB 5,000–6,000 ($150–$190).

Moreover, legally practicing CAM physicians face competition not only from conventional practitioners who rely on pharmaceuticals to address the same health problems, but also from various illegal and semi-legal "informal healthcare" agents who charge less for their services (healers, unlicensed centers of traditional medicine, at-home massage therapists, MLM companies, and others).

Concluding the overview of the market for services of CAM physicians, we would like to focus on the issue of estimating the number of such professionals. Unfortunately, most of them are not included in detailed public records. Official statistics covers only doctors who have a formally recognized medical specialty: reflexologists, manual therapists, and among nursing staff—massage therapists. The basic form of federal statistical monitoring of the status of medical and pharmaceutical personnel contained no data on doctors engaged in other traditional medicine practices even at the time when such practices were licensed. Accordingly, the government neither collected nor considered such data. Another potential source of information on the number of CAM physicians—registers of members of professional associations—is also obviously incomplete, since the associations do not cover all professionals practicing in Russia.[98]

Expert estimates are usually based on the number of people who have completed special training to provide CAM services. However, this technique, which is not very effective even when it concerns conventional medical professionals, can hardly serve to determine the number of complementary and alternative medicine practitioners. This is because in practice, the pre-requisites for obtaining authorization to engage in medical practice (mandatory professional development and certification every five years) result in the situation when not every person trained at some point as a reflexologist may legally practice reflexology at present. Besides, such doctors often work as multidisciplinary specialists combining leech therapy, reflexology, chiropractic, and conventional medical practices. In fact, expert estimates reflect the potential number of individuals that can provide CAM services, rather than the actual number of active practitioners for whom a specific type of traditional medicine has become their main occupation.

According to the estimate of Olesya Yurchenko, as of 2004, there were 25,000 reflexologists, 13,000 homeopaths, 10,000 manual therapists, 500 leech therapists, 450 apitherapists, and 1,500 herbalists in Russia (Cit. ex: Sadykov, 2013, p. 57). However, there is a several-fold

---

98 For example, as of November 2014, the list of members of the United National Register of Osteopaths contained only 402 persons; of them, forty-five percent were practicing in St. Petersburg and about fifteen percent—in Moscow (the Register is available at the organization's website: http://enro.ru; data as of November 2014).

difference between these figures and official statistics or the results of a simple extrapolation of data obtained in the course of our fieldwork to Russia as a whole. For example, according to Rosstat, there are about one and half thousand reflexologists in Russia (1,453 in 2013 and 1,244 in 2005). Based on information about the number of homeopaths in Perm, we can assume the overall figure for Russia to be 1,200–1,500 homeopaths. Obviously, such a gap in figures can mean that a considerable part of CAM physicians practices illegally and does not publicize their activity. However, it is unlikely that there are ten times as many shadow professionals as legal specialists of the same profile.

Further we shall discuss the status evolution of four most popular areas of CAM in Russia, focusing on their integration into legitimate medical practice. I will attempt to dwell on the attitude of the state towards them, the resources for consolidating the professional identity of the specialists, and the extent of activity. In each case there will be an individual history of recognition by orthodox medicine and the state.

*Homeopathy*
In the Soviet Union, this area of CAM existed with varying success, and its proponents had to prove their method's right of existence in applied medicine. Mass anti-homeopathy campaigns were held in 1938 and 1968. On the eve of the collapse of the Soviet Union, due to the efforts of the republican medical authorities, the green light was given to the development of homeopathic pharmacies and clinics on a self-financing basis, as well as training of pharmaceutical staff for such pharmacies. In 1994, the Scientific Council of the Russian Ministry of Health and Medical Industry proposed to approve homeopathy as a method of formal healthcare, because this "would allow controlling more precisely the provision of homeopathic care to the population".[99] Based on this decision, a year later the Russian Ministry of Health and Medical Industry adopted the well-known and rather laconic order No. 335 of 29 November 1995 *On Applying the Method of Homeopathy in Healthcare Practice*. It still remains the principal official document recognizing the existence of homeopathy in Russian healthcare.

---

99   Resolution No. 26 of the Board and Bureau of the Scientific Council of the Russian Ministry of Health and Medical Industry dated 27 December 1994.

A curious detail—the document approved a regulation on the physician using the homeopathic method, but not on the homeopath. The application of this method imposed certain constraints on the physicians—they had to have an appropriate state certificate of education (postgraduate courses) and were obliged to upgrade their skills at special courses in homeopathy every five years.

The following sixteen years (from 1996 to 2012) homeopathy was among the occupations subject to licensing. The guidelines for licensing traditional medical practices clarified that no permit was required if the physician was not practicing classical homeopathic approaches, but simply prescribing homeopathic compounds "based on the clinical diagnosis" (Karpeev, Kiseleva, 2003).

The order of 1995 not only allowed using homeopathy in treatment—it ensured the reproduction and development of this CAM area through the establishment of a relevant scientific and educational infrastructure. However, the Russian regulatory framework provides neither for the position nor for an educational or clinical specialty of "homeopath"; homeopathy is not represented in the list of medical services. The *Russian Classifier of Occupations* (in the previous and current versions) mentions homeopaths, but does not place them in the same group with conventional medical specialists. In short, although treatment of patients by homeopathic remedies is allowed in Russia, the legal framework for the emergence of a corresponding medical specialty is quite unfavorable.

If a physician decides to engage only in homeopathy, it is very difficult to stay within the boundaries of legitimate medical practice: he has to pass dual certification—in the basic specialty and homeopathy—and also somehow resolve the issue of licensing; there is no place for him in public health facilities due to the lack of a relevant specialty and positions, and setting up a private practice involves lots of hassle (Grigorieva, 2009).

Such a regulatory framework, as well as considerable marketing efforts of pharmaceutical companies producing homeopathic remedies (Heel, Boiron Lab., Edas, Materia Medica, and others) have produced two opposite approaches to applying homeopathy in treatment.

On the one hand, doctors of different specialties, not necessarily certified homeopaths, extensively prescribe homeopathic compounds within formal healthcare. Physicians often prescribe such remedies to avoid vulnerable patients (children, pregnant women) developing adverse side effects from taking allopathic drugs. Centers for alternative medicine often make similar prescriptions after electroacupuncture and remedy selection according to Voll. Opponents of homeopathy criticize this practice in the context of the general struggle against "humbugmycins"—drugs with unproven therapeutic properties, very popular in Russia.

On the other hand, there is a small group of doctors that have broken with formal healthcare and adhere strictly to Hahnemann's classical tradition, which clearly rejects allopathic medicine. They consider the above practice to be "pseudo-homeopathy" or "sort-of-homeopathy". The costs of maintaining a private practice, substantial time invested in work with patients (a consultation with diagnosis lasts several hours), the need to make drugs to order—all these factors determine the high price of their services[100] and, respectively, the narrow range of potential customers.

Another consequence of the inconsistent legal status of homeopathy is the development of informal practices that do not comply with the established requirements for this occupation: in combination with healing, in the form of "energy-informational" or particular "Orthodox" homeopathy.

During our fieldwork in the Kama area we saw the following picture: the services of homeopaths are available only in the regional center. Outside of major cities homeopathy as a medical practice is not represented, except for prescriptions and pharmacy sales of popular remedies like Oscillococcinum and the occasional use of Heel homeopathic preparations in neurological practice. Perm has two homeopathic pharmacies where you can get medical advice. Homeopaths also consult at several private clinics and health centers. Combining different kinds of CAM practices is common (homeopathy plus reflexology, bioresonance diagnosis and therapy, leech therapy, and massage). We estimate the total number of homeopaths in the regional center at about twenty. However, members of the local online forum teron.ru agree that there are few "real" or "classical" professionals among them, and it is meaningless to search for a good doctor in Perm. Some of the conventional physicians we interviewed spoke well about homeopathy. However, they emphasized that it was a complex art requiring professional skills. According to them, that was the reason why homeopathy was underdeveloped in Russia.

I believe the position of classical homeopathy in Russian healthcare is shaky and insecure. Under the existing legal framework, this area of CAM is reduced to the practice of conventional doctors prescribing

---

100   A session costs from RUB 1,500 to RUB 15,000 ($47–$470).

homeopathic remedies. The environment for consolidating the position of homeopathy as a profession is unfavorable. Finally, the conceptual idea of treating with ultralow doses of a medication are far more vulnerable to criticism by evidence-based medicine (e.g., Shang A. et al., 2005) and modern natural sciences than the foundations of some other CAM branches, such as acupuncture, manual therapy, phytotherapy, and leech therapy.

*Reflexology*
The method of acupuncture, originating from traditional Chinese medicine, started integrating into Soviet healthcare in the mid-1950s. Official documents show that the two processes of recognizing reflexology—extending access to budgetary resources and securing the right of a particular professional group to engage in this practice—were simultaneous and interconnected.

In 1957, following contacts between representatives of Soviet medical science and Chinese experts in oriental medicine, acupuncture was included in the curriculum of Soviet medical schools. Order No. 106 of the USSR Ministry of Health dated 10 March 1959 *On Applying the Method of Acupuncture in Inpatient and Outpatient Health Facilities* stated the need to "radically prevent individual cases of inappropriate use of acupuncture, as well as its application in private practice". For this purpose, the government imposed restrictions on the application of this method ("physicians with relevant training authorized to practice acupuncture shall be allowed to do so only in inpatient and outpatient health facilities") and introduced centralized training at specialty courses and at the workplace. However, only forty-five days were given to master the art of acupuncture, and authorization was granted to doctors of basic specialties (neurologists, general practitioners, surgeons, pediatricians, and psychiatrists).

A decade later the health authorities stepped up the process of formalizing reflexology as an official medical practice. The word "reflexology" appears in regulatory acts only in 1967. Orders of the USSR Ministry of Health of 1971, 1973, and 1976 set the following tasks: organize acupuncture sections within scientific medical societies (neurologists and psychiatrists, physiotherapists and balneologists, general practitioners); establish the main scientific methodological center and leading Research Institute of Reflexology; set up reflexology departments at postgraduate medical education institutions; open acupuncture rooms in clinics and hospitals (by 1980, a total of 181 such rooms should have been opened). Since 1981, acupuncture sessions were held in physiotherapy treatment rooms, and doctors practicing only this treatment were classified as physiotherapists.

In the late 1990s, this method was monopolized within one medical specialty. By Order of the Ministry of Health No. 364 of 10 December 1997, reflexology was included in the nomenclature of medical and pharmaceutical specialties. Initially, neurologists and physiotherapists were entitled to apply for the position of reflexologist, but later this was narrowed down only to physicians with neurology as their basic specialty. Order of the Ministry of Health No. 38 of 3 February 1999 approved regulations on the treatment room and ward of reflexology, as well as staffing and equipment standards, thus paving the way for the full-scale development of this occupation within healthcare.

Simultaneously with formalizing reflexology as a separate medical specialty, official documents expanded the range of methods based on the notion of acupuncture points. Differentiation of acupuncture techniques in Russia peaked in the 1990s. If in Soviet times regulatory documents mentioned only acupuncture and sometimes moxibustion, the 1996 list of traditional medical practices already included four types of diagnosis and eighteen therapies differing by the technique of stimulating acupuncture points with the aim of regulating the body's functional systems. Guidelines for licensing traditional medical practices (2003) distinguish "over thirty reflexology techniques depending on the instrument and the treatment modality" (Karpeev, Kiseleva, 2003).

Reflexology became an area of CAM included in the *poryadok* on medical rehabilitation. Reference to it in this document means that in certain cases the state undertakes to pay for the services of reflexologists. In other words, despite the lack of conclusive (in terms of evidence-based medicine) statistical evidence of the efficacy of the impact on acupuncture points (e.g., Madsen, Gøtzsche, Hróbjartsson, 2009), the use of reflexology techniques as complementary ones became generally accepted medical practice in Russia.

Note that the Russian regulatory framework for medical practice assigns reflexology a role among complementary therapies for neurological diseases. Regulations allow using this method to address various health problems, but the basic specialty of such doctors (neurology) largely determines the clientele and the profile of the diseases. Therefore, among reflexologists predominantly those undertake to treat a broad variety of diseases (including alcohol and tobacco dependence) who position themselves as followers of traditional Chinese medicine, work in clinics of alternative medicine or maintain their own private practice, often without registering a legal entity. In most cases, our informants-neurologists expressed a positive attitude towards reflexology, even if they did not practice it themselves. However, their words reflected the perception of these methods as alternative ones, different from orthodox medicine.

How developed is the current market of professional reflexology services in Russia? According to Rosstat, as of 2013, Russian healthcare institutions employed a total of 1,453 reflexologists. The Russian Professional Association of Reflexologists has about 1,400 registered members,[101] including seven from the Perm Territory. Permstat reported that in 2012 the Perm Territory had only twenty-two reflexologists; moreover, their number was half of that recorded in 2007.[102] Obviously, these figures cover only legitimate licensed professionals complying with all relevant regulations and do not reflect the activity of physicians operating in the shadow sector. The latter include, among others, neurologists trained in acupuncture, who occasionally provide such services within the walls of their healthcare institution or on the side—in private clinics and at health resorts.

Of the surveyed localities, such professionals practiced only in the cities. Not all private clinics, including centers of alternative medicine, provide reflexology services. According to informants, most neurologists at the Perm regional clinical hospital know and apply acupuncture techniques. Moreover, the local professional association—Association of Reflexologists of the Perm Territory, established in 1983—is quite active in Perm. The health authorities of the regional center also made attempts to

---

[101] As of 15 May 2015, the Association had 1,394 members. *See* Russian Professional Association of Reflexologists (website).
URL: http://www.acupro.ru/chlenstvo/reestr_spetsialistov.

[102] For comparison: the website of the Russian Ministry of Health provides the following figures of healthcare personnel in 2012: Reflexologists in Russia—907; in the Perm Territory—9 (URL: http://old.rosminzdrav.ru/docs/mzsr/stat/47/Resursy_i_deyatelynosty_uchrezhdenij_zdravoohraneniya_I_chasty_%28Med._kadry%29.doc). In other words, the statistics of Rosstat and the Ministry of Health do not match.

develop this area of CAM by administrative methods. In October 1998, after the default in Russia, the city health department sent an information letter to the chief doctors of the subordinate healthcare institutions suggesting to step up the work of reflexology treatment rooms on a fee basis "due to the reduced number of hospital beds, inadequate supply of drugs, and the poor financial situation of Perm residents". It also encouraged "to ensure sufficient workload for the reflexologists."[103] In medium-sized towns up to four reflexologists practice acupuncture—most often they do it as a part-time job, being employed at the same time as neurologists at public healthcare institutions.

Such services are not very popular among patients. Thus, an informant working as neurologist in a district center, who used to practice acupuncture ("treated the peripheral nervous system and tobacco dependence") but gave up this occupation, communicated that patients came to him once a month to get rid of smoking and once every six months with neurological problems. According to another informant—a reflexologist in a medium-sized town—clients are few and their range is limited, since not everyone can afford such treatment.

Consequently, reflexology in Russia is currently one of the best integrated into official medicine CAM occupations. Although it does not comply with the principles of evidence-based medicine, in Russian healthcare it occupies a place on a par with other medical specialties. However, the work of a reflexologist is linked to the expertise of a neurologist and refers mainly to the field of medical rehabilitation. Along with the objective inconvenience of this method for the patient, this factor limits the development of the legitimate services market.

Against this backdrop, the persistence of acupuncture practices "based on Eastern philosophy" (as opposed to orthodox medicine) is not surprising. The entourage of the alternative method proves to be more attractive to customers. The idea of stimulating acupuncture points underlies the emergence of independent "informal healthcare" markets unrelated to the services of professional reflexologists: markets for health devices for home use and "computer-aided diagnosis of the body".

---

103 Letter of the Municipal Health Department of Perm to the Chief Doctors of Healthcare Institutions No. 07-574 of 13 October 1998 *On Expanding the Use of Reflexology Methods in Healthcare*.

*Manual medicine*
Practices designated by the expression "manual therapy" give a vivid example of the semantic differences in its meaning. These differences result from the segregation of professionals providing CAM services. Based on common sense, a manual therapist is a person who treats by mechanically applying hands to the human body. In this sense, an ordinary massage therapist, a village bonesetter, a classic Western osteopath, and an exotic visceral chiropractor represent the same craft. However, the history of recognition of manual therapy in Russia, as well as in the leading Western countries, demonstrates competition between the followers of different manipulative techniques, who build around them integral and isolated knowledge systems (schools) protected from the intrusion of outsiders. Chiropractic and osteopathy are globally the most popular and reputable among them.

In the 1970s, medical scientists in the USSR started studying and implementing into medical practice manipulative methods of treating spinal disorders that were developed in Europe. Particularly popular were the works of the Czech Professor Dr. Karel Lewit and his colleagues, whose efforts, according to their Russian followers, "had created manual medicine, which took the best from chiropractic and osteopathy relating to the spine".[104] Official documents of the Soviet period refer to manual therapy as a complementary method for treating early stages of osteochondrosis and joint injuries; later documents mention treatment of spinal and limb joint disorders. Guidelines for licensing traditional medical practices (2003) attributed manual therapy to traditional medicine and gave a broader definition of its scope of application: organic and functional disorders of the musculoskeletal system (Karpeev, Kiseleva, 2003).

In 1988, when the country already had about a thousand physicians trained in manual therapy, the USSR Ministry of Health issued Order No. 617 establishing a methodological and educational infrastructure for the development of this branch. A network of manual therapy rooms—one room per 100,000 population—was set up in clinics and hospitals. The Ministry of Health recommended selecting doctors for the postgraduate courses "primarily from among neurologists, orthopedic traumatologists, neurosurgeons, and exercise therapy physicians."

---

104 Vasilieva L. F. *On the Death of the Teacher*. Russian Association of Manual Medicine (website). URL: http://rosmanter.com/%D0%BD%D0%BE%D0%B2%D0%BE%D1%81%D1%82%D0%B8.

Ten years later manual therapy became a separate medical specialty available to doctors specializing in neurology or traumatology and orthopedics (the list was later expanded to include pediatrics and internal medicine). The network of manual therapy rooms was significantly expanded to one room per 15,000 population. From the standpoint of the authorities, securing manual therapy within formal healthcare was necessary to cut off physicians without relevant training from this practice: "doctors trained at commercial institutions provide unskilled medical care, which results in a large number of health complications, including the disability of patients" (Order of the Russian Ministry of Health No. 39 of 10 February 1998).

As a result of formal manual therapy being "reduced" to manipulations of the spine and joints, practices of manual manipulations of the patient's body to treat a wider range of disorders started formalizing into separate professional occupations requiring special education and qualifications. Currently, osteopathy, craniosacral therapy, applied kinesiology, and visceral chiropractic are developing as separate branches of CAM in Russia. Each branch has its own terminology built on imported and adapted foreign original techniques. At the same time, the legal framework enabling integration into formal healthcare forces the practitioners of these CAM techniques (except osteopaths) to obtain a medical degree and permission to work as manual therapists, if they want their practice to be completely legitimate.

To others than supporters of particular techniques, fundamental differences between them are hardly distinguishable. Moreover, since there are no established definitions here. It is noteworthy that according to the physicians directly involved in shaping the professional field of manual therapy in the Soviet Union, these schools use essentially the same methods for dealing with lesions of the musculoskeletal system; the only difference is in the definitions and the conceptual rationale for the doctor's manipulations (Ivanichev, Lewit, 2010).

These schools have different degrees of recognition by the state, but, unlike manual therapy, they were mainly perceived as areas of alternative medicine. Of them, osteopathy has the most successful history of lobbying in contemporary Russia. This branch managed to completely break away from manual therapy. In 2012, the position of osteopath was added to the *Nomenclature of Positions of Medical and Pharmaceutical Personnel*; in 2013, the health authorities approved specialty *31.08.52.*

*Osteopathy. Osteopath* in the system of higher medical education, and reference to it was made in the nomenclature of medical services. At the time of writing the book, the only barrier separating osteopathy from the camp of branches of medicine fully integrated into formal healthcare was the lack of medical specialty *Osteopathy*, and, accordingly, licensed medical activity. However, this barrier complicated the training and activity of osteopaths. And at the end of 2015 this medical specialty was finally included in the nomenclature.[105]

Although the lobbyists of osteopathy insist on its fundamental difference from other manual treatments, the boundaries of the profession are in fact still blurred. Osteopathic services are provided by manual therapists, neurologists, massage therapists, reflexologists, and other specialists engaged in medical rehabilitation. Private educational institutions that train osteopaths provide educational services not only to manual therapists but to anyone interested, and the curricula are far from the standards of conventional medicine. Osteopathy centers often make public presentations and advertise their services by contrasting them to orthodox knowledge, for example: "Unlike physicians of classical medicine, osteopaths do not split the body into a dozen separate, almost unrelated, functional systems."[106] Finally, some osteopaths oppose integration into official medicine, not wanting their system of knowledge to be "brushed up". According to the Russian Craniosacral Academy, "due to the compromise with allopathic medicine, the graduates and teachers of Russian osteopathic schools often no longer understand the difference between contemporary osteopathy and manual therapy."[107]

The other branches of manual medicine in Russia (applied kinesiology and visceral chiropractic) are also struggling to enhance their identity and be recognized by the state in the form of approved independent specialties.[108] However, they are much less successful than osteopathy. In the absence of a clearly defined legal status, a stake on "informal healthcare" agents—massage therapists, healers, and just people keen

---

105 The Order of Russian Ministry of Health No. 700n of 7 October 2015.
106 Osteopractika Center of Smirnov A.E. (website). URL: http://www.osteodoc.ru.
107 The Russian Craniosacral Academy (website).
 URL: http://cranio-acad.ru/cranio/istoriya.
108 For example, the goal of the Interregional Professional Kinesiology Association (established in 2011), as declared on its official website, is "government recognition of kinesiology as an independent profession in Russia".
 URL: http://www.rusmpak.com/o-mpak.

on personal health improvement—proves to be a more effective way of developing the schools. For this reason, the professional associations admit to membership and serve not only physicians or people with a medical background, but anyone who is interested.[109]

Upon integration into Russian formal healthcare, manual therapy was also separated from medical massage—a related service market. Pursuant to the regulations of the 1990s–2000s, the latter is attributed to traditional medicine.

According to official statistics, manual therapists in Russia are even less numerous than reflexologists—858 persons in 2013 (910 in 2011). These data differ significantly from the figures published on the websites of professional associations, schools, and in other publicly available sources. Thus, about 400 people were registered in the Unified National Register of Osteopaths (as of November 2014), and about 150—in the register of the Russian Association of Manual Medicine.

In 2012, the Perm Territory, according to Permstat, had only fourteen professional manual therapists. However, the number of professionals registered with the Perm Territorial Association of Manual Therapists was much higher—forty-six.[110] The website of the Association informs that its President has been teaching manual therapy at the Perm State Medical Academy since 1994. During this period "he has trained over 100 manual therapists, who are now working in the Perm Territory and beyond it." It appears that most manual therapists in the Kama area either do not work in line with their training or practice informally at home or in private clinics, so they are not captured by official statistical reports. Some members of the regional association of manual therapists participate also in associations of osteopaths and are popular and expensive specialists. There are altogether about twenty well-known osteopaths in Perm.

Of the localities surveyed in the course of fieldwork, manual therapists practice in Perm and medium-sized towns, mostly at health resorts. Perm's private medical clinics and wellness centers also offer the services

---

109   For example, the Professional Visceral Therapy Association (previously, the Visceral Chiropractic Association) unites about two thousand members skilled in manipulations of internal organs. Among them are physicians, traditional healers, and people practicing personal health improvement.
URL: http://visceral.ru/visceral/?page=2.
110   Data as of May 2015. Perm Territorial Association of Manual Therapists (website). URL: http://manual59.ru/doctors.html.

of osteopaths and the more exotic craniosacral therapists and specialists in the massage of internal organs (in one case a visceral chiropractor positioned himself as "expert in deep touch massage"). The borderline between such experts and traditional healers-bonesetters, who also sometimes call themselves *manual'shchiki (manual therapists)*, is blurred. Usually they have a medical background, but do not comply with the regulatory requirements regarding licensing and certification of professionals.

In general, as in the case of reflexology, the path of manual therapy to formal healthcare involved limiting the scope of the methods and securing the right to use them for a small group of professionals with higher medical education and particular postgraduate training. As a result, some manual practices remain outside the legal framework. A diversity of schools of manual techniques is a specific feature of this CAM area. These schools adhere to the idea of holistic medicine, oppose themselves to the surgical and medical treatment of Western biomedicine, and offer their services on the "informal healthcare" market.

*Naturopathy (natural therapy)*
CAM disciplines attributed to manual medicine are not unique when it comes to problems with defining the subject area. Logically, naturopathy should include any treatment by natural cures and factors. However, experts in using particular remedies—leech therapists, phytotherapists or apitherapists—are more common among practicing physicians than naturopaths (natural therapists).

Guidelines for licensing traditional medical practices defined natural therapy as a branch of traditional medicine representing "a set of treatments using remedies of natural (plant, mineral, animal) origin allowed to be used in Russia according to the established procedure" (Karpeev, Kiseleva, 2003). The Guidelines emphasized the distinction between natural therapy and dietetics based on vegetarian foods, as well as the practice of taking dietary supplements. The document contributed to the confusion in defining the subject area of naturopathy—it attributed treatment by natural cures administered to acupuncture points (namely, leech therapy and bee sting therapy according to acupuncture principles) to reflexology, which was subject to separate licensing. Another guidance document included leech therapy, apitherapy, phytotherapy, mineral therapy, shilajit therapy, and treatments using remedies of animal origin in natural therapy. At the same time, the document stated that "in Russia, natural therapy is part of national healthcare subject to state licensing; however, its definitions and terminology still remain to be clarified." Consequently, natural therapy was distinguished from naturopathy, which was understood as a set of non-standardized, scientifically unsubstantiated methods of treatment by natural cures (*Applying the Terms Naturotherapy and Naturopharmacy in Healthcare Practice,* 2000).

The legal status of physicians providing services in this field is much less definite than that of reflexologists and manual therapists, formally recognized as medical professionals, and even than that of homeopaths. In line with the general logic of formalizing medical specialties, representatives of naturopathic branches of CAM also strive to secure a monopoly on the application of their methods.

Thus, the Coordinating Council of Russia's Hirudotherapists aims to substantiate an independent clinical discipline *Hirudotherapy* and the medical specialty *Hirudotherapist*. The authors of the methodology guide on phytotherapy emphasized the need to distinguish phytotherapy, "which must be based exclusively on scientific facts and operate with standardized drugs", from non-professional herbalism (*Phytotherapy,* 2006).

However, the existing regulatory framework facilitates the integration of various forms of natural therapy into Russian healthcare only as complementary therapies which any physician may apply when necessary. Naturopathic methods as complementary treatments are used mainly at spa facilities and in medical rehabilitation, where they are applied on a par with other natural factors (mineral waters, peloids, special climate, physiotherapy). The legal framework prevents formalizing them as individual professional occupations assigned to particular professional groups.

After licensing of traditional medicine was abolished in 2012, the borderlines between different natural therapy practices became even more blurred. Under licensing, the physicians were required to undergo special training—every five years advanced training and professional development in phytotherapy, leech therapy, and apitherapy. Currently, this requirement is not clearly outlined in official documents.

The adherents of naturopathic methods refer to the relevant methodology guides and instructions approved by the Russian or USSR Ministry of Health as their basic documents. Thus, a guide on hirudotherapy were issued in 1989; the guide *Hirudo-Reflexology in the Treatment of Patients in the Acute Period of Ischemic Stroke*—in 1999; the guide *Using*

*Hirudotherapy in Healthcare Practice*—in 2002. Methodology guides on phytotherapy were issued in 2000. The followers of apitherapy even refer to the *Instruction on Applying Apitherapy (Treatment by Bee Venom) Through Bee Stinging* approved way back in 1959.

In the *Nomenclature of Medical Services* phytotherapy is placed in Section 20—Treatment by exposure to climatic factors (water, air, etc.), along with other wellness services. Leeching is listed in Section 14—Nursing or care for individual anatomical and physiological elements of the body. It is also mentioned in documents standardizing nursing—along with other simple medical services, such as cupping. Bee sting therapy is not included in the list of medical services at all.

Including naturopathic methods as complementary ones in conventional clinical practice does not prevent the development of alternative medicine schools on their basis, where the purely pharmacological substantiation of the therapeutic effect of natural cures is replaced or supplemented by esoteric ideas and popular concepts, which adherents of orthodox medicine consider pseudoscientific. For example, the St. Petersburg Academy of Hirudotherapy claims having discovered that leech bites reduce the level of chaos in the human body, influence the state of the meridians and acoustic pulses that affect all human organs and systems, and change the structure of water.[111]

So, natural therapist, phytotherapist, hirudotherapist, apitherapist, litotherapist (specialist who treats with stones and minerals), etc. are the self-designations that professionals use to communicate with each other and the patients. No particular physicians have a monopoly on practicing naturopathy, but the methods per se are not forbidden. Due to the lack of clear regulations, the borderline between practicing naturopathy as part of official medicine and the services of "informal healthcare" agents is very blurred. This is also reflected in the supporting educational infrastructure—courses in phytotherapy and leech therapy are accessible not only to doctors of all specialties, but also to people without a medical background. Finally, people without any special education—herbalists, beekeepers, and healers—also practice treatment and self-treatment using natural remedies.

---

[111] St. Petersburg Academy of Hirudotherapy (website). URL: http://academia-hirudo.ru/index.php?option=com_content&view=article&id=12&Itemid=12.

Let us now consider the situation with various naturopathic services within CAM that are provided by physicians.

To start with, their presence in public healthcare institutions is minimal. In the surveyed localities of the Kama area, we encountered them mainly at health resorts, and also at private clinics specializing in CAM, and wellness centers not licensed to engage in medical activity.

Combining various medical and wellness practices is typical for people providing services in this field. Most often, we came across combinations where classic medical practice (general practitioner, gynecologist, neurologist, physiotherapist, etc.) was the main occupation, and naturopathic services generated additional income from a part-time job or illegal private practice.[112] Judging by the responses of the informants, the reason for this is low demand for natural therapies, which prevents doctors from making a living off them.

In particular, leech therapy, being the most popular natural therapy in Russia, has many contraindications. Leeches are applied only to adults. The procedure is quite unpleasant for the patients, and few of them can endure a full treatment course. In addition, there is widespread concern among potential clients that the inferior quality of the leeches or their repeated use can result in dangerous infections.[113] For example, according to the information provided by the staff of a surveyed resort, no more than five percent of the guests book leech therapy sessions; of them, eighty percent undergo such treatment at the resort on a regular basis—annually or every other year. Apitherapy—a painful procedure which also has contraindications—attracts about ten percent of the guests. Thus, the range of clients is very limited.

---

112   For example, in one case, the head of the neurology department of the city hospital applied leeches on a private basis. In another case, a gynecologist provided leech therapy services by appointment, renting a room at the local beauty parlor.

113   Producers of medicinal leeches believe such concerns are not groundless. Altogether there are about a dozen breeding factories in Russia that supply approximately five million leeches a year. However, leech breeding is a demanding business, and the market is full of leeches cultivated without observing the process specifications, thus exposing patients to a potential risk. Leeches, either wild-caught or cultivated in ordinary pond water, are sold under the guise of "factory-bred" for half the price. See *Danger: "Wild" Leech*. International Medical Leech Centre (website).
URL: http://leech.ru/ru/pages/132.htm.

Another typical feature of the Russian market for naturopathy services is the fact that it is largely driven by the producers of naturopathic remedies: leech breeding biofactories, manufacturers of dietary supplements and herbal combinations. Not only do they support the professional associations of CAM physicians, but also arrange their training.

To conclude, naturopathic branches of CAM are applied as complementary treatments in the health resort sector and in medical rehabilitation, thus determining their integration into formal healthcare. However, this does not result in the formalization of respective medical specialties. Excluded from the system of licensing medical practices, they are gradually losing their distinction from "parent" healing practices, which emerged in Russia in the 1990s–2000s. I believe that without a government infrastructure supporting reproduction of knowledge and professional training, the future of phytotherapy, leech therapy, apitherapy, and other treatments by natural factors as independent professional occupations is uncertain, since it is contingent entirely on consumer preferences and the efforts of producers of naturopathic remedies.

*Shadow practices*

Admitting CAM methods to medical practice and securing the right to apply them for healthcare professionals through establishing statutory requirements for this activity has a reverse side. Many agents providing complementary and alternative medicine services cannot comply with these requirements. The monopolization of this field forces them out into the shadow sector. As mentioned in Chapter 1, the supervisory authorities do not have the adequate resources to fully control compliance with the established statutory principles. For this reason, such "informal healthcare" professionals feel quite comfortable operating illegally. They continue successfully working until by chance (scheduled inspection, emergency, political situation or coincidence) they come to the attention of the supervisory authorities. We shall now consider what I believe to be the major cases of shadow practices in contemporary Russia.

*Massage*

Massage is one of the most widespread and affordable "informal healthcare" services in Russia. Due to its mass proportions, it becomes virtually immune to punishment by the supervisory authorities. Let us see how this is done.

From the standpoint of officials, massage the purpose of which is health improvement is a medical service. Therefore, an organization or a private massage therapist must obtain a medical license. Licensing regulations effective in the 1990s–2000s attributed medical massage to the *Traditional Medicine* section. However, the *Nomenclature of Medical Services* (2011) classified different types of massage predominantly on the basis of anatomy, i.e. distinguishing it by parts of the body (general massage, hand, foot, face massage, etc.) and groups of diseases. In other words, the language of healthcare administration makes no differentiation by massage technique (oil, honey, clay, aromatherapy, acupressure), purpose (anti-cellulite, cosmetic, sports, warming) or sphere of traditional medicine from which the massage originates (Ayurvedic, Thai, Tibetan). The anatomical approach allows broadly interpreting any massage as medical. The outcome is the appearance of such documents as the special information letter of the Russian Ministry of Health No. 17-2/10/2-1005 of 20 February 2013 clarifying that Thai massage is also subject to licensing. The letter stated: "The key factor in classifying Thai massage as medical massage is the nature of the service itself, the manipulation implying that the staff must possess relevant medical qualifications, knowledge, and skills to avoid causing damage to the health of patients."

The licensing requirements in this case are less stringent than for many other medical practices: it is sufficient for a massage therapist to have secondary rather than higher medical education, be a certified specialist, and take refresher courses every five years; the equipment is minimal. Complying with these requirements is no problem for any healthcare center. In actual life, however, people practicing massage on a fee basis mostly work in the beauty and wellness industry and at home rather than in healthcare institutions. They obtain no special work permit from the state. Given that one of the general licensing requirements for medical facilities is that its head must have higher medical education and experience of working in healthcare, a beauty parlor or a fitness center have little chance of getting a license, even should they wish to.

Besides, many masseurs and masseuses have neither the required nursing education nor a professional certificate in medical massage.[114] They improve their skills through the widespread shadow infrastructure of short-term courses, self-education (literature, video lessons), and apprenticeship. The state system of training massage therapists as part of medical education cannot stand up to the competition of private centers that flexibly adapt to changing customer demands and the fashion for particular types of massage.

Moreover, a whole segment of the massage market booming in recent years,—traditional Asian massage (Thai, Balinese, Ayurvedic, etc.)—initially falls into the "informal healthcare" area, since the main stake in the competition for the client here is made on the authenticity of the employees who received traditional education abroad. As our informants said, "real Thai girls work here", "you cannot teach a Russian all this in a month". However, to obtain a license in Russia they need a Russian-type certificate of education. Considering that applying for a license also implies obtaining a work permit from the Russian migration authorities, companies arranging the work of such foreign professionals prefer to stay in the shadow.

Many representatives of the beauty and wellness industry are simply not aware of the need to obtain a license, thinking that an employee's certificate issued by some private massage training facility is sufficient. Those market agents that have studied this issue in an attempt to avoid problems with the supervisory authorities refer to the contradictions between the departmental acts of the Russian Ministry of Health and the national classifiers which provide for non-medical types of massage.

Based on the logic of the previous version of the *All-Russian Classifier of Services to the Population* effective prior to 2014, massage could be attributed to consumer services provided by public baths, showers, and saunas, or to "hairdressing and beauty services" provided by community

---

114  Outside of big cities, beauty salons have difficulty finding an employee with a medical background and valid certificate, which is required not only for massage but for many cosmetic services as well. This is how the administrator of such a salon in Kungur describes the problem: "We spent over a year searching for a cosmetologist, placed ads. But it is difficult to find a professional with a medical background. (…) A nurse, at least, who would know how to use a syringe."

facilities. In turn, the *All-Russian Classifier of Products by Economic Activity* distinguishes between medical activities and sports and recreational activities ("activity in order to improve the physical condition and provide comfort") and includes massage rooms in the latter category. For this reason, numerous unlicensed market agents tend to substantiate their position by claiming that they are offering "wellness", "rejuvenating", "relaxation" massage or "body care" rather than "therapeutic" massage.

Legal advisors often refer to the resolution of the Federal Commercial Court of the West-Siberian Federal District of 2008,[115] which reversed the judgment of the commercial court of the Khanty-Mansi Autonomous District on holding a businesswoman providing massage services administratively liable for working without a medical license. The ground for the reversal was failure of the trial court to establish whether this massage was a medical or a sports and recreational service. In another appellate ruling,[116] the court of the Khanty-Mansi Autonomous District confirmed the need to determine the medical nature of the massage. This meant that the controlling officers had to confirm that the specific service was a medical intervention aimed at prevention, diagnosis, treatment of diseases, and medical rehabilitation.

Therefore, in order to put a stop to illegal unlicensed massage practice, the supervisory authorities have to prove that the massage in question is actually of a medical nature. What arguments do they use? First of all, they refer to the *Nomenclature of Medical Services*, which makes things easier for them by classifying types of massage according to anatomy. So, if a salon's price list or advertising mentions a type of massage coinciding with the description of a medical service from the nomenclature (e.g., "back massage"), this is sufficient to initiate administrative proceedings. Moreover, the customers themselves may testify that they went to the salon for health reasons. In most cases the court accepts such argumentation as convincing. However, there are also cases in law enforcement practice when the arguments of the prosecution proved insufficient.

---

115  Resolution of 18 September 2008 No. F04-5348/2008 (11771-A75-29) on case No. A75-1332/2008.
116  Appellate Ruling of the Court of the Khanty-Mansi Autonomous District—Yugra of 2 October 2012 on case No. 33-4315/2012.

The bank of decisions of the Commercial Court of the Perm Territory[117] for 2010–2014 contains fifty judgments on the administrative liability of sole proprietors for providing unlicensed massage services in beauty salons, spa and fitness centers. The defendants were either the owners of the facilities or massage therapists subleasing premises. However, the standard punishment (a fine of four thousand rubles) does not contribute much to preventing this shadow practice. For example, the massage therapists—sublessees of the Vitamin Sports Center in Lysva were held liable twice (in 2011 and early 2013) for working without a medical license. At the time of our fieldwork, a masseur was also working at the Center, and also without a license. The selective attitude of the supervisory authorities to unlicensed massage is striking. Court hearings of the above fifty commercial cases resulted in the administrative liability of five entrepreneurs from Perm, four—rom Lysva, four—from Kungur, fourteen—from other towns of the region, and twenty-three (i.e., about fifty percent)—from Berezniki. Such statistics can hardly be explained by anything other than a targeted interest of the Berezniki prosecutor's office in the local beauty salons.

Comparing law enforcement practice concerning unlicensed massage provided by "informal healthcare" agents and formal healthcare facilities, we can conclude that the former find it easier to avoid problems with the authorities. Public and municipal healthcare and social institutions are in general more often held liable for lack of a medical license than private companies from the beauty and personal care sector. Roszdravnadzor regularly inspects such organizations, and they keep internal documentation (job descriptions; staffing schedule; list of fee-based services; employment contracts and salary records; service registers; timesheets, etc.) where massage is mentioned; therefore, it is easier to prove their guilt. At the same time, their violations are usually situational (i.e., applied for a license but had not received by the time of the inspection), concern various aspects of medical care (not only massage), and are due to the lack of budgetary resources for compliance with licensing requirements.

The clients themselves are not concerned that a massage therapist may be unlicensed. In the opinion of an ordinary consumer, the legitimate medical massage provided in conventional health facilities is inferior to the

---

117 The Bank of Decisions of the Commercial Courts. URL: http://ras.arbitr.ru.

services of informal agents. Long queues, entry coupons, waiting lists, low skills, and poor service—this is how our informants in general described the massage services in the local polyclinic.

However, in the free market a massage therapist has more chances to earn a good reputation with clients, not least because he or she is more motivated. Even those whose main employment is with a public clinic, demonstrate more responsibility and attention in their side jobs. References of satisfied customers are the main tool in disseminating information about them in the localities. Rumors of good massage therapists who can "fix the back", "cure scoliosis", etc. spread quickly.

Since customers do not view massage as potentially hazardous to the health, they see no sense in rigid regulations. The society finds nothing wrong with occupations illegal in terms of law as long as there is no direct damage to the health. This approach is also common among those who theoretically should be against illegal massage services—municipal officers and physicians. For example, the head doctor of a health facility believes that no license is needed if massage is done "in private".

Who are those "informal healthcare" agents that provide therapeutic massage services? The first category is professional massage therapists employed at conventional health facilities. According to the Russian Ministry of Health, overall 20,712 massage therapists were working in the country in 2012.[118] They are among the staff of virtually every district or city clinic, as well as health resort facility. Making money on the side off duty by giving massage at their own or the patient's home is generally accepted practice. However, as all the stakeholders understand the illegal nature of such services, an outside observer can hardly record such work. The management of health facilities assured our research team that none of their staff massage therapists "moonlight", because "they have no time" and "they are overloaded with work". In the meantime, local residents indicated the contrary.

The second category is purely business agents working in the beauty and personal care sector, in centers of alternative medicine, fitness centers and sports and recreational facilities, as well as at home. Judging

---

118 *Statistics on Resources and Activity of Healthcare Organizations.* The Russian Ministry of Health (old website). URL: http://old.rosminzdrav.ru/docs/mzsr/stat/47/Resursy_i_deyatelynosty_uchrezhdenij_zdravoohraneniya_I_chasty_%28Med._kadry%29.doc.

by the information obtained in the surveyed localities from publicly available sources, we can assume that the number of such agents exceeds the total figure of massage therapists employed at healthcare institutions, per official statistics.

As already mentioned, you will not encounter the word combination "medical massage" in this sector. However, the massage services are mostly advertised precisely as therapeutic, aimed at addressing health problems. For example, an advertisement claims that the aromatherapeutic treatment "back gua sha" "cleanses the meridians" and can help "cure over 400 different diseases" (including diabetes mellitus, hypertension, gastritis, uterine fibroids, etc.). Patients also perceive the services of massage therapists expressly as treatment. Thus, in one beauty salon we were referred to another one, where a masseuse was "treating many children, with scoliosis and other disorders". A resident of Kungur informed us that his wife was frequenting a massage parlor where the masseuse "examines her, prescribes a course of treatment, and treats".

In most cases, the masseurs and masseuses are self-employed economic agents, also when they provide services at the premises of beauty salons or fitness centers. They rent a room in such organizations and work by appointment. Thus, should the prosecutor's office suddenly show interest, the administrator of the facility can always say that the owner is not directly involved in the work of the massage therapists and is not responsible for them, even if the price list features various types of massage.

In conclusion, we should note one more aspect of including massage services in "informal healthcare". In practice, the word "massage" implies various types of manual manipulations of the human body. In many cases, they are inseparable from the practices and ideas of different branches of alternative medicine. For example, Thai massage is promoted as a technique based "on the concept of invisible energy flows in the human body". Healing techniques may also be called massage (in this case the interviewees referred to a special "energy massage").

*"Comprehensive computer-aided diagnosis"*
The development of this branch of "informal healthcare" should be considered against the backdrop of one of the problems of formal healthcare. Sick Russian citizens regularly face the inadequate availability and commercialization of modern diagnostic tests and consultations of medical

specialists. Public health facilities outside of major cities have no relevant equipment and personnel because these are not envisaged by the per capita provision standards, and private medicine is underdeveloped. For this reason, patients from the province have to travel to the regional center or the closest major city to clarify a diagnosis or identify a disease early. The practice of medical "business tours" to the province became a response to this problem. Teams of visiting medical specialists from regional public hospitals occasionally consult at local clinics on a fee basis. And urban residents are forced to turn to private clinics and LLCs established under the auspices of public health facilities to pass timely a scarce diagnostic test.

In short, the range of free opportunities for high-quality diagnosis is limited, while there are generally accepted and legal practices of getting such services for money. At the same time, ordinary Russians are flooded with media communications about the importance of preventive examinations and the rapid development of medical technology, which has reached unprecedented levels. The media pressure urges them to check their health even when there are no obvious signs of disease.

All this creates a favorable environment for the emergence of forms of pseudo high-tech diagnostics. Here are their typical features:

- Versatility, relative cheapness, and convenience for the client; at a convenient time, within a period from half an hour to one and a half hours, the client is offered to get full information about the state of all organs and systems of the body at a price comparable to that of one ultrasound examination in a clinic
- Use of mobile hardware systems connected to a personal computer and registered as medical equipment
- Reliance on methods, the use of which prior to 2012 was subject to licensing as traditional medicine practice (electroacupuncture according to Voll and other)
- Medical entourage; professionals in white gowns, with a medical degree, medical certificates and diagnosis

In the opinion of conventional medicine, such practices rely on scientifically unsubstantiated methods of quantum, vegeto-resonance or bioresonance therapy, as well as the ideas of acupuncture implying that human hands and feet have biologically active points that reflect the state of a person's health. From the perspective of the government, this service is a type of conventional functional diagnostics, and must therefore meet all the requirements for medical activities, including licensing and restrictions on advertising. This position was repeatedly expressed in the decisions of the health supervisory authorities and the prosecutor's offices.

Representatives of MLM companies and independent entrepreneurs not engaged in the sale of goods provide such comprehensive diagnosis services. For the former (Chapter 2 focused on them), the diagnosis is primarily a marketing tool for persuading customers to buy their products. In this case, its cost constitutes only a minor part of the patient's expenses. For example, an informant had the following proportion: examination—RUB 2,000 ($63); subsequent course of treatment—RUB 12,000 ($380). The latter "work off" the cost of the hardware and software, which can reach impressive amounts ($3,000 and more). Both categories try to engage real physicians to perform the diagnosis.

In the surveyed localities, such diagnosis was carried out at clinics of alternative medicine, MLM offices and also, outside the regional center, in the form of specific touring. Such touring is interesting by a combination of the most obvious regulatory violations and pronounced appearance of conventional medical activity. We shall examine it in more detail.

In the areas of our fieldwork, "guest performers" in 2012–2013 visited every district center on average twice a year, and medium-sized town—once or twice a month, staying in every place from one to two days. The procedure cost in the range from one to two thousand rubles ($60–$130). On average, they served about a dozen customers daily. During the first visits the number of clients can be two or three times as high;[119] but then people lose interest. Many are disappointed; they get the feeling "they are being defrauded". However, some locals perceive such a diagnosis as a worthy replacement for the classical clinical examination, especially if it takes place at their usual polyclinic: "For a thousand rubles they checked everything, absolutely everything—weight, joints, blood vessels, heart, eyesight, hearing, and made an ultrasound of all organs".[120]

---

119 These figures were obtained from informants. Media sources of other regions, with reference to statements of the prosecution, reported higher numbers. For example, in 2012, about 200 people made preliminary appointments with visiting "diagnosticians" in one of the districts of the Tomsk Region. See *The prosecutor's office forbade the company from Moscow to perform medical diagnosis in the Tomsk Region.* NIA-Tomsk. 28.02.2012. URL: http://www.70rus.org/more/15107.
120 Informant: female, about 60 years old, local resident, medium-sized town.

Advertising presents the service as a technological innovation, now also available to residents of the provinces. It is emphasized that such diagnosis allows identifying a disease before its outbreak, i.e. revealing invisible changes that have not yet manifested themselves as symptoms.

The "guest performers" set up their work according to the following scenario. Besides leasing premises and announcing their upcoming visit through the newspapers, they make appointments by telephone in advance. In one case, the director of the municipal institution, where the diagnosticians were leasing an office, managed the appointment list. If potential customers show little interest, the visit may be cancelled or shortened. A health professional or a doctor together with an IT specialist receive the patients. Local health facilities are the favorite venues for the diagnosis. Visiting diagnosticians rent there the assembly hall or a vacant room for a day or two (sometimes for longer periods). Where they cannot manage to secure access to a health facility, the "guest performers" stay at local educational and leisure institutions (municipal libraries, supplementary education centers for children, etc.). Visiting diagnosticians often hold consultations over the weekend when the facilities are closed.

Everything is done to minimize the chances of attracting the attention of law enforcers and being held liable for illegal medical activities. The advertisements usually contain no information either on the entity or the medical license, with the only contact data being a mobile phone number. Patients are received by appointment made in advance, which is intended, inter alia, to cut off suspicious customers.

In a way, an outstanding entity is Ritm-M LLC. Field "computer-aided examinations of the whole body" by method of segmental thermoalgometry (a type of acupuncture diagnosis) are conducted in the name of this company. The company is registered in Moscow, with representatives operating in the regions by power of attorney or under contracts. Judging by announcements in the local press, during the past five years Ritm-M has been occasionally surfacing in district centers throughout the vast territory of Russia—from the Altai Territory and Tomsk Region to the Arkhangelsk Region and Krasnodar Territory. Law enforcement bodies are chasing it all over Russia. Whenever prosecutors came to investigate, the "guest performers" disappeared into thin air, and the head doctors of the central district hospitals where they leased premises were reprimanded. In many cases, there were no lease contracts, i.e. the Moscow specialists were working by private agreement with the management of the local hospitals.

The prosecutors claimed that the entity was advertising and providing medical diagnostic services without an appropriate license. The position of the prosecution on this case has been repeatedly upheld in commercial courts of different levels. Ritm-M, however, does not consider such computer-aided diagnosis to be a medical service, and therefore prefers to defend its position in court rather than accept penalties, albeit minor.

The search for the manufacturer of the equipment leads to RUNO Medical Company LLC, whose leaders have developed and patented the variational thermo-algometry method. The company manufactures two types of products: the RUNO diagnostic system and the STAM "health scanner". The RUNO system was registered and included in the State Register of Medical Devices; the "health scanner" is positioned as a "household appliance based on the same principles as the RUNO system", but intended for home use by people without medical education.[121] STAM costs RUB 73,000 (over $2,000); this includes a "device for assessing thermo-pain thresholds", licensed software and its support. It is unlikely that at such a price anyone would use the device personally at home. Another option is leasing the device on a monthly basis. The first installment amounts to RUB 10,000 and includes the cost of the equipment and the lease payment for the first month (about $300). The individuals wishing to use the device for business purposes must register on the company's website and complete training.

We have described in detail the promotion of the variational thermo-algometry device, because this is a standard pattern in the market of equipment for "comprehensive computer-aided diagnosis". Between the producer/distributor and the consumer of the service based on the ideas of alternative/traditional medicine, there is an intermediary represented by the elusive "touring" diagnostician who operates a device leased for ten thousand rubles.

*Speleotherapy (halotherapy)*
In the global perspective, we see a two-sided process of the medicalization of the Russian beauty and personal care industry. On the one hand,

---

121 RUNO Medical Company LLC (website).
URL: http://runomed.ru/sale/market_stam.php.

the medical corporation aided by the government machine appropriates the exclusive right to work in a successful business sector, declaring piercing, massage, tattooing, and many beauty treatments to be medical services. On the other hand, the industry participants themselves include the nice word *wellness* in their lexicon. They exploit the health concerns of the consumers, presenting their services as recreational or even therapeutic.

The largest market here is massage, which was described earlier herein. Another booming segment of the wellness industry, which substitutes the services of healthcare institutions, are salt rooms. Speleotherapy (or halotherapy) has a history of developing as a branch of recreational medicine. The *Nomenclature of Medical Services* attributes it to a type of physiotherapy or treatment by natural healing factors. However, it was people engaged in speleology and the salt mining industry rather than medical professionals who spurred its development as an independent therapy. Another important feature: treatment by the healthy air of salt caves and their emulations (rooms equipped with air ionizers and lined with natural materials) has become a popular trend specifically in the former Soviet Union.

The first speleotherapy clinics on the basis of salt mines, pits, and natural caves date back to the second half of the twentieth century. In 1969, a permanent commission on speleotherapy was set up under the International Union of Speleology. In the USSR, the first pilot clinic opened its doors in 1968 at the Solotvyno salt mine No. 8 in the Transcarpathian Region of Ukraine. In 1977, an underground speleo-hospital was established in the Kama area at the BKRU-1 mine in Berezniki. Basically, these two centers were at the origin of the main competing branches of salt aerosol treatment. In 1989, the director of the former, Pavel Gorbenko, discovered and patented a method for generating an artificial therapeutic microclimate similar to that of Solotvyno. The method is called *Halochamber*. At present, the St. Petersburg Institute of Preventive Medicine (alias the National Institute of Health)[122] established by Gorbenko promotes the ideas of "a unique domestic technology—halotherapy" as part of naturopathy in the Russian market of equipment for salt chambers. The latter center serves as a basis for developing speleoclimate therapy as a field of

---

122  St. Petersburg Institute of Preventive Medicine (website). URL: http://www.nih.ru.

science and the business of creating speleoclimatic chambers manufactured from sylvinite rocks of the Upper Kama salt deposit.

Based on our field research in the Kama area, we can assert that speleotherapy today is quite a widespread service. Many health resorts have salt rooms. In recent years, the business of providing halotherapy services also outside health facilities has been rapidly developing. Thus, at least twenty independent unlicensed salt chambers (rooms) are operating in Perm in addition to the halotherapy services at health resorts and other health facilities. Many of them considerably indicate on their websites and in advertising that the service is no medical activity. However, in terms of Russian legislation this is definitely not the case, which is evidenced by law enforcement practice.

Halotherapy is quite a risky business for a small entrepreneur because it requires significant investment ($10,000–$30,000). A steady flow of customers is needed to recover the invested funds. The easiest way to attract customers is to sell the service as a therapeutic one. The salt rooms are mostly popular with mothers whose children have asthma or other respiratory diseases. The best option for the salt room owner is a doctor's referral. In one case, a businesswoman made a round of the local health facilities and advertised the services of her new business. However, there were no health professionals among her staff. She herself had started the business primarily due to the health problems of her own child.

The notion of curing with air saturated with salt aerosol also drives the production and sales of appliances for home use—salt lamps, natural air ionizers, etc. Here, the ideas of halotherapy are often supplemented by esoteric concepts of minerals having special energy and therapeutic properties.

***

To summarize, the market for CAM therapeutic and diagnostic services, or, according to the terminology accepted in Russia, traditional medicine services, is currently exposed to opposing factors. I believe it would be imprudent either to talk about its development and the consistent professionalization of CAM occupations, or just to see purely negative trends. The situation differs depending on the branch and individual therapy.

Some are quite successful and are recognized by the state as part of conventional medicine; others, on the contrary, lose their positions. For example, the osteopaths managed to establish their own professional identity and service market after splitting off from manual therapy. But the homeopaths cannot find their place in healthcare, although it has become common practice for conventional internists and pediatricians to prescribe homeopathic remedies.

In one way or another, the key factor for doctors of traditional medicine is neither consumer demand nor the objective process of the medical community and the population realizing the advantages of CAM methods. The key factor is the position of the state that establishes a regulatory environment allowing such specialists to work on a par with other medical professionals. This position, in turn, is largely determined by the professional communities' lobbying efforts and the general complex struggle of medical corporations for resources.

It is also important to understand that besides the desired outcome (formal recognition of the specialty, access to the support infrastructure of medical practice, and a guaranteed customer flow), the process of integration into formal healthcare has a reverse side. Many agents cannot comply with increasingly stringent regulatory requirements for professional occupations and are forced out into the field of illegal activities. And there, in the free market environment, they may prove to be even more successful than in a formal health facility. As we saw in the cases of massage, computer-aided diagnosis, and halotherapy, this shadow segment of therapeutic and diagnostic services continues to exist, because the attention of the supervisory authorities is situational and selective. As for the patients, the availability of a medical license means less to them than a doctor's good reputation.

## 4.3. All diseases of the nerves: Psychotherapy as an alternative to orthodox medicine

Two and a half decades ago, owing to the TV *Health Sessions* of Anatoly Kashpirovskiy, many Russians regarded psychotherapy as an almost universal treatment for all diseases. As this psychotherapist himself said, he had learned "to use psychological influence to cure people from a variety ...of previously incurable diseases." Although the surge in interest in paranormal treatment and extrasensory perception in Russia is usually associated with his name, Kashpirovskiy and his followers have repeatedly emphasized that his method is based purely on suggestion rather than any supernatural powers or abilities.[123]

Russians have long lost the strong faith in the healing powers of suggestion and auto-suggestion they had in the early 1990s. However, the services of psychologists, psychoanalysts, and psychotherapists for treating a wide range of diseases that are within someone else's competence (i.e. within the competence of particular medical specialists) are still in demand.

In contrast to traditional healing based on paranormal phenomena, quite scientific methods are used here to work with the patient's consciousness but their scope is extremely expanded. For example, some specialists in neuro-linguistic programming promise to cure cancer, asthma or diabetes. Psychologists applying Bert Hellinger's family constellations method undertake to eliminate the "systemic" causes of grave incurable diseases, and hypnotists attempt to cure by hypnosis organic paralysis, disorders of the sense organs, and infections (including HIV). Various psychological schools and centers promote autogenic training, "attitude change", and "self-persuasion" methods as the main way to improve health. Finally, numerous specialists offer to treat alcohol, drug, tobacco, and gambling addiction using the so-called "coding" (*kodirovanie*), although they have no legal right to work in this field (only addiction psychiatrists are authorized to apply such treatment in Russia).

There are two principal ways in which psychologists participate in treating people. The first one is by directly providing diagnostic and therapeutic services (consultations, treatment), and this will be the focus of our discussion in this section. The second way is by teaching people certain original techniques of applying psychological skills to overcome diseases. This implies transferring ideas and knowledge that anyone concerned can master. Such services are provided by centers for psychological help, training, self-actualization, and personal development that are often related with certain healing systems, popular teachers (Mirzakarim Norbekov, Vadim Zeland, Alexander Sviyash, author of the book with an indicative name—*There Is No Health in the Drugstore; It's All in Your*

---

123 The official website of Anatoly Kashpirovskiy.
URL: http://www.kashpirovskiy.com.

*Head*, and many others), as well as traditional and modern religious and spiritual teachings. The development of their schools in Russia shows that making esoteric studies or alternative medicine practices look respectable is easier if you position yourself as a psychologist or psychotherapist rather than a healer or spiritual teacher.

Let us see how the attitude of the state (stipulated in laws and regulations) creates barriers, which oust the treatment services of psychologists into "informal healthcare".

The Russian health system assigns psychologists a secondary role of supporting the patient, although in some cases it is mandatory. Psychologists are included in the teams of medical and social workers which are formed to treat patients in some medical fields, for example, in oncology, palliative care, and psychiatry.

However, in fact, medical psychologists have an ambivalent status. Along with the nurses, they are on the lower rungs of the informal hierarchy of positions in health facilities and in fact play second fiddle to the doctor. "Their training is problematic, the status in medical institutions is not defined, and functions are vague,"—this is how representatives of the profession assess the situation (Rusina, 2011, p. 24; Berebin, 2012).

Because of this attitude, psychologists who wish to work with patients engage in private non-medical practice. In this field, it is much easier to comply with regulatory requirements than in a medical institution. However, the temptation is also higher to become informal, i.e., to engage in illegal business activities, and versatile, i.e., to undertake treatment of the "psychological foundations" of a wide range of diseases.

According to the authorities, only people with specific medical training and background may engage in *treatment*. Thus, only a psychiatrist specially trained in psychotherapy may be authorized to practice psychotherapy. In public health facilities, psychotherapists are also in most cases playing second fiddle to the psychiatrists, as they are part of the psychiatric service.

Regulatory acts also enshrine the monopoly of addiction psychiatrists (i.e., psychiatrists who have completed separate training in the specialty *Narcology*) to treat addictions. Fighting drug addiction as a medical problem is in the competence of the public addiction treatment service. The wording of articles 54-55 of the Law *On Narcotic Drugs and Psychotropic Substances* protects the service against the attempts of alternative agents to treat drug addicts. In particular, the Law stipulates that the state guarantees drug addicts relevant addiction care and social rehabilitation. Addiction care includes prevention, diagnosis, treatment, and medical rehabilitation.[124] The law expressly states that only medical organizations licensed to engage in such activity may provide addiction care, and only state and municipal health facilities, which may be neither privatized nor transferred under fiduciary management, are authorized to provide actual treatment. There is a special clause stipulating that only methods not prohibited by Russian legislation, as well as duly registered medicines and medical devices, shall be used for diagnosis and treatment.

The nuances of licensing medical activities in Russia impose additional restrictions (services may be provided only under a particular specialty and at the address indicated in the license). Since the field of psychiatry and narcology are monopolized and rigidly regulated by the state, it is difficult to avoid violations outside of state institutions.

However, the psychiatrists we communicated with claimed that in practice the government was hardly doing anything to prevent the shadow practices of psychologists and psychotherapists. On the illegal commercial service market, conventional techniques are combined with "absolutely odious ones", prices are considerably inflated, but a patient can get anonymous treatment. This circumstance takes potential patients away from the public psychiatric and addiction treatment services.

At some point, the government took situational measures to eradicate the practice of combining psychotherapy with obviously unscientific treatments in public health facilities. In 1996, the Russian Ministry of Health and Medical Industry issued special order No. 245 *On Streamlining the Application of Psychological and Psychotherapeutic Methods* (repealed in 2007). The Order instructed the heads of subordinate institutions and government bodies to prevent mass healing sessions banned in 1993 by the *Fundamental Principles of the Legislation of the Russian Federation on National Healthcare* and actively oppose the proliferation of paranormal doctrines and practices in psychotherapy.

What is the picture that emerges from our observations in the Perm Territory?

---

124 In 2013, an innovation was introduced into health legislation, by which "socio-medical rehabilitation" was split into medical rehabilitation and social rehabilitation. Non-medical organizations are allowed to provide services of the latter type.

On-site consultations and appointments is the most interesting format of professional psychological services within "informal healthcare". This work is organized similarly to itinerant trade in health products and "computer-aided diagnosis": frequency—once a month or every few months; prior advertising in the local media; rent of premises in public places for several hours; and established "touring" routes.

Visiting psychotherapists work mainly in medium-sized towns and large cities. They are rare guests in rural areas, including the administrative centers of municipal districts, due to the insufficient number of customers. At the same time, residents of such districts travel to the closest cities to visit them, usually to be "coded" against alcoholism. They do it at their own expense or at the expense of their employer. In one of the districts we heard stories about a "forward-thinking" director of a major agricultural enterprise, who sent employees—drivers, mechanics—at his own expense to Kungur or Perm to be "coded". Medium-sized towns attract visiting psychotherapists mainly from Perm, where those have a regular practice, and from the neighboring regions.

The regional center, in turn, receives visitors of a higher level—popular psychologists and psychotherapists who have established their own schools and hold mass sessions rather than individual consultations. Thus, during our fieldwork in 2013, Rushel Blavo, specialist in music therapy; Vladislav Hajiev, representative of Norbekov's institute; and Marina Krymova, psychologist and esoteric, visited Perm. Such "guest performers" have their own, albeit small, audience. They use the mass sessions primarily as an advertising tool to engage people in costly training courses and seminars.

Outside the regional center, visiting psychotherapists extensively offer addiction treatment as the most popular service. Treatment of alcohol abuse at the time cost from RUB 2,500 to RUB 8,000 ($80–$250), and tobacco addiction—from RUB 2,000 to RUB 3,000 ($63–$95). There are many so-called "coding" techniques. Some claim they work "according to Dovzhenko", others offer their original techniques.

From the medical standpoint, such methods constitute one or another form of mediated emotional stress psychotherapy. In terms of sociology, "coding" was a phenomenon specific to post-Soviet countries and linked with the charismatic doctor Alexander Dovzhenko, whose popularity peaked in the 1980s (Chepurnaya, Etkind, 2006). Proponents of evidence-based medicine oppose the application of "coding" in narcology.

They consider this technique to be placebo therapy and give it such sarcastic characteristics as "scientifically decorated shamanism" or "mystical rituals performed on the patient's psyche" (Avtonomov, 2014; Aleksandrov, Korolev, Aizberg, 2008; Soshnikov et al., 2011).

Despite criticism, the national fame of Dovzhenko himself, whose method was admitted to Soviet medical practice in 1984, and the promised easy way to overcome addictions (in one session) triggered the emergence of a specific market of expensive services. Market players include traditional healers using the word "coding" to explain their techniques; public addiction treatment facilities offering on a fee basis stress psychotherapy combined with drug therapy (Torpedo, Esperal); and private shadow and semi-shadow entrepreneurs. A review of commercial ads shows that at least twenty-five centers and private practitioners offer some sort of "coding" services in Perm.

Besides addictions, visiting psychotherapists also treat stuttering, enuresis, headaches, and other neurological disorders. They tour the surveyed cities regularly (generally, once or twice a month), sometimes for many years. It appears they have divided the market within the Perm Territory. Thus, one psychotherapist visited eight municipalities in the northeast of the region, and the other—six municipalities in its southern and central part. One interviewed psychotherapists said the following about his competitor: "No, he is a good doctor, and we share the market in Chusovoy." We identified five regularly visiting specialists in Chusovoy, and three in Kungur. On average, they receive from ten to twenty patients per day.

Let us consider in more detail the touring activity of Ramil Shamsiev. In three days, the psychotherapist from the Sanomed Medical Diagnostic Center (Neftekamsk, Bashkiria), a follower of Kashpirovskiy, managed to hold his "therapeutic sessions" in six localities of the Perm Territory, covering up to two settlements a day. In each one he stayed for four hours renting premises at the local cultural center or hotel. He came regularly once a month. The venues of the sessions also did not change. They included both privately owned buildings and municipal cultural and recreational facilities. According to informants from among the local residents of Kungur, Shamsiev received from fifteen to twenty patients a day. Most of them were over 45, but there were also young people.

The sessions were advertised in advance in the local newspapers. The advertisements presented Shamsiev as a "certified doctor, psychotherapist, cardiologist, functional diagnostician, and hypnotist of the international category." The scope of services included treatment of a wide range of diseases, including alcohol and drug addiction, excess weight, smoking, gambling addiction, defects of speech (stuttering), and enuresis. In Bashkiria itself, the local diocese of the Russian Orthodox Church is set against the Sanomed Center.

The most frequent violations common for such "guest performers", as well as in-patient psychotherapy centers, are either absence of a medical license per se or lack of a license for a particular medical activity which they practice and advertise. In some cases, a license is available, but it is no longer valid. Usually, a private psychotherapist-"encoder" holds a license for psychotherapy but not for addiction psychiatry. Probably, this is because they first engaged in this commercial practice in the 1990s, when the requirements for professional education in the relevant specialty were less stringent. However, most often, it is the Antimonopoly Service that attempts to prosecute them for the improper advertising of their services rather than the authorities responsible for supervising the provision of medical care.

# 5 Religious institutions: Health concerns and commerce on health problems

How is it possible to discuss the involvement of religious organizations in maintaining the health of people? Most often this is done in the context of the impact faith has on health. Today this is one of the most popular topics of study in various scientific disciplines. In the 1990s–2000s, medical professionals and psychologists demonstrated an increased interest in quantitatively measuring the impact of religious beliefs and spirituality on the mental and physical condition of an individual (Koenig, King, Carso, 2012). For us, the evidence of the therapeutic effect of faith in this context is not relevant. We are interested in another issue: how do religious organizations and, in a broader sense, spiritual teachings and movements substitute or complement the health system, if at all?

In this context, we should consider at least several aspects of the way religious institutions contribute to maintaining the health of the population.

First, there is the regulatory aspect of the issue. Religions are comprehensive regulatory and philosophical systems. As such, they establish for their followers principles of everyday life and attitude to the body, which true believers must observe. Specific rituals and prohibitions (permanent or temporary restrictions on eating certain foods, daily routine, body care procedures, ban on alcohol and tobacco, regulation of sexual relations, etc.) shape a way of life that affects human health. For example, the teachings of the Quran contain quite stringent requirements for a proper way of life, which by themselves contribute to maintaining health: appropriate diet (halal, ban on rotten food and overeating) and hygiene in everything. Our Muslim informants particularly emphasized this point.

In addition to general life principles, there are individual regulations that govern the interaction of a believer with formal healthcare. Among them are the rejection of alcohol-containing drugs or blood transfusions, abortion ban, the requirement to be examined by a doctor of the same sex, etc. Such conditions turn a religious person into a patient who needs a special approach. In certain cases (in closed religious communities avoiding communication with the outside world), people do not visit healthcare institutions at all. However, complete rejection of healthcare services by a believer is unacceptable for the state and may trigger a court decision banning the religious organization.[125] Religious institutions also voice their opinions on methods of alternative medicine. So, faithful followers of a religion consider any actions in respect of their own health through the prism of their doctrine.

Second—and this is most often remembered in the context of the relationship between health and religion—the priest helps a sick person to cope with the ailment psychologically; to develop the right attitude and acquire mental health, which in the religious worldview is key to the well-being of the body. In addition to the psychological function, spiritual institutions directly offer believers ways to deal with diseases that are alternative to conventional medicine. Health here is viewed as a gift bestowed by God, and disease—as a trial or punishment for sins. Prayer, blessed objects, rituals, communication with healers and righteous people—all is used to influence the physical condition through healing the spirit, or, as those who participate in such practices sometimes formulate, to influence "the true cause of the disease." These practices force us to recall that the religious and scientific worldviews are essentially opposite. So, even if a religious doctrine provides for segregating the areas of competence with modern medicine and cooperating with it, ultimately, religious institutions inevitably oppose themselves to scientific knowledge when it comes to addressing health issues.

Moreover, mass religions with a long history have developed their own "medicines"—knowledge about the human body and treatment practices based on religious dogmas. Historically, Islamic, Buddhist (Tibetan), and Vedic (Ayurveda) medicine precede Western medicine. In today's world, they are maintained and supported as forms of traditional medicine

---

125 According to the Law *On Countering Extremist Activities*, likely harm to the health of people is an indication of extremist activity (Art. 9–10). In 2013, the regional court of Novosibirsk declared the Elle Ayat religious group (originally from Kazakhstan) extremist and banned its activity. Adherents of this movement established centers, where for a fee they promised to cure from all diseases. Proceedings were initiated following the death of several people who refused to take medication in favor of treatment based on the doctrine. In 2012–2014, courts in Bashkiria, the Chelyabinsk Region, and the Altai Territory banned groups of the Orda religious movement (related to the Ata Zholy movement, Kazakhstan) on charges that they engaged in pseudo-healing activities that were detrimental to people's health.

to which not only believers but anyone dissatisfied with the formal health system may turn.

Third, along with other NPOs, religious organizations serve if not as an alternative, then as a supplement to public healthcare due to their social activity, of which helping the sick is a part. They engage in fundraising, spiritual and psychological support, medical services, and patient care.

Finally, one further aspect that is often overlooked by researchers regards the economic component of the activities of religious organizations. Along with ideas and rituals, they offer consumers various health products, thus competing in "informal healthcare" markets with other suppliers of medicinal gifts of nature as well as handicraft and industrial goods.

Each of these aspects allows us to consider the scope of the activities of religious organizations as a segment of "informal healthcare". However, it is hardly possible to give a detailed and comprehensive description of this segment in one chapter (and even in a separate book). I will, therefore, focus on several points which I consider most important. For that purpose, I will rely on nationwide data as well as the findings of out fieldwork in the Perm Territory. Since the issues we address are not a priority for domestic religious studies, even a fragmentary description may be useful for further research in this area. It is preceded by a general characteristic of the religious situation in Russia, which is necessary to determine research priorities.

Compared to other "informal healthcare" practices, religious practices are among the most mass ones, this being determined by the number of believers in Russia. The most common way to estimate the number of believers is associated with the religious self-identification of the people. The results of the surveys on this issue vary depending on the wording of the questions and answers, sampling, data processing technique, and other factors (see Table 5). In one way or another, the surveys show that from sixty to ninety percent of the Russian adult population declare their religious affiliation.

Table 5. Religious Identification of Russian Adults: National Survey Results (2011–2013)

| Self-identification | NRU HSE Center for Studies of the Civil Society, 2011 (Mersiyanova, Korneeva, 2013) | Public Opinion Foundation (FOM), 2013[126] | Levada Center, 2013[127] | Sreda, 2011[128] | RAS Institute of Socio-Political Research (ISPRRAS), 2012 (Sinelina, 2013) |
|---|---|---|---|---|---|
| Orthodox | 70 % | 64 % | 68 % | 50 %[129] | 84 %[130] |
| Muslims | 8 % | 6 % | 7 % | 4 % | 5 % |
| Other Christian denominations | 1 % | 1 % | 2 % | 1 % | 0 |
| Other | 1 % | n/a | < 2 % (Judaism, Buddhism) | 1-2 % (Judaism, Buddhism) | — |
| Atheists (non-believers) | 16 % | 25 % | 19 % | 13 % | 6 % |
| No answer (don't know) | 4 % | 4 % | 4 % | 27 %[131] | 3 % |

126  *Values: Religious Commitment. How Many Russians Believe in God, Go to Church, and Pray their Prayers?* Public Opinion Foundation (website). 14.06.2013. URL: http://fom.ru/obshchestvo/10953.
127  *Russians on Religion.* Levada Center (website). 24.12.2013. URL: http://www.levada.ru/2013/12/24/rossiyane-o-religii.
128  *Religion.* Sreda Research Service (website). 04.05.2011. URL: http://sreda.org/opros/v-boga-veryat-82-rossiyan.
129  Overall, 50% of respondents identified themselves as Orthodox. At the same time, 42% declared belonging to the Russian Orthodox Church (ROC), 1%—to the Orthodox Church unrelated to ROC (Old Believers' Churches, Russian Orthodox Autonomous Church (ROAC), Ukrainian Orthodox Church of the Kiev Patriarchate (UOC-KP), and others), and 7% do not belong to any of the Orthodox Churches.
130  The survey question "What is your religion?" had two response options: "Orthodoxy"—82% and "Old Belief"—2%.
131  The wording of the response: "I believe in God, but practice no specific religion."

Survey data on the share of the dominant religion—Russian Orthodoxy—demonstrate the largest discrepancies (from a half to three-quarters of the adult population). This may be due to the features of post-Soviet religiosity. Instead of religious affiliation, the respondents tend to talk about their cultural or national identity, i.e., about belonging to the Orthodox or Islamic culture.[132] Non-institutionalized forms of religiosity—esoteric and occult teachings—are also common in Russia, although their proponents often claim to be affiliated with Orthodoxy or other traditional religions (Belyaev, 2009). In this situation, sociologists shift their attention to whether the believers share the religious doctrine and participate in the life of the church (Chesnokova, 2005; Prutskova, 2012).

The gradation of believers by involvement in the life of the religious community and their understanding of the religious doctrine is important for our research. Is this understanding deep enough to avoid doing something that a priest may consider a delusion, sin or even blasphemy? The latter is manifested, for example, in the fact *whom* an Orthodox person addresses in prayer when ill—an icon or God.

Those for whom religious affiliation only plays the role of a cultural and ethnic code in the Orthodox environment are often referred to as *zakhozhane* (church-passers instead of churchgoers). They turn to religious rituals only occasionally, often doing so for health reasons. However, their understanding of the mechanisms and nature of the impact that faith has on disease will differ, sometimes dramatically, from the canonical teaching. There will be more paganism in it than Christianity. Thus, blessed water becomes for them a tool in household magic, which the priest would call sorcery. As one of our informants said, "there are lots of people in Orthodoxy whose mentality is semi-pagan."[133] Practicing believers are more likely to treat diseases in line with the official doctrine of their religion.

Of the available expert estimates of the number of practicing believers in Russia, those made a decade ago by Filatov and Lunkin (2005) seem the most credible: Orthodox (ROC)—3–15 million; the Old Believers—50,000–80,000; Catholics—60,000–200,000; Protestants—over

---

132 For example, according to a survey of the mid-2000s, 77% of the respondents in the Yaroslavl Region declared themselves Orthodox, whereas 58% answered that they were believers (Sinelina, 2005).
133 Informant: female, 40–50 years old, Orthodox activist, medium-sized town.

1.5 million; Jews—30,000; Muslims—no more than 2.8 million; Buddhists—no more than 500,000; and authoritarian new religious movements (NRMs)—no more than 300,000 people. Orthodox believers are much less involved in the life of the religious community than the adherents of other Christian denominations. This is how Kofanova and Mchedlova (2010) rank religious activity in Russia: the most active are Protestants followed by Catholics, the Orthodox, and Muslims, with Buddhists being the least active. Besides Protestants, small religious movements, such as the Old Believers or some new religious movements implying fixed membership, also form active and strong communities.

To characterize the religious situation in Russia we must say a few words about the diversity of religious associations and the problems of their typology. The socio-political vocabulary has a fixed expression "traditional religions of Russia"—this implies Orthodoxy, Islam, Judaism, and Buddhism.[134] Accordingly, all other doctrines automatically fall into the category of "non-traditional", even though their history in Russia may extend back over a century or more (for example, Catholics, Baptists or Lutherans). They have to prove their right to exist in the country by appealing to the law on freedom of conscience, the secular nature of the state, international recognition, or cultural traditions of the local social/ethnic groups.

At the regional level, political expediency, the position of the authorities, and the lobbying efforts of religious organizations may determine whether a denomination is considered traditional. Thus, an Interdenominational Advisory Council has been functioning in the Kama area since 1998 by analogy with the Interreligious Council of Russia. However, the regional council includes representatives of seven rather than four religious denominations, which are thus positioned as "traditional religions of the Kama area".

Problems also arise when talking about Orthodoxy: in everyday language and sometimes even in theological discourse it is synonymous with the teachings of the Russian Orthodox Church, although this largest Orthodox denomination is not unique in Russia. There are also Old Believer churches and communities, the Russian Orthodox Autonomous

---

134 In the logic of government, representatives of the four traditional religions are those with whom the authorities can engage in dialogue, also on public health policy issues. For example, they were included in the Government Commission on Public Health established by Dmitry Medvedev's Order No. 1864-r of 8 October 2012.

Church, the Russian True Orthodox Church, and others. Unless otherwise stipulated, when I herein write about Orthodox organizations or communities and activists, I also mean those of the Russian Orthodox Church.

Small religious and spiritual associations of relatively recent origin are usually referred to in Russian religious studies as new religious movements (NRMs).[135] This notion is used for lack of a better term, although its content raises many questions (*New Religions in Russia: Twenty Years Later*, 2013). In fact, the characteristic of NRM serves only as antithesis of the notion of traditional religion. In public discourse, other definitions are more often used to emphasize the contrast with traditional religions—sect and destructive cult. However, the legislation contains no such term as sect, and its current use differs from the historical one. It is safe to say that the Russian Orthodox Church presently ensures its semantic content in the Russian media.

With some exceptions, the religious situation in the Kama area is in line with the national one.[136] Parishes of the Russian Orthodox Church were present in all the surveyed localities, but the activity of parish life differed from place to place. Muslim communities, which rank second in the region by the number of formally registered local religious organizations, are formed mainly by local ethnic groups (Tatars and Bashkirs), and in the cities—also by migrants from Central Asia and the Caucasus. A special regional feature is the rapid development of various Protestant denominations—primarily Pentecostals and Neo-Pentecostals—in the 1990s–2000s and the continued existence of traditionally strong Old Believer communities. A detailed description of the local situation is given in Appendix 2.

Proceeding from this, I hereinafter give priority to the Russian Orthodox Church as the largest church dominant in public discussions, whose scale of activity in "informal healthcare" is significant for the research. Other religions should be viewed primarily as a source of ideas and rituals for fighting diseases that are relevant for certain ethnic groups (as in the case of Islam) or for the adherents of these religions (mass

---

135 As of the mid-2000s, Russia had about seventy-five principal NRMs of various ideological orientation (Balagushkin, Shokhin, 2006).
136 According to a 2011 sociological survey (Mersiyanova, Korneeva, 2013), the religious self-identification of the population in the Perm Territory is generally in line with the national trends: Orthodox—71% (RF—70%); other Christian denominations—1 (1); Muslims—5 (8); other—1 (1); atheists—17 (16); undecided—5 (4).

churches and Protestant denominations). Small religious associations, even if the scale of their actual participation in "informal healthcare" is minor, are interesting in terms of the variety of alternative opportunities they can offer a potential patient.

Before proceeding to the description, we should clarify what we mean by "informal healthcare" agents in the case of religious and spiritual institutions. This may be the religion in general with its teachings, governing bodies, and the network of organizations and institutions. This may be a specific cleric, head of a community or local religious organization (LRO). Finally, a public or commercial structure affiliated with a religious organization (publishing house, trade or production company, charity fund, cooperative, etc.) may also be an agent. Such a distinction is meaningful, because it allows considering the ideological differences among agents representing one religion that are significant in terms of the attitude to health. Differences are most pronounced in the Orthodox environment, which at first glance seems ironic, since the Russian Orthodox Church is distinguished from other denominations widely represented in Russia by a unity of command and rigid vertical governance.

## 5.1. The attitude of religious organizations to conventional and alternative medicine

In the recent past, most of Russia's major religious associations have developed and adopted documents stating their position on relevant social issues. These documents in general demonstrate a similar approach to conventional medicine and formal healthcare which consists in their full support, except for decisions relating to principal bioethical issues (abortion, euthanasia, reproductive technologies, and genetic engineering). Such documents recognize the merits of medical practice; emphasize the need to combine medical and pastoral patient care; stress the importance of disease prevention; warn against alcohol and drug abuse; and reject alternative medicine.

The Russian Orthodox Church has conceptually developed and outlined these issues in *The Basis of the Social Concept* (2000).[137] The Russian Protestant movements have stated a more or less unified official

---

137   *The Basis of the Social Concept of the Russian Orthodox Church.* Document adopted by the Bishops' Council of the Russian Orthodox Church (Moscow, 13–16 August 2000). The Moscow Patriarchate (website).
URL: http://www.patriarchia.ru/db/text/141422.

approach to medicine in a document titled *The Social Position of the Protestant Churches of Russia*, which was prepared in 2003 by the Advisory Council of the Heads of Protestant Churches in Russia and reissued in 2009.[138] *The Foundations of the Social Concept of Russian Judaism* developed by the Congress of Jewish Religious Organizations and Associations in Russia is an attempt to formulate a unified position of the Jewish communities.[139]

Organizations representing Russian Muslims have so far produced no unified approach paper on social issues. This may be due to the absence of a single governance center of the Muslim communities (there are several spiritual directorates in Russia) and conflicting relations between associations and groups. In their attitude to official medicine, as well as any other aspects of social life, the followers of Islam rely directly on the Quran and the hadiths. Their current interpreters speak about the need to observe the prescriptions of official medicine. In practice, people coming to a mosque to be cured by faith are sent to a regular hospital after prayer.

Some sharia restrictions—it is forbidden to consume alcohol and unclean food products; an unrelated man and woman may not remain alone with each other, etc.—could make a Muslim a difficult patient. However, the clarifications of Russian and foreign preachers, religious scholars, and sharia institutions are, with some exceptions, friendly to modern medicine. They allow using prohibited means/methods to treat patients in complex or desperate cases or because such practices are widespread and common.

Only some new religious movements completely reject the health system. Mainly isolated communities forbid their adherents to visit doctors and take medicines. In a milder form, leaders of closed NRMs "do not recommend" their followers to get treatment in healthcare institutions, as this is interpreted as weakness of the spirit and lack of faith in the divine healing power.

---

138 *The Social Position of the Protestant Churches of Russia.* Document adopted by the Advisory Council of the Heads of Protestant Churches in Russia. Moscow, 2009. Second edition, supplemented. The Advisory Council of the Heads of Protestant Churches in Russia (website).
URL: http://www.g-protestant.com/documents/docs/article/81397.

139 *The Foundations of the Social Concept of Russian Judaism.* The document reflects the position of the Congress of Jewish Religious Organizations and Associations in Russia. 2003. Russian Archipelago.
URL: http://www.archipelag.ru/agenda/strateg/konfess/conception/judaism.

An interview with a former follower of Vladimir Beloded—leader of the closed community Family of the Children of God in the Perm Territory—shows how such soft bans can function:

> Beloded's policy was very subtle. He said, "You are free. If you feel unwell, let Heaven help you. Mother of God, all will help you. But if you are weak in faith, if you still rely on the help of the Devil, then, of course, go see a doctor." I personally nearly died from appendicitis.[140]

One of the largest closed religious communities in Russia—the Church of the Last Testament (followers of Vissarion in the Krasnoyarsk Territory—about forty villages)—does not reject hospitals and medication but offers "self-healing" and "attainment of Truth" instead. To prevent potential accusations of depriving the settlers of medical care, the organization's website declares that many of the believers have either a classical medical background or are traditional healers "who provide care on site."[141]

NRM followers may reject healthcare services for many reasons: they do not accept modern civilization in general; they are convinced that physicians can inflict harm; or the methods of treatment are inconsistent with their religious principles. Besides prayer, the range of alternative means includes methods of traditional medicine, dietary restrictions (vegetarianism, raw foodism, and fasting), breathing and physical exercises. The teachings of some NRMs are based on their own health techniques. Such religious organizations, even if they do not restrict the access of their adherents to medical care in the event of illness, reject the preventive function of healthcare where doctors receive the right to monitor and supervise the life of a healthy person. Hence home births and rejection of vaccinations and regular checkups.

For example, Rodnovers (*Rodnovery*) are convinced in the parasitism of many social institutions, including healthcare. This also affects the attitude to medicine—they widely believe that vaccination is the West's method of sterilizing the Russian nation, that drugs serve only to enrich the pharmaceutical companies, and so on. Instead, they practice raw foodism and herbalism. Anastasians (*Anastasiytsy*)—the Ringing Cedars

---

140  Informant: female, 40–50 years old, medium-sized town.
141  The Church of the Last Testament (informal website).
     URL: http://vissarion.chat.ru/church/information.html.

of Russia social movement—also practice traditional medicine and vegetarianism in their family homesteads and avoid, if possible, any contacts with formal healthcare.

Some NRMs reject only certain types of medical care. Jehovah's Witnesses are known to refuse transfusion of blood and its components for religious reasons. Up to the 1950s, they were also forbidden to get vaccinations. However, they accept other types of medical care (are admitted to hospitals and visit doctors, if necessary). Scientologists—the followers of Ron Hubbard's doctrine—are not against medicine in general. They oppose only psychiatry which they call pseudoscience and accuse of ill-treating mental patients and doing business on antidepressants. Throughout Russian regions they organize exhibitions titled *Psychiatry: Industry of Death*.[142]

It is important to understand that not only marginal NRMs oppose medical science and reject healthcare services, primarily evading preventive care. In the Muslim educational literature, Prophetic and conventional medicine are often contrasted. In the Russian Orthodox Church, the attitude of ordinary priests and parish activists to Western medicine is sometimes completely different from the official position of the Church. Some of the clergy we spoke with were skeptical of medicine and preferred traditional remedies to pills. According to our medical informants, cases of refusing to give birth in hospitals that they personally were aware of concerned specifically families of Orthodox priests.

One more aspect is the personal attitude of some zealous Christians. For active believers, prayer may be a more relevant method of fighting disease than going to a doctor or taking drugs. Some people are convinced that one must first go to Church and only then to hospital. We encountered them both in the Orthodox and the Protestant environment. Finally, just like in the other social groups, there are people among the believers who do not trust current pharmacology and advocate traditional methods.

As an illustration let us consider the attitude to vaccination in the Orthodox environment. The official view of the Russian Orthodox Church on vaccination is moderate. In particular, the Church and Community Council on Biomedical Ethics of the Moscow Patriarchate and the Russian

---

142  In 2011 such an exhibition was held in Perm. *See* Scientific antipsychiatry (website). URL: antipsychiatry.ru/index.php?i=content&mode=news&t=7973.

Society of Orthodox Doctors in 2009 issued a joint statement declaring vaccination a necessary current measure for preventing infectious diseases, the rejection of which can trigger grave consequences.[143] Expressing concern that some vaccines are produced using fetal tissue obtained from abortion, the authors of the statement, nevertheless, advocated their use where no "alternative (ethical)" vaccines were available. At the same time, the belief that any vaccination is harmful is common among ordinary priests. Not only do they abstain from vaccination in their own families, but also communicate this attitude to their parishioners. The anti-vaccination movement is also quite popular among the Orthodox laity. An Orthodox church shop may sell revelatory brochures of Galina Chervonskaya and her followers containing horror stories about vaccination next to the brochures of the Society of Orthodox Doctors on the benefits of vaccination, with buyers showing more interest for the former publication.

So, Russia's leading religious communities proclaim their support of official medicine and declare cooperation with the health system part of their social policy, although not all their clergy and parishioners share this position.

How do religious organizations in practice collaborate with the health system in Russia? Note that there is an unspoken rule for health officials to maintain official contacts only with representatives of the traditional religions. In the surveyed settlements—only with the Russian Orthodox and Muslim clergy.

Pursuant to Russian law, a patient is entitled to demand that a priest be admitted to him/her in hospital. During interviews, physicians, clergy, and officials often mentioned that exercising this right was the only form of collaboration between health facilities and religious organizations they were aware of. Other possible options, if any, were mentioned as isolated cases.

This was at odds with the nationwide picture that was emerging in media. This may be due to regional specifics—the frequency and diversity of interaction formats may depend on the position of the regional authorities and the influence of local religious organizations. Judging by these criteria, the Perm Territory cannot be considered a region where the religious influence on local life and policy is strong.

---

143 The Moscow Patriarchate (website).
URL: http://www.patriarchia.ru/db/text/964218.html.

What is the situation nationwide? Since 2003, the relations between the Russian Orthodox Church and the Ministry of Health have been administratively formalized. The Ministry of Health established a special commission to implement the cooperation agreement. In 2011, a new cooperation agreement was signed with the Ministry of Health and Social Development on a broad range of issues: from the participation of religious representatives in rulemaking and joint public health programs to spiritual education of medical students and "the creation of conditions for the functioning of Orthodox religious organizations and Orthodox social services" in the institutions subordinate to the Ministry.[144]

In recent years, similar agreements have been concluded at the regional level between regional health ministries and the diocesan administrations of the Russian Orthodox Church. In regions with a large share of Muslim population, cooperation between the regional health authorities and local Muslim organizations has also been administratively formalized. It is noteworthy that in this case the authorities prefer multilateral agreements, emphasizing the equality of traditional religions. Thus, in 2008, a General Agreement on Cooperation was signed in Tatarstan between the Muslim Spiritual Directorate of the Republic of Tatarstan, the Kazan Diocesan Administration of the Russian Orthodox Church, and the Ministry of Health of the Republic of Tatarstan.

In practice, the Russian Orthodox Church collaborates with health institutions mainly in three formats. First, priests provide religious services to patients in health facilities. According to orthomed.ru, as of April 2013, there were altogether forty-two places of worship in Moscow hospitals (chapels, churches, and indoor temples). Second, hospital patients are one of the target groups for sisterhoods and charity organizations. In 2013, eleven such organizations were operating in Moscow, with the largest and best known of them being the Sts. Martha and Mary Convent of Mercy.[145] The St. Dmitry Nursing School—a publicly funded institution issuing state diplomas—trains sisters of charity in Moscow. Finally, priests

---

144 *The Agreement on Cooperation Between the Russian Orthodox Church and the Ministry of Health and Social Development of the Russian Federation* of 8 July 2011. The Moscow Patriarchate (website).
URL: http://www.patriarchia.ru/db/text/1556321.html.

145 The Convent has about one hundred sisters. It provides visiting nurse care; has its own outpatient clinic; and serves in several public health facilities, including the Sklifosovsky First Aid Research Institute.

assist doctors in preventive work regarding childbirth and addictions. They talk to patients in "spiritual offices" opened at antenatal clinics and polyclinics; take part in joint events with doctors at schools and colleges, etc.

All these formats were underdeveloped in the surveyed localities of the Perm Territory. Four hospital chapels functioned in Perm. In the other localities, we did not see any premises at public health facilities that were specially dedicated for religious needs. Educational events were usually held outside medical premises, and the participating doctors acted on their own initiative. For example, the Ecology of Pregnancy club school at the Church of the Holy Prince Vladimir in Perm functioned this way.

Outside of the regional capital, any interaction between health facilities and religious organizations, except for the above-mentioned admission of priests to bedridden hospital patients (which can hardly be called actual collaboration), is even more limited. Our informants were not particularly concerned about the cooperation of healthcare institutions with religious organizations. This is how the head doctor of a central district hospital described the situation:

> *Informant*: The Orthodox Church, Muslims—only a positive attitude to both churches; no objection whatsoever. As for the rest—Baptists and others—I simply keep them out.
> *Interviewer:* Don't you have any such people among the staff? Such religions are quite popular among medical personnel.
> *Informant*: We had such a woman. But I had a conversation with her and explained that she should not impose anything on the patients. Her personal life should not interfere with work.
> *Interviewer:* Does not the Orthodox priest request a chapel or prayer room to be opened at the hospital premises?
> *Informant*: Well, I simply don't object when relatives invite a priest to the hospital, ask to administer the last sacraments or something else... Both the Orthodox priest and the imam have free access to the patients. We create no obstacles for them.
> *Interviewer:* Do they themselves ever come up with initiatives to hold some joint actions? Against abortion, for example?
> *Informant*: No. We simply don't have such strong-minded priests.[146]

In addition to collaborating with health institutions, religious organizations attempt to work directly with physicians. They formulate rules for doctors on how to treat people properly so as not to violate religious canons and prohibitions. They take the basic rules of medical conduct from the Holy

---

146 Informant: male, about 50 years old, head doctor of a central district hospital, district center.

Scriptures: the Bible, the Quran, and the Torah. However, this is not enough. National and local religious organizations work out special Orthodox, Christian, and Muslim codes and guidelines for doctors as part of their community work.[147]

Non-profit associations of Orthodox physicians exist in some Russian cities. The Russian Society of Orthodox Doctors was registered in 2009. It aims to improve medical care by providing both spiritual assistance and gratuitous healthcare services. The Society engages in religious and educational activities among doctors and patients; holds conferences, and publishes a journal. However, its activity is not particularly noticeable in the Perm Territory. In any case, the representatives of the social service department of the Perm diocesan administration informed us that they had encountered no members of the Society of Orthodox Doctors.

The Protestant churches of Russia are also extensively working with health professionals and medical students. Like in the Orthodox environment, public associations of people working in the health system also emerge here. For example, the Russian Union of Evangelical Christian Baptists cooperates with the medical community through the Christian Medical Association of Russia,[148] which declares "fostering a new generation of Christian physicians" its priority. However, officials oppose such ambitions, fearing the promotion of "non-traditional religions" at the workplace.[149]

Let us now consider the attitude of religious organizations officially supporting conventional medicine to alternative therapies. They invest a lot of effort to fight some "informal healthcare" agents. This concerns not

---

147 For example, the Code of Professional Ethics of the Russian Orthodox Doctor was adopted in 2012.
148 The Christian Medical Association of Russia (website). URL: http://mxap.ru.
149 In 2007, there was a much-publicized conflict in Perm between the administration of the Perm Medical Academy and Nadezhda Garyaeva, a professor of the Academy and one of the leaders of the local New Testament Church. Garyaeva was accused of using her official position to promote creationism at the sessions of the students' scientific club on the topic *The Origin of Man: Truth and Fiction. See* court decision on this case. Slavic Center for Law and Justice. URL: http://www.sclj.ru/court_practice/detail.php?SECTION_ID=156&ELEMENT_ID=1386.

only their direct competitors in the market of ideas (other spiritual teachings), but also those agents that work in the market of therapeutic services.

The intellectual core of this struggle in the Russian Orthodox Church is the St. Irenaeus of Lyons Center for Religious Studies (President Alexander Dvorkin). Generally, competing with "non-traditional" religions and spiritual teachings for the minds and souls of the Russians, the Russian Orthodox Church in fact becomes the main social institution for evaluating alternative health practices in the country. Extensive missionary literature is dedicated to exposing health management methods related to non-Orthodox ideas and beliefs—from appeals to magicians and questionable use of prayer to yoga and wushu. The Russian Orthodox Church also names dangerous some popular psychological teachings, self-regulation and health schools, although they have nothing to do either with religion or paranormal phenomena.[150]

The Russian Orthodox Church expressly warns against occult-magic practices (healing, psychic therapy, sorcery) that "subject the will and consciousness of people to the power of demonic forces".[151] In my view, such concern is out of proportion with the scope and importance of such practices in the contemporary Russian society. However, such focus is understandable in the context of the religious worldview, for which the existence of hostile spiritual beings is as obvious as material things, and the Church is the age-old protector from these forces. It is not by chance that interviewed clergy often responded to questions about witch doctors by instructing the interviewer to avoid them at all costs. At the same time, some of our informants readily resorted to the help of babushkas (herbalists, bone-setters), if those were not using magic.

---

150   Thus, a list of "well-known destructive totalitarian sects and groups having a significant number of relevant features, as well as occult centers and movements operating in the Russian Federation, Ukraine, and Kazakhstan" (prepared by the participants of the *Totalitarian Sects and the Democratic State* conference organized by the ROC Novosibirsk Diocese in 2004) received extensive publicity. The list includes about 400 organizations and groups, not all of them being religious organizations. There are health doctrines and centers, esoteric psychotherapeutic schools, and even direct sellers of health products, including Herbalife.

151   *The Basis of the Social Concept of the Russian Orthodox Church*. The Moscow Patriarchate (website) URL: http://www.patriarchia.ru/db/text/141422.

However, most witch doctors in rural areas nevertheless resort to prayer, consider themselves Russian Orthodox, and heal using their "gift", i.e. supernatural abilities rather than just herbs or massage. Therefore, the priests, in their own words, must be vigilant. Practicing healers try to manipulate clerics to enhance their own influence: "They try to entice the priest—invite him to sanctify the house, take communion."[152] Priests also regularly deal with parishioners seeking blessing to visit a healer or requesting holy water for magic rituals.

Other Christian churches and denominations also focus on fighting against magical methods of healing and oriental health systems. For example, Baptist missionary literature in Russia claims that alternative medicine relies on Eastern philosophy and religion, and "at least seventy percent of its branches are associated with the explicit or veiled use of satanic forces" (Plett L., 2008, p. 257). Besides "sorcery and magic methods of treating diseases", the cited book includes most of the other practices in dangerous types of alternative medicine, namely, hypnosis, yoga, autogenic training, acupuncture, iridology, biofield therapy, phytotherapy,[153] and homeopathy ("it is rooted in black and white magic"). Curiously, treatment by holy water widely practiced in Orthodoxy is also regarded here as sorcery.

However, the Protestant communities at the grassroots level have no rigid bans on alternative medicine, and do not regard it as a serious relevant problem. Rather than punishing members of the congregation that turn to healers, fortune-tellers or psychics, pastors try to persuade them. Thus, according to one of the pastors, if a person has turned to faith, he is accepted with all his sins. They excommunicate no one and never scold people for going to fortune-tellers; they simply explain that it is wrong to do so.

Like Christianity, Islam disapproves of healing associated with occult practices. The Quran expressly prohibits turning to sorcerers who communicate with jinn. Moreover, not only turning to sorcerers is considered a sin, but the very belief that sorcery can somehow help people. However, judging by the words of Ramzan Kadyrov, Head of the Chechen Republic, who stated the need to ban the activities of witch doctors and

---

152   Informant: Orthodox priest, about 70 years old, medium-sized town.
153   The danger of phytotherapy is seen here in the fact that herbs are harvested in the new moon phase, considering the lunar calendar, using charms, spells, etc.

magicians in Chechnya,[154] traditional healers are thriving in Muslim areas no less than in the Orthodox environment.

Thus, a brief overview of the attitude of religious organizations to official medicine in Russia allows to characterize it as benevolent neutrality, especially if it concerns the attitude of mass denominations. The latter are also natural enemies of alternative therapies associated with occult practices. Criticism of the health system or rejection of medical services are inherent only to religious associations that have chosen the strategy of opposing modern civilization. Such teachings often have a strong element of healing, and addressing health issues is an important aspect of the religious doctrine. We shall now proceed from the declared positions to the specific resources that religions offer their adherents as unique means to fight diseases.

## 5.2. Treatment arsenal: Religious ceremonies, rituals, and practices to address health problems

*Russian Orthodoxy*
For Orthodox Christians, church is a place where they seek not only spiritual support but also help in addressing health issues. For baptized Russians that are not practicing believers, health problems are often an occasion to recall their religion and go to church at times other than the two major religious holidays (Christmas and Easter). Relying on faith to fight disease is a common way for churchgoers to care for their loved ones who are not very religious. A "must" in all our interviews with clergymen and active parishioners was a story about someone coming to church to get rid of a disease (often, but not necessarily, cancer) and getting relief.

The Orthodox culture has some established faith-based health practices. Moreover, they are perceived as an alternative to conventional medicine, even if the Orthodox doctrine positions them primarily as care for the soul.

Physical illness is a mandatory topic of discussion with the priest (spiritual father, monk), and the ceremonies he performs serve to eradicate its spiritual cause. The most important one is confession. Second, there are special services (prayer services), which the priest performs for

---

154 *Ramzan Kadyrov Called on Wizards and Sorcerers to Stop Anti-Islamic Activity.* Islam Today. 11.02.2013. URL: http://islam-today.ru/article/7240.

domestic purposes, including health problems; ordered prayers for good health—one-time and recurrent; and extreme unction. Currently, there is a practice of ordering daily prayers (*sorokoust*) for good health (for forty days, six months, and a year), although traditionally this was prayerful remembrance of the deceased.

Further, holy wells (which can be found in many settlements) and religious processions are very important for believers in fighting against disease. An informant regularly participating in religious processions not only in her native town but also in other districts and even regions said that the power of a religious procession was in overcoming oneself, one's weaknesses and fears through enormous physical exertion. This is a kind of test as to whether an individual truly believes in God, and God loves him. If faith is true, God will always give the strength to overcome this trial. She started resorting more often to this practice when "the ultrasound found something nasty" in her body.[155]

Another common practice is veneration of certain saints and icons believed to specialize in curing particular ailments. People turn to them if they have one or another disease. Information on numerous Orthodox websites clarifies this issue. Thus, one should pray to the *Vsetsaritsa* Most Holy Mother of God icon for a cure from cancer; to the Sign *(Znamenie)* Mother of God icon—from blindness and cholera; to the Reverend Alexander Svirsky—from paralysis; to the Wonderworker Simeon of Verkhoturye—from pains in the legs; and to the Martyr Vitus—from epilepsy. Such lists exist in large numbers not only on the Internet and in religious literature intended for the general reader, but also in the churches. In the Perm Territory, we visited a church where a poster was pinned to the door with a list of saints, "on whom the Lord has bestowed special grace to cure diseases and assist in other needs." The priest was skeptical about such instructions. He said they had appeared in his temple because of yielding to the requests of the parishioners.

Some of the saints are especially popular. The reason for this is easier to find in sociology rather than in theology. A vivid example is the St. Matrona of Moscow, who lived in the first half of the twentieth century and was canonized as a local Moscow saint in 1999. During her lifetime, she was famous as a healer; and even today, hundreds of pilgrims flock daily to the Pokrovsky Convent, where her relics lie, and ask her to cure

---

155   Informant: female, 50–60 years old, Orthodox activist, medium-sized town.

them from various ailments. In the middle of a weekend day in October 2013 we counted about three hundred people in the queue to the relics and another two hundred—in the queue to Matrona's miracle-working icon. People with grave diseases, those who wish to conceive a child, as well as those seeking to resolve domestic problems come to ask her for help. Matrona's cult, full of pagan superstitions, is flourishing today in Russia much to the displeasure of theologians. Online information about St. Matrona is also available on numerous websites dedicated to paranormal phenomena, which the Russian Orthodox Church refers to as occult.

Even though worshipping sacred objects (miracle-working icons, relics) is an integral part of Orthodox life, the attitude of some priests to it is controversial. They associate it with certain negative trends, such as the believers ranking temples by degree of sanctity, or the temples artificially stimulating the influx of visitors by promoting miracle-working icons, holy wells, and relics. Thus, one of the informants was rather irritated by the activity of those parishes that have popular shrines or sacred places—by advertising their special features, they distort the believers' faith. As such promotion is the most effective way to attract people, monasteries and temples compete in marketing healing artifacts, and the number of sacred objects in Russia is growing exponentially.

Worshipping sacred objects is inextricably linked with the institution of testimony—people's stories about the miracles they had experienced. Indeed, if we are to speak of the healing properties attributed to sacred objects and holy places, they exist in the public opinion precisely because of such stories (and not due to authority, scientific knowledge or statistics). The more witness accounts, the more convincing the healing powers and the more people believe to get relief from their diseases thanks to the object of worship. This institution is of an ongoing nature—not only is it a mandatory element in the canonization of saints,[156] but even outside this

---

156 "Working miracles in life and death" is a mandatory criterion for canonizing saints in the Russian Orthodox Church. Evidence to this effect is collected on the level of diocesan commissions and is an obligatory aspect of church life. However, as the secretary of the Synodal Commission on the Canonization of Saints noted, "descriptions of miracles submitted to the Commission in many cases can hardly be called miracles at all. Moreover, every miracle requires convincing evidence 'from insiders' and 'from outsiders', which means that it has to be examined by the religious authorities and physicians (in the event of being cured from a terminal illness)". See Maksimov M. *Preparing Documents for the Canonization of Saints*. The Synodal Commission on the Canonization of Saints (website).

procedure, it is a measure of the saint's popularity with the ordinary people.

Official and unofficial (people's) websites of major monasteries and convents often contain pilgrims' life stories depicting the miracles they experienced. On the website of the Pokrovsky Convent believers are thanking St. Matrona of Moscow for helping to "cure vasoneurosis and heart failure", "heal a child from meningitis", "exorcise demons and lead to faith", "get rid of headache and secure a job in three days", "find a husband and buy an apartment, cure pus abscesses, and cervical extropion", and so forth.[157]

In one of the surveyed monasteries, evidence is recorded by hand in an ordinary ledger, which is kept in the church. An informant said that only a minor part of such evidence was recorded in the book, since not all pilgrims were aware of its existence and not all of them revisited the monastery. In one way or another, those who are psychologically prepared to see a miracle demonstrate this ability more often. Most of the people who had experienced help from the monastery's sacred objects and confirmed it were participants of excursions organized by a resort close to Perm. This was facilitated by the fact that the holiday-makers were focused on health issues. In addition, the persuasion skills of the tour guide also played their role. During the bus ride to the monastery she prepared the pilgrims for a certain perception of what was happening. Recorded evidence includes accounts of successfully resolved family problems (including relatives stopping drinking), cured headache and pain in the joints and the back. Such records reflect the desire to experience a miracle, and their style is like that of the letters patients write to the *HLS Bulletin*. They would hardly survive the scrutiny of strict logic or medical expertise; nevertheless, they become part of the personal experience that people share with their friends and other believers, strengthening their faith in the healing power of the sacred artifacts.

In addition to sacred objects with curative properties, healing services under the banner of the Orthodox faith are also in demand in Russia. The theological understanding of the relationship between the physical and the spiritual is often too complicated for the *zakhozhane*; therefore,

---

URL: http://kanonkom.ru/docs/protoierey-maksim-maksimov-podgotovka-materialov-k-kanonizacii-svyatyh.html.

157  The Pokrovsky Convent (website). URL: http://www.pokrov-monastir.ru/?include=static&page_id=142.

they see no difference between what a cleric is doing and magical practices. The public opinion is very responsive to miracles performed here and now. Due to this, various forms of occultism and pagan worshipping of "Orthodox healers" develop on the basis of Orthodoxy. In Christianity, the art of healing (curing from diseases) is considered a miracle bestowed by God on very few people. The apostles and some of the saints have been recognized as healers. Therefore, for the Russian Orthodox Church, the people who currently call themselves Orthodox healers are quacks, and the clergy that promote healing are sectarians.[158]

The case is more complicated when it comes to monastic hermits engaged in healing. Some elders (*startsy*) in the monasteries of Togliatti, Penza, Saransk, Borovsk, and other locations practice healing by the liturgical spear. Although the Moscow Patriarchate does not particularly welcome this activity, it does not prohibit it. Pilgrims from all over Russia come to see the elders. Usually, the elders themselves charge no fee for the treatment, but the monasteries accept offerings. Businesses on arranging pilgrimage tours thrive around such healing.

The rite of exorcism (exorcism prayer—*otchitka*) is another curative rite for which the Russian Orthodox Church has mixed feelings. The prayer is based on the texts from the Euchologion of Peter Mogila. It is applied to patients suffering, among others, from mental and neurological disorders. The Internet contains stories of people suffering from cancer, arthritis, and other grave diseases being subjected to exorcism in Russia. The ritual may be performed both in person and in absentia, i.e., in the absence of "the possessed". The lists drawn up in the Internet by supporters of Orthodox exorcism indicate about a dozen monasteries in Russia that perform the ordinance for those suffering from evil spirits. At the same time, its opponents point out that exorcism is an adopted catholic rite and that in 1997 Patriarch Alexy II condemned the increasingly frequent practice of exorcism services. According to Alexey Osipov, Professor of the Moscow Theological Academy (2000), "exorcising is an occur-

---

[158] For example, Metropolitan Raphael (Prokopyev), head of the True Orthodox Church, whom the Moscow Patriarchate of the Russian Orthodox Church does not recognize, promotes healing practices. There are also pseudo-Orthodox cults with an emphasis on healing: religious groups of mother Fotinia Svetonosnaya (Lightbringer) *Resurrecting Rus,* the worshippers of the adolescent Vyacheslav from Chebarkul, etc.

rence of the same spiritual order as some developments currently widespread in the non-Orthodox West, such as the so-called Pentecostalism, Charismatic Movement, New Age Movement, and the so-called psychic therapy in the secular environment. All this cripples human souls and bodies."

Archimandrite Herman (Chesnokov) of the Trinity Lavra of St. Sergius, who has the blessing of Patriarch Alexy II to exorcise, is currently considered the most famous Russian Orthodox exorcist. He performs this rite in church three times a week for a mass gathering of people (in an overcrowded church), including visitors from afar. To cast out demons, a person is required to attend the exorcism service three times, with a confession before and a communion after the ritual. In addition to the story of the commandments and sins of modern man, the sermon preceding the rite[159] condemns sorcery, recourse to healers and psychics, and "coding" from alcoholism. It gives a naturalistic and medicalized description of how the demons affect certain human organs: "With their spiritual burden they pressure our body, squeeze our veins and blood vessels. The blood pressure immediately increases. Thus, the demons affect all our organs: the heart, lungs, kidneys, arms, and legs. Wounds appear on the legs, and venous thrombosis begins. The cunning demons cause cardiac asthma and dictate their will through hallucinations" (Archimandrite Herman, 2006, p. 24).

Interviews with representatives of the clergy revealed that Orthodox exorcism was not confined to isolated cases. On the contrary, it emerges as a regular practice requiring courage and sacrifice from the priest ("I would never undertake it; this is the lot of solitary monks leading a highly righteous life"). However, not only the select few are capable of exorcising ("any priest can do it"), and many people need it. Our interviewees were aware of this practice. One of them even mentioned that his father (also a priest) had attempted to exorcise. No rites of exorcism are performed at the Verkhnechusovskaya Kazanskaya Trifonova Convent; however, a constant flow of pilgrims wishing to get rid of demons or drive them out of their relatives visits the grave of Archpriest Nikolai (Rogozin)

---

[159] The sermon is outlined in a brochure published in 2006 with a circulation of 100,000 copies.

there. During his lifetime, this priest was famous for helping "people possessed by evil spirits".[160]

For us, the rite of exorcism is interesting by the fact that it vividly demonstrates the position of religion alternative to conventional medicine. Physical diseases here are not simply regarded through the prism of human sinfulness. They are directly interpreted as the interference of foreign spiritual entities, which doctors *mistakenly* take for diseases. Thus, one of the informants declares, "There is such a disease as epilepsy. Medicine does not recognize it, but this is when a person is possessed by demons."[161] Another one insists, "If we speak about psychiatric problems, not all of them are associated with mental disorders. No amount of drug therapy can cure them."[162]

We have depicted the situation in the religious life of an Orthodox believer, some elements of which (rites, attributes) traditionally replace or supplement the functions of healthcare. Not all such practices conform to Church canons. The extensive use of some of them can be explained only by strong elements of paganism in the worldview of Russians who consider themselves Orthodox.

The issue of "Orthodox medicine" as such is even more complicated, if we are to understand it as a set of knowledge and practices alternative to conventional medicine aimed at treating the body rather than the soul. This notion exists in the current Russian language, but it has different interpretations. According to the official position of the Russian Orthodox Church, it is the same classical medicine based on natural sciences where the doctor additionally helps the patient to cope with illness by relying on faith, since all diseases have spiritual roots. An educational brochure contains the following definition: "Medicine, which in its understanding of the origin and nature of diseases, in addition to natural science relies on Christian doctrinal provisions and considers them in the treatment and prevention of diseases" (*When Diagnosed...*, 2012, p. 20). In practice this looks as follows: Orthodox believers get treatment in public hospitals, but at the same time "resort to all available Church means of

---

[160] The biography of the priest published by the Convent contains stories of casting out demons (*"Write down good deeds on copper, but resentment on water..."*, 2011).
[161] Informant: male, 30–40 years old, Orthodox priest, district center.
[162] Informant: male, 60–70 years old, Abbot of an Orthodox monastery.

helping the sick", such as prayer, extreme unction, daily church prayer services, fasting, holy water, etc. (*When Diagnosed...*, 2012, p. 45).

However, some Orthodox activists and doctors also share the concept of "Orthodox medicine" as a specific system of traditional methods of treatment. This interpretation is applied to alternative treatment ideas and schools adapted and adopted by Orthodox agents of "informal healthcare". Judging by the literature exhibited on the stalls of church shops and Orthodox fairs, the most popular branches of alternative medicine are currently homeopathy, phytotherapy, and aromatherapy.

Some of our informants from church shops practiced Orthodox aromatherapy in the form of "using church incense and essential oils to heal the body and soul." Such ideas are promoted in the publications of Orthodox doctor Konstantin Zorin. The Ukrainian herbalist and healer Evgeny Lebedev also has followers among Russian Orthodox believers. His books (*Let Us Cure Cancer, Let Us Cure Everything,* and others) are available in the shops of some parishes of the Russian Orthodox Church, although clergy in Ukraine repeatedly warned against "treatment according to Lebedev."

Orthodox homeopathy originates from the ideas of the Holy Martyr Metropolitan Seraphim (Chichagov), who at the end of the nineteenth century developed a method of treatment based on the homeopathic law of similarity and recipes of traditional medicine. Unlike classical homeopathy, he prepared drugs mostly from non-poisonous plants growing in Russia. The surge of interest in Chichagov's heritage in the 2010s is associated with the activities of Ksenia Kravchenko, author of the technique *Self-Healing Under the System of the Holy Martyr Seraphim Chichagov*. Her approach is based on limiting the amount of consumed liquid and taking iodine and anthelmintics. Physicians have repeatedly declared this to be quackery. Kravchenko's lectures became popular after a video of them was posted on the website of the Trinity Lavra of St. Sergius. However, the official representatives of the Russian Orthodox Church many times publicly declared that Kravchenko's system has nothing to do with the works of Chichagov.

Religious life is more closely linked with folk medicine in the Old Believers' version of Orthodoxy, although they do not position it as particular "Orthodox medicine". In addition to prayer, extreme unction, and veneration of the saints, Russian Old Believers resort to the help of community members skilled in folk methods of treatment, which have survived due to traditionalism, especially in rural areas. Such methods include herbal therapy relying on ancient handwritten books of herbal remedies combined with prayer books, as well as bonesetting ("kneading the head", "kneading the bones").

In general, the Orthodox environment is very responsive to all kinds of health doctrines and original techniques based on the ideas of folk medicine, even though they differ from the official position of the Russian Orthodox Church on the relationship with formal healthcare. In one way or another, parishes actively participate in "informal healthcare"; by providing spiritual support, the Church also partially replaces conventional medicine. This may be a consequence of the specific religiosity of Russia's current population, which the local Orthodox organizations tend to accept rather than try to remedy the situation.

On the one hand, virtually all informants from among the Orthodox clergy and church staff emphasized the idea that turning to God for help in the event of health problems or any other worldly difficulties must involve constant spiritual work. They were very critical of using faith to resolve health and other everyday problems—a practice typical for the *zakhozhane*.

On the other hand, we must admit that the priests themselves partly encourage and support this attitude, as it allows them to attract more people. In the dilemma between the correct understanding of the religious doctrine by the believers and the well-being of the parish, they opt for the latter. The missionary factor also underpins their loyal attitude to semi-paganism—any appeal to the Church is regarded as the first step on the way to faith. Probably that is why the subject of faith healing is emphasized in educational literature and in the sale of religious items and presented in a simplified form. Due to such simplifications, holy water and other consecrated objects are presented as remedies in the style of collected recipes of alternative medicine.

For example, the educational brochure *The Foundations of the Orthodox Faith*, on sale in all church shops of the Perm Diocese, informs: "Drink holy water in the morning, on an empty stomach, but where necessary (in case of a serious disease or grave life circumstances), drink it at any time of the day or night... You may add small amounts of holy water to food or take medicine with it. Before giving pills to a patient, wash his face with holy water and make him drink it. It goes without saying that this should be done with love and fervent prayer to the Lord for the patient's recovery" (*The Foundations of the Orthodox Faith*, 2010, pp. 99–100). Where consecrated products are standardized and sold in large quantities, like in the Trinity Lavra of St. Sergius—one of the most visited Russian monasteries,—every item is accompanied by an "instruction for use", turning it into a remedy for believers. Thus, the souvenir packaging of a shawl for women labeled "Shawl consecrated at the monastery of St. Sergius of Radonezh the Wonderworker" recommends to "put it on with prayer in the event of ailments of the soul or body and apply it to sore spots."

*Islam*

Reading the Quran is the main practice of fighting disease that Islam offers its believers. According to the doctrine, the Holy Book of Muslims is itself a means of healing, as recorded in its text: "And We send down in the Quran that which is a healing and a mercy to the believers" (Surah 17. Al-Isra, verse 82). As our informants mentioned, treatment with the help of the Quran proceeds from the meaning and the significance of this collection of sacred texts: "If you read the Quran, you will be healthy. That is what is written there. If you do not read the Quran, you will not be healthy."[163]

In case of illness, it is recommended to read or listen to some Surahs (chapters) of the Quran. Not only imams recite the Quran; any devout Muslim observing all rules of Islam may do it. The righteousness of the reciter is more important than his official position. One of our informants explained that "if a righteous, that is a purified person prays for others, Allah helps him."[164] Therefore, in the surveyed localities, it is customary for Muslims to seek prayer support in health problems not only in the mosque, although this is also common. One can also turn to a familiar righteous person. Accordingly, healing practices in the form of reciting the Quran are not prohibited in the villages. This is a contrast with Orthodoxy, where faith healing outside the temple without participation of a priest is usually regarded as sorcery.

However, imams with an extensive knowledge of the teaching of the Prophet are still considered the best reciters. In Kungur, residents and visitors from other towns often come to the mosque expressly for the local

---

163 Informant: male, 60–70 years old, mullah, medium-sized town.
164 Informant: male, about 30 years old, mosque employee, Perm.

imam muhtasib to pray for them to be cured. He says that he helps anyone who addresses him, including Orthodox believers.

In Islam, the evil eye and the influence of evil spirits are considered, among other reasons, to cause diseases, especially mental disorders and conditions that cannot be precisely diagnosed by conventional medicine. Special rituals, such as reciting selected verses of the Quran and performing ablution, are intended to counter the harmful effects of sorcery. Only specially trained theologians engage in driving out the jinn and breaking the evil eye.

Besides, the doctrine of Islam has a special section of medical knowledge. It is called "Prophetic medicine", or "medicine of the Prophet", and is based on the sayings (hadith) of Muhammad on health maintenance strategies and therapies. It contains advice on nutrition, purification, treatment, etc. In Islamic countries and regions, Prophetic medicine is currently regarded as folk (traditional) medicine. To meet the needs of those who want to receive treatment in compliance with the doctrine, a certain infrastructure has developed around it: special Islamic clinics; private hijama (bloodletting) professionals; educational literature and courses; mosque and online shops selling oils, balms, ointments, and other remedies made from black cumin seeds, sets for performing hijama, as well as books of recipes.

We did not expressly compare the situation in the Perm Territory with other regions; however, a review of publicly available sources indicates that this specific sector of goods and services is far less developed in the Kama area than in areas with a dominant Muslim population.

In Bashkiria, Tatarstan, and the North Caucasus republics, consultations on issues of Prophetic medicine supplement regular medical services in private clinics positioning themselves as Muslim ones. Wellness facilities and centers of alternative medicine also offer hijama, or bloodletting with the help of vacuum cups (wet cupping), which is promoted as a method for treating many diseases (including cancer, infertility, diabetes, and hypertension). In Kazan, Ufa, Grozny, Makhachkala, and even Moscow, one can easily find someone through friends, newspaper ads or social networks who would perform bloodletting at the patient's home. Many providers advertise that they do it for free or at no fixed price ("at your discretion", " at the pleasure of Allah"). A fee-based manipulation costs up to two thousand rubles ($63). Patients generally require that hijama specialists have a medical background and sterile instruments. Due to the magnitude of bloodletting services in the Chechen Republic, special regulatory measures were adopted in 2013 to control the activity of such specialists. Those wishing to engage legally in hijama therapy at the patient's premises must be certified by the Center of Islamic Medicine.[165] Media reports stated that over thirty people had been certified as of the end of 2013. Muslim exorcism is also practiced. As for driving out jinn from the possessed, the best-known facility in Russia is the abovementioned Center of Islamic Medicine in Grozny, designed to accommodate up to 150 patients a day.[166] Prayer recital and other methods of Prophetic medicine are used here to unjinx, break the evil eye, and treat psychiatric disorders.

In the Kama area, Islamic medicine is offered on a much more modest scale. In the surveyed localities, ads contained no reference either to hijama services or to the sale of remedies from black cumin seeds. A representative of the Muslim community in Perm mentioned the existence of hijama practitioners who visit their patients. They work without a fixed fee (for gratitude), but only through acquaintances. They do not advertise their services, understanding their illegal nature. In Perm, hijama courses are organized by the Ural office of the Professional Visceral Therapy Association. The therapy here is presented without any reference to Islam, but simply as "one of the most ancient methods of treating various diseases, which was known before our era."[167] The Perm Muslim community also has a specially trained imam who drives out demons, but he does not publicize his activity either. Our informants in Kungur and Lysva pointed out that enthusiasm for Prophetic medicine was typical of fundamentalists, whereas local Muslims were rather passive in terms of faith and in matters of health limited themselves to prayer.

*Protestantism*
Hardly any widespread Orthodox healing practices (using special rituals, consecrated objects, holy places, and religious attributes) are applied in Protestantism. Prayer is the main support in case of ailment. This practice

---

165 Salamova Z. *Folk Healers Will Have to Obtain a Permit to Perform Bloodletting.* ChGTRK *Grozny.* 11.12.2013. URL: http://grozny.tv/news.php?id=3275.
166 Imam and theologian Daud Selmurzayev, Head of the Center, also holds the position of Deputy Minister of Health of the Chechen Republic.
167 The Ural office of the Professional Visceral Therapy Association (website). URL: http://visceralperm.ru/xidzhama.

is most common and significant for Protestants. Collective prayer for the health of certain people is an essential part of religious life. It is used both on a community level and within one Church/denomination across the region or nationwide.

Pentecostalism also widely resorts to healing sessions held by preachers—both local and visiting.[168] Treatment methods include collective prayer, anointing, and laying on of hands. The sessions take place both in person, at large gatherings of people, and using modern means of communication (television and Skype). This practice is inseparable from the doctrine, which asserts that the miracles of the time of the apostles, described in the Gospel, can take place in our days; and such miracles are evidence of the presence of Jesus, and his care for the people. Thus, just as in Orthodoxy, personal testimony of miraculous deliverance from disease during healing sessions is widely practiced by Pentecostals. However, our informants emphasized in interviews an important point of Christian faith—it is the Lord that heals people and not the preachers, pastors or members of the community.

Healing sessions are especially popular in charismatic movements. Liberal Pentecostal denominations, for example, believe that the gifts of the Holy Spirit, such as healing, prophecy, miracle-working and glossolalia (speaking in tongues), can occur in the life of believers today, and strive to prove it daily. Charismatic communities in Russia develop mainly through fighting against drug addiction and alcoholism; therefore, getting rid of addictions is the main miracle of which they testify.

*Other religions and spiritual teachings*
Compared with the Orthodox, Muslim, and Protestant communities, other religious associations in Russia and the Kama area are far less numerous. Accordingly, the scale of their involvement in maintaining the health of the population is also significantly smaller. For their adherents, however, when needed, they can replace or supplement formal healthcare. For example, Catholic practices of fighting diseases include intercessory

---

168 A well-known preacher from Nigeria visited Chusovoy and Lysva during our fieldwork there. However, not only foreign guests hold healing sessions. Ivan Komarov, an Evangelist from Barnaul, is also active in this respect. Formerly Director General of OJSC Altai Airlines, he currently leads the Interdenominational Health Ministry Christ the Healer. He is also the organizer of a network of "healing rooms" in Pentecostal churches throughout Russia and abroad. *See* his website: http://ya-iscelen.com.

prayers, pilgrimages to holy places,[169] and exorcism. A religious Jew can order a special prayer in the synagogue for the recovery of the sick ("Mi Shebeirach"); a particular pulse diagnosis practice is also based on the Torah.

The situation with Buddhism is more complicated. Like other world religions, it has its own body of ideas and practices aimed at maintaining health and fighting diseases. It is Tibetan medicine. Its specialists rely on the medieval treatise *rGyud-bZhi* (*The Four Tantras*) and comments to it. The Buddhist Tibetan Medical and Astrological Institute currently operating in the north of India is the world center for preserving and promoting Tibetan medicine. Medical professionals are also trained at some Buddhist centers (temples) that have medical schools. Practicing doctors (emchi) work in monasteries; in Russia, there are such monasteries in Buryatia, Tuva, and Kalmykia.

At the same time, numerous clinics, centers, and private entrepreneurs operate all over Russia under the guise of "Tibetan medicine". Some of them are internationally certified and, among other things, train doctors; others are dubious healers. Considering in addition the enormous amounts of educational literature and the use of certain Tibetan methods in other alternative health practices, we can safely say that Tibetan medicine currently exists separately from Buddhism. Besides, legal and shadow markets of educational and instructional literature and media; medical services; education; phyto bars; herbal teas; and tours to Tibet have developed around it. Buddhist religious organizations are to a lesser extent agents of Tibetan medicine than the numerous business entities unrelated to them or sharing other religious values. For example, at some point, an Ayurvedic salon close to the Perm Society for Krishna Consciousness was organizing sessions of a visiting doctor of Tibetan medicine in Perm.

Within one chapter we cannot give a detailed description of the numerous healing ideas and practices that new religious movements and spiritual teachings, which have emerged in Russia in the past twenty to

---

169 One of the most famous pilgrimage destinations is the French town of Lourdes. It is believed that there, on the site where there was an apparition of the Virgin Mary in the nineteenth century, a spring appeared, the water from which can now cure physical ailments. However, the scale of Russian Catholic pilgrimages to Lourdes is small. At the same time, travel agencies specializing in Orthodox pilgrimages also arrange tours there.

thirty years, offer their followers. However, we can identify some general trends that determine their participation in "informal healthcare".

New spiritual teachings of Eastern origin (with followers also in Perm) often have a pronounced health focus. In such cases, health approaches are a foundation of the doctrine (which, in turn, distinguishes them from the major world religions). For example, Maharishi's teaching about transcendental meditation appeals to the well-known wisdom that all diseases of the nerves. The Maharishi Vedic approach to health offers disease prevention, "instant relief and progress toward normal functioning of physiology."[170] The central practice in the teaching of Bhagwan Shree Rajneesh (Osho) is dynamic meditation, which "considers man himself as a disease" and opposes medicine, which "considers each disease in man separately" (Osho, 2000, p. 1). The Chinese syncretic teaching Falun Gong (Falun Dafa), which creatively revised the idea of qi energy, promises its followers exceptional health and development of supernatural abilities through spiritual practices and physical exercises.[171]

Meditation and yoga-based health techniques developed by the preachers and spiritual leaders of various neo-Hindu and neo-Buddhist movements are practiced not only by the followers of the guru. Their ideas are popular among a much wider audience due to mass publications of literature intended for the secular reader, special seminars held by spiritual health centers, etc.[172]

To expand their influence and engage new adherents, NRMs strive to convey to the public the value of their teachings through secular entities—non-governmental organizations, cultural centers, schools of personal development, and charity foundations. This strategy is used by the Hare Krishnas, who firmly occupy in Russia the niche of agents of the traditional Indian (Vedic) culture with such of its elements as astro-psychology, yoga, and Ayurveda. Due to their efforts, Ayurveda, the ancient Indian system of medicine, is associated with certain religious beliefs, although supporters of a purely medical approach to it also exist in Russia.

---

170   Maharishi Vedic Education Development Corporation (website). URL: http://www.transcendental-meditation.globalgoodnews.com/04-tm-health.html.
171   Falun Dafa (website). URL: http://en.falundafa.org/introduction.html.
172   *See, e.g.*, the website announcing therapy and meditation groups, and psychological trainings organized by Osho's followers in Russia: http://oshogroups.ru/index/a/0.

In Perm, for example, Ayurveda courses were organized by the Aurama salon affiliated with the local Society for Krishna Consciousness.

New spiritual neo-pagan and syncretic teachings that cannot rely on the authority of the most well-known traditional health systems but wish to distance themselves from contemporary medicine invent their own unique pseudo-ancient health remedies. For Anastasians, the "Ringing Cedar" from the Siberian taiga is such a remedy. Besides, the method of farming promoted by Vladimir Megre makes it possible "to get rid of absolutely all diseases", because "illness as such is the removal of man from the mechanisms of nature that take care of his health and sustenance" (Megre, 2009, p.12). Amid the Rodnovers, the Slavic system of spiritual healing *Jiva* is popular. It draws on the ideas of Reiki, and was developed by Vladimir and Lada Kurovskie (2010), a Ukrainian couple, who call themselves the high priest and priestess of the community *Rodovoye Ognishche Slavyanskoy Rodnoy Very* (known as Ancestral Fire).

*The economic aspect of healing practices*

The arsenal of treatment methods that religious organizations and spiritual teachings offer to the population varies not only by its ideas but also by the way "informal healthcare" agents communicate with the customer (patient). It includes rites performed by the clergy or pious believers; techniques applied by specially trained people (healers, emchi, etc.); and practices that a believer can engage in on his own. In the last case, the believer can rely on pastoral care and the support of the religious community, as well as educational literature and health products recommended by the doctrine, which are supplied by the religious organizations and their affiliated businesses.

It is more difficult to capture and describe the economic aspect of this variety of healing practices than the ideological one, not to mention measuring it, as market categories are not applied to the activity of religious organizations. When we are not talking about *goods and services*, it is logical to assume the gratuitous nature of such activity. Ultimately, however, the believer does not get help for free, but incurs certain expenses. What are these expenses, except for the obvious cost of religious literature and health products?

Most religious organizations in Russia charge their followers no fee for helping to fight diseases. Moreover, such fees may seem blasphemous: "You see, I don't heal anyone. I am just a pastor. If someone asks for help, I pray for him, but it is God that heals. And if God heals, how can I ask money for this?"[173] However, the organizations themselves exist on regular voluntary contributions of all members of the community—generally ten percent of the believer's income (tithe). The amount of the tithe ultimately depends on the individual's devoutness, as the community has neither the resources nor the authority to verify his income. Anyway, it is impossible to determine the share of health-related donations in an adept's total contribution.

The Russian Orthodox Church is an exception. Here, the tithe principle is not observed, but it is customary to fix a price for special services and rites that the priest performs. In addition, the specific features of Orthodox ceremonies imply substantial sales of candles and other required items (crosses, icons, prayer books, oil, incense, and bottles for holy water). In the absence of the tithe, ordinary parishes generate their income mainly from selling candles and goods in the church shop and from the priest performing upon request prayer services and religious rites.

Precise information about the income and expenses of Russian Orthodox parishes is publicly unavailable, and the state of church accounting at the grassroots level raises doubts about the very existence of such information. Expert estimates made by Mitrokhin (2001) and Edelstein (2000) as of the beginning of the 2000s produced the following breakdown of the income part of parish budgets: the largest share was attributable to candle sales (60–70 percent of the total turnover of the church); 20–30percent—to religious rites and services; and 10–15 percent—to the sale of goods in the church shop and donations during the service. Large and famous churches have a higher proportion of income from performing religious rites. An external observer, however, cannot distinguish the specific amounts that believers donate for health purposes.

To avoid accusations of engaging in business activities, the internal regulations of the Russian Orthodox Church require that the prices for goods and services of a local religious organization be referred to as "recommended donations". The amounts are established at the level of the diocese; however, we encountered varying figures in the Perm Territory. In one church, two different price lists were pinned on the wall, both referring to the same order of the Perm Diocesan Administration. In some

---

173  Informant: female, 40–50 years old, pastor of a Pentecostal community, district center.

cases, there may be no fixed price at all. This is more acceptable for both poor rural parishes (since not everyone can afford to pay) and "guest" temples with a busy flow of visitors (since some of them can afford to pay a lot more). At the observation sites, prices for religious rites and prayer services ordered in the event of illness varied as follows (in rubles): note for good health—3–5 ($0.1–$0.2) per name or 10 rubles for a note with several names; forty-day prayer—120–160 ($4–$5); year-long prayer—250–600 ($8–$19); and extreme unction—100–200 ($3–$6). As we see, there is no generally accepted idea of the value; the prices are rather symbolic if we compare them with the costs a patient incurs when turning to doctors of conventional or alternative medicine.

As for the services of healers using alternative methods under the banner of religious or spiritual teachings, no generally accepted market prices apply to them either. Here, voluntary donations are also common, when the patient himself determines the amount of compensation depending on his income, devoutness, and the effect of the therapy on his health.

Finally, participation in religious healing practices is associated with hidden indirect costs, which are the higher the more value the practice has for the believer. Thus, pilgrimages to popular monasteries, holy wells, and "power places", as well as trips to attend the healing sessions of well-known preachers are associated with high transport costs, payments to intermediaries, and significant time investment.

## 5.3. Social service as a form of religions' participation in healthcare

At first glance, the social work of religious organizations aimed at helping the sick is unrelated to "informal healthcare". First, such activity fits into the legislative framework, and shadow practices are few here. Second, in most cases alternative medical practices are not applied here. Third, religious social work more often includes support activities—fundraising, nursing, and home care—rather than actual medical services.

Nevertheless, we are interested in this aspect of religious life for two reasons. Historically, prior to the emergence of public healthcare, religious organizations provided medical care in the Christian world. Patient care institutions (hospitals, almshouses) were established at monasteries and convents. And today, many forms of religious charity are intended to compensate for the gaps in the provision of public healthcare, and missionary work is inextricably linked with medical charity. In other words, to a certain—albeit small—extent, denominational structures act as providers of healthcare services and make medical care more accessible.

In addition, the social service of the churches is sometimes a substitute for the treatment that public healthcare for whatever reason cannot provide. This is the case with treating dependence on psychoactive substances. In Russia, such ailments are exclusively within the competence of one field of professional medicine—narcology. However, the state of the national addiction treatment service and the nature of the dependencies recognized as diseases are such that even after a course of treatment, primarily pharmacological, the patients are not cured. Therefore, customers are of the view that rehabilitation centers and associations of people suffering from addictions that are run by religious organizations and formally provide only spiritual help and engage in social rehabilitation, indeed *treat* alcohol and drug addicts.

Community service is organized differently in Russian religious organizations, and their contribution to healthcare also varies. The emphasis on charity of the church is typical primarily of Christian denominations, where it is inextricably linked with missionary work. We focused on the organizations that are most often represented in the surveyed localities— Russian Orthodox parishes and Protestant communities.

The publicly available online Social Service Database of the ROC (http://social.miloserdie.ru, hereinafter referred to as the Database) established in 2011 by the efforts of the Synodal Department for Church Charity and Social Service is currently the main source of information on the social work of the Russian Orthodox Church. However, it may be used to estimate the scope of the social work with reservations, because information is entered in the database as reported by the temples and at the initiative of the leaders of the diocesan and parochial social institutions. Accordingly, the database sometimes reflects the desired situation rather than the reality, or vice versa. Some facts are not recorded. Thus, some initiatives mentioned by our informants in the parishes of the Perm diocese were lacking in the database.

Anyhow, the site of the Department for Church Charity and Social Service of the ROC reports that the Church has over 3,400 religious social institutions, projects, and initiatives in Russia. Impressive absolute figures are disappointing when compared with the total number of Orthodox religious organizations. Researchers estimate that approximately only every tenth parish engages in social activity (Oreshina, Prutskova, Zabaev, 2013). In other words, community service in the Russian Orthodox Church is currently underdeveloped.

There are several reasons for this. The local communities are weak and fragmented. The situation in the ROC is affected by the bitter legacy of the Soviet period. As Filatov (2005) indicates, that time was marked by the emergence and establishment of a certain type of religious behavior which did not envisage any participation in the communal life of the parish. Another factor is the general attitude of the clergy to avoid interfering in the sphere of competence of the government. Performing mandatory religious rites is the top priority for the clergy. Despite the social doctrine of the ROC[174] formulated in 2011, most clergymen perceive anything beyond liturgical service as a compulsory additional assignment. The specific financial relations within the ROC also have a negative impact. The parishes have virtually no funds to support social projects, and centralized competitive allocation of money for such purposes is underdeveloped. Besides, volunteer initiatives in Orthodox parishes are further hindered by one of the fundamental principles of church life in the ROC—the need to obtain permission for every action from a higher rank in the form of a blessing. Knorre (2012, p. 98) notes that due to this, church staff most often do not dare to undertake anything "without a blessing". Under such rules, the main advantage of non-government social service—the spontaneity and selflessness of volunteer work—is lost.

The extent of social activity significantly varies from parish to parish. It depends primarily on the personality of the priest and the degree of the community's consolidation. Our observations confirm the trend captured by researchers of the contemporary Orthodox parish in Russia. A strong community is interrelated with the priest's style of leadership and his endeavors in organizing non-liturgical activities in the parish (Zabaev, Prutskova, 2013; Filatov, 2005). The life of the parish depends very much on the charisma and authority of the priest and his ability to build relations with the benefactors (sponsors) that provide the material base. However,

---

174 *On the Principles of Organization of Social Work in the Russian Orthodox Church.* Document adopted by the Bishops' Council of the Russian Orthodox Church on 4 February 2011. The Moscow Patriarchate (website).
URL: http://www.patriarchia.ru/db/text/1401894.html.

the welfare of the church does not determine the activity of the parish in the social sphere. On the contrary, it often happens that the additional resources raised due to the church's popularity, the existence of sacred objects, and the large flow of *zakhozhane* are invested in line with business logics back in the material base (construction of new buildings, reconstruction and renovation of the temple, landscaping, and enhancement of the priest's living conditions) rather than in gratuitous social projects.

Let us consider what forms of community service in support of the sick the ROC nevertheless has. Over the past few years, the number of initiatives aimed at developing social work in the Orthodox parishes, including patient care, has markedly increased. However, higher figures in the Database may be partially due to the more active process of filling in the data. According to Table 6, in the period from 2011 to 2015, the Database showed that the number of sisterhoods increased more than four-fold; schools of sobriety—almost six-fold; self-help groups for addicts and co-dependents—almost eight-fold; medical units—three-fold; almshouses (of which some hold licenses for medical activities, and the rest enter into agreements with healthcare institutions)—nearly two-fold. Organizations that do not require substantial funds for the establishment and operation demonstrated the highest growth. The social activity of the parishes is very unevenly distributed across regions. About half of all self-help groups for addicted people run by Orthodox churches (71) were in Moscow (21) and the Moscow Region (17).

Table 6. The number of certain types of Orthodox organizations (church social services) providing patient care (2011, 2015)

| Type of Orthodox organization (church social service) | 2011[175] | 2015 (at 9 Feb. 2015) |
|---|---|---|
| Almshouses | 21 | 38 |
| Hospitals | 2 | 5 |
| Self-help groups for addicted people | 9 | 71 |
| Medical units | 16 | 50 |
| Sisterhoods | 51 | 227 |
| Schools/courses of sobriety | 8 | 47 |

The most common format of patient care in Orthodox social service is the sisterhood that provides visiting nurse care at the patient's home or at major medical clinics. Sisters of charity also patronize children in social institutions of the closed type, as well as homeless, elderly, and poor people. In addition to catechetical activity (explaining, providing spiritual literature, preparing for communion, etc.), where possible, sisters of charity help the patients financially and physically; they buy food and medicine and care for bedridden patients.

With regard to medical care provided in organizations of the ROC, altogether fifty medical units and five hospitals were registered in the Database at the beginning of 2015. The units mainly imply free medical consultations provided by parishioners with a medical degree (at least five of them are homeopaths). Members of the regional societies of Orthodox doctors hold such charity consultations. They usually do it at the society premises. It is often specified that such consultations are held orally, i.e. the doctor makes no written prescriptions. In fact, such medical activity is illegal (it is conducted without a license, without observing sanitary standards and regulations, without statistical reporting, without maintaining medical records, etc.). However, formally, consultations are provided on a voluntary basis by employees of public healthcare institutions.

There are also several medical centers at monasteries and convents that provide medical care. According to the Database, the Hope

---

175 Database figures as of beginning of April 2011 are quoted from Knorre (2012).

(*Nadezhda*) medical center at the Holy Trinity St. Seraphim-Diveyevo Convent (Nizhny Novgorod Region) operates a 50-bed hospital for monastics, which has a surgery, medical ward, dental office, and pharmacy. Another medical center at the Holy Trinity New Golutvin Convent in Kolomna was established by and at the expense of the convent with the active participation of the Kolomna Orthodox Medical Society. The nuns of the convent—"experts in therapy, neuropathology, homeopathy"—consult patients. The official website informs, "Doctors use different methods of treatment: herbal medicine, allopathic and homeopathic medical supplies, and, what's the most important, conversation about Church Sacraments in which the medicine is given by God."[176] We did not manage to find the medical license of the center.

By contrast, full-fledged legal medical institutions that are called Orthodox and belong to the Russian Orthodox Church are integrated into formal healthcare and present no alternative to it. Their emergence and development may be perceived as a desire to establish an in-house healthcare structure, which would allow controlling the quality of medical services provided to the clergy and other ROC employees and the conformity of such services to Orthodox canons. The Central Clinical Hospital of St. Alexis, Metropolitan of Moscow, in Moscow is the most famous and largest Orthodox Hospital. In 2013, the St. Elizabeth clinic providing outpatient care opened its doors in Perm. However, the history of its establishment marked by scandals tarnished the reputation of the Perm diocesan administration more than it served to address the practical tasks of social service or the provision of medical care to the local clergy.[177] As a matter of fact, the term "social service" is not quite relevant in the case of such medical institutions, because they operate under compulsory health insurance. They differ from ordinary health facilities only by the status of the founders and the fact that healthcare services are supplemented by the spiritual help of a priest. Medical centers funded solely by the

---

176  The Holy Trinity New Golutvin Convent (website).
URL: http://novogolutvin.ru/en/obedience/med/medical.html.
177  On favorable terms under a long-term lease agreement, the Perm authorities transferred the building of a former maternity hospital historically associated with the Assumption Monastery to a company affiliated with the Perm diocese. The company—Jordan—was supposed to set up an Orthodox clinic there. However, for a long time the building was not used as intended—some premises stood vacant, some were subleased. Finally, the regional administration of the Federal Antimonopoly Service and the prosecutor's office had to intervene.

church and sponsors are an exception. The most well-known, if not the only, such example is a small 35-bed charity hospital of the Blessed Saint Xenia of Petersburg, which is jointly financed by the parishes of the St. Petersburg diocese.

Schools of sobriety, self-help groups for addicts and co-dependent people, and rehabilitation centers for drug addicts are the ROC's contribution to the fight against alcoholism and drug addiction. As of 2014, thirty-three rehabilitation centers were included in the List of organizations collaborating in the rehabilitation of drug addicts with the Coordination Center for Combating Drug Abuse of the Department for Church Charity and Social Service of the ROC. However, the Department's website mentions over sixty rehabilitation centers. The societies/schools of sobriety and self-help groups practice collective prayers (often reading the Akathist in front of the *Inexhaustible Chalice* icon of the Mother of God); conversations with relatives; courses conducted by the priest with the participation of invited narcologists and psychologists; vows to abstain from alcohol; educational and joint leisure activities (choral singing, etc.). The temperance movement, where alcoholics take a vow of abstinence from alcohol—an important pre-Soviet social tradition of Orthodoxy—is currently re-emerging in Russia due to the enthusiasm of individual priests, such as Archpriest Igor Bachinin from Ekaterinburg.

If we turn from the nationwide situation to what is happening on the micro level, in individual localities, the participation of the Russian Orthodox Church in addressing socially important health-related problems will be hardly noticeable.

The Community Service Department was established at the Perm diocesan administration quite recently, and at the time of our fieldwork (2013), it was only attempting to organize systematic work in this field. The department oversaw fifty-five poor and large families; it held one-time charity events to raise funds to operate sick children and purchase school supplies for children from low-income families. According to the Database (as of 17 March 2015), a total of about thirty church social institutions are operating in the Perm Territory. They include five posts for collecting and distributing clothing and other in-kind donations; five soup kitchens; five groups of mercy; two asylums for pregnant women and mothers with children; four youth associations (clubs); two retirement homes (almshouses) for seven and twenty-seven people; a school for sisters of charity on the basis of the Perm College of Medicine; a rehabilitation center helping children with cerebral palsy and autism; a community for people with total or partial hearing loss; an orphanage; and a temporary shelter for the homeless.

Non-liturgical church work in the parishes of the surveyed localities is mainly limited to educating children and the youth and providing occasional help to the poor. Almost all parishes run Sunday schools and summer camps for children. The diocese also has a network of youth military-patriotic clubs, with martial arts tournaments held between them. Financial aid is a more complicated issue. On the one hand, the temples regularly collect donations for nationwide or diocesan purposes—for victims of natural disasters, sick children, etc. On the other hand, there are virtually no mechanisms for the church to provide charity support to the members of the local community. Usually, help is given to the families of churched parishioners as needed; however, this is rather a manifestation of community and rural solidarity than religious education. In addition, the parishioners sometimes bring to church things (clothing and shoes) they no longer require and leave them for the poor. Whoever needs the things may take them, but except for one church in Perm, nobody purposefully delivers them to any social institutions. Thus, the temple is just the site, but not the organizer of charitable activities.

In general, the priests are not ready, willing or able to organize social work. The most common reasons for this that our informants named were lack of resources, poverty of the parishes, and the high workload of the priests. Some informants sincerely did not understand why the church should do anything besides prayer services and pastoral work with the parishioners. Some voiced the opinion that addressing social problems was not a task for religion, for example: "The government is just waiting to shift the burden of social work on the Church."[178] Priests also mentioned having to deal with human vices, communication difficulties, and a parasitic attitude when providing charity. Thus, community service was discouraging in terms of result and effectiveness. Problems exist both from the side of those asking for help and the laity involved in community service:

> ...Unfortunately, I have been repeatedly deceived... This undermines faith in people, and it is hard to take. Sometimes, you confide in a person, help him,

---

178  Informant: Orthodox priest, 60–70 years old, medium-sized town.

and then find out that he was cheating and just wanted to defraud the priest... I had my fingers burned several times, and I am now somewhat suspicious of requests.[179]

As for fighting the dependence on psychoactive substances, the most common method of dealing with alcoholism that the ROC offers a believer is a weekly rite of blessing the water and praying for those suffering from alcoholism and drug addiction with the Akathist to the Mother of God in front of the *Inexhaustible Chalice* icon. Very rarely the liturgical service is supplemented by some social activity on fighting addictions. An example is the Perm Holy Trinity St. Stephan Monastery—the Church's actual center for publishing, missionary, and social activity in the region. There, prayer services in front of the *Inexhaustible Chalice* icon are accompanied by conversations about alcohol and drug addiction. They are held by monk-priest Alexander Usachev, a trained narcologist and representative of the local society of Orthodox doctors. We found the only example of a parishioners' grassroots self-organization at the temple of St. John the Baptist in Kungur. Several female enthusiasts from families of alcoholics united to read the *Inexhaustible Chalice* Akathist; the status of the association was "a group of activists". About forty people joined the group during the first year of its existence. They work without any outside support but quite consistently, with the participation of the priest and a psychologist from the drug treatment clinic. In addition to prayers and discussions, anonymous psychological counselling is arranged here. Group members attended a seminar in Ekaterinburg; they collect literature and hygiene products for the local drug treatment hospital. As one of the women organizers explained, they united to "understand ourselves, to help other people... She has a drinking husband, I—a brother."[180]

However, social service associated with supporting addicted people is definitely not a priority for the ROC on the local level. Doctors from the narcological centers said they saw no initiatives from Orthodox organizations in this field. The priests, in turn, told us that alcohol and drug addicts were a very difficult social group for missionary work.

In sum, the social activity of the Russian Orthodox Church is largely subordinated to the tasks of catechesis and religious education, which explains the priorities of the individual areas of social work. Free care to

---

179   Informant: Orthodox priest, 30–40 years old, Perm.
180   Informant: female, 40–50 years old, Orthodox activist, medium-sized town.

patients is not among them. Moreover, the priorities of Orthodox religious organizations on the micro level astonish at times by their irrelevancy to the population's real problems. Instead of addressing alcoholism, drug addiction, and the social adaptation of the poor, we saw them engage in distributing pamphlets exposing the Dulles plan and raising funds for new church bells.

Against this background, Protestant churches occupy a promising niche for missionary social work on the local level. Volunteering[181] is more developed in this environment, and the evangelization policy is very active. These two factors enable performing locally appreciable social work using minimum resources. "People in difficult life circumstances" are the principal target audience of Protestant organizations. Of the vulnerable categories of the population, they choose to patronize the most stigmatized ones, those who rarely get public support,—drug addicts, alcoholics, the homeless, and HIV-positive people. Accordingly, prison and rehabilitation work are a priority.

Actual medical service intended for non-stigmatized patients is less developed in Russia's Protestant communities, including because the administration of public health facilities opposes it. However, isolated projects in this field nevertheless exist. The best-known Baptist endeavor is the missionary health program based on the Agape Medical Center established by the American missionary Dr. Bill Becknell. The Adventists have a special notion—"medical social service". Although Russia is not included in the scope of activity of the Adventist Development and Relief Agency (ADRA), there are several medical facilities in Moscow and Ryazan financed by the Adventists that provide free services to the poor.

Fee-based medical service courses and health centers emerging here and there in Russia are another interesting form of Adventist activity. It exists at the intersection of social work and the health business. One of such centers is operating in the Perm Territory. It is called The Living Source (*Zhivoy Istochnik*) and is located in the Perm District. Established in 2009 in the form of a limited liability company, this facility is in fact a resort for adherents with focus on a healthy lifestyle. It hosts the Abundant Life (*Zhizn s Izbytkom*) health camp and courses where the participants can familiarize themselves with the "Divine healing program, foundations

---

181 According to the estimates of Mersiyanova and Korneeva (2013), self-identity as a believer and affiliation with the Protestants or Catholics is the strongest factor underlying the potential engagement of contemporary Russians in volunteering.

of anatomy and physiology, weight-reduction and anti-stress programs," and learn to practice massage, "hydrotherapy", vegetarian nutrition, etc.[182]

However, it is work with addicts that is the hallmark of the social work of Protestant organizations in Russia; and here, Pentecostals are in the lead. In the past twenty years, they have established an extensive network of rehabilitation centers (RCs) for drug addicts and alcoholics. There is no precise information of their numbers; the website of the Associated Russian Union of Christians of Evangelical Faith (Pentecostals) states that Churches of the Union support over three hundred and fifty rehabilitation centers. According to rough estimates, about thirty RCs of various capacity (able to accommodate from five to fifty people at a time) operate in the Perm Territory. Some of them are united into branch networks. The website of the regional drug treatment center mentions thirteen NPOs involved in rehabilitation; of them, ten organizations with twenty-five RCs in the region are associated with Protestant churches.

Christian rehabilitation centers are an interesting and ambiguous phenomenon in the social life of contemporary Russia which requires special study. I will focus here only on the common features of such entities, which are a prime example of "informal healthcare".

In some Russian towns, cardboard or paper sheets with laconic inscriptions promising "free, confidential, and anonymous" deliverance from drug and alcohol addiction, and a phone number are an integral part of outdoor advertising. Such sheets appear on bus stops, trees, walls, and fences. They are often joined by ads (obviously originating from the same home printers) offering the assistance of freight handlers and laborers. This is a standard presentation of RC services for the public, though it may be complemented by billboard and media advertising.

RCs rely on the "Twelve-step" model, which implies that drug addicts and alcoholics receive support from people just like themselves who managed to "call it quits". The Russian Orthodox Church does not welcome such methods, considering them "sectarian", but the narcologists we interviewed believe such methods are effective precisely due to their "sectarian" nature. Through personal example and very emotional religious practices, the Pentecostals manage to convince addicts of the need

---

[182] The Seventh-Day Adventist Church. Euro-Asia Division (website). URL: http://adventist.ru/2012/04/13/liderskiy-kurs-meditsinskogo-sluzheniya.

to stop taking psychoactive substances and the possibility to do so, provided they turn to God. Social rehabilitation includes counselling, reading spiritual literature, work therapy, and psychological guidance by members of the religious community. Usually, the rehabilitation cycle in such centers lasts from three months to a year and consists of several stages with a different level of restriction on the addict's freedom of movement. For this reason, the organization has several sites/premises. The informants said that a noticeable influx of people wishing to get rid of addictions is observed in the autumn and winter season due to the arrival of the homeless.

The rehabilitation centers have the official status of autonomous non-profit organizations or charitable foundations. They are formally independent of the churches and often do not use the name of the parent organization to conceal their religious affiliation and avoid claims from the authorities. However, they are closely associated with the communities. In some Christian evangelical churches, the rehabilitation center network is that basis on which the religious organization develops, and new congregations emerge. For example, in Lysva, the charitable foundation Independence (*Nezavisimost*) appeared in 2009, whereas the affiliated local religious organization of evangelical Christians Exodus (*Iskhod*) was registered only in 2012; at the time of field research, the Adonai Church was non-existent, and the community developed around the Adonai Charitable Fund, which managed the Lazar Rehabilitation Center. Many members of such communities are converted former drug addicts and their families. They form the core of social service and promote the RC. Our informants always stressed in the interviews that participation in the life of the religious community was purely voluntary, but the addicted people needed the constant emotional and psychological support they received in church in order not to "crack".

The local community disseminates information about the rehabilitation centers affiliated with their religious organization and works with the co-dependents (relatives). Organizations with a branch network of several RCs have an advantage. They can send people to other localities and even regions. Our informants believe this gives the opportunity "to make a new start". Various umbrella organizations (coalitions, associations, and programs) created nationwide by individual churches or their alliances facilitate the development and establishment of new RCs. Usually with the assistance of similar foreign organizations they replicate the RCs methods and approaches; arrange training for those involved in the rehabilitation work; and establish their own systems for certifying rehabilitation techniques to provide the evidence base needed for the legality of the centers' operation. At the time of field research, the most prominent coalitions in Russia were the Iskhod therapeutic community for drug addicts, the Russian coalition of Christian rehabilitation programs Teen Challenge, and the Union of Civil Initiatives.

Rehabilitation centers allow the religious communities to build relations with the local authorities, which used to perceive them only as sectarians rather than social partners. Charitable foundations enter into agreements with the regional offices of the Federal Drug Control Service and the Federal Penitentiary Service, and social agencies. They also participate in anti-drug campaigns organized by the local law enforcement authorities. All this contributes to their legitimation. In the Perm Territory, some religious centers are involved in the publicly funded program to issue certificates for free social rehabilitation of drug addicts. In Lysva, the local administration engaged in dialogue with such organizations, because at some point they became the most prominent socially oriented NPOs in the city. According to the estimates of the local authorities, a total of 700–800 people from the very bottom of the society passed through their rehabilitation centers in 2012.

Where do the RCs get funding? Some of them charge relatives for the addict's stay at the center (information obtained in fieldwork indicates amounts varying from four thousand to twenty-five thousand rubles per month, which is equivalent to $130–$800). Very few rely on the public funds allocated for the certificates to drug addicts in the Perm Territory. For those who do not charge fixed fees, the rehabilitees' labor is the main source of income. In addition to work at the rehabilitation center itself, this includes hired labor at local farms (if the center is in a rural area), log house building, construction, loading-unloading, and other unskilled labor. Thus, the rehab center generates business, which can be not only self-supporting, but also profitable.

This approach to occupational therapy, as well as the need to pay for rehabilitation, discourages locals from seeking assistance at the RCs. A female informant admitted she gave up the idea of sending her relatives to such a center when she realized that "rather than being treated, our boys will be used there as unpaid workforce." The statistics of complete recovery from addiction in such centers is quite modest (generally, the RCs indicate a figure of 20%–30% as the proportion of fully recovered rehabilitees). The active opposition from Orthodox sect fighters is yet another unfavorable factor for the RCs. Despite all this, Pentecostal NPOs maintain leading positions in the Russian market of treatment services to drug addicts, which they achieved through their active social work, particularities of the religious practices, and drawbacks of the public addiction treatment system.

Speaking about religious organizations operating in the addiction treatment market, we should mention one more project; it is unrelated to the Christian doctrine. Followers of Ron Hubbard's teaching, known for their rejection of official psychiatry, launched the Narconon anti-drug detoxification program in Russia in the 1990s and established a network of fee-based rehabilitation centers. Their technique, based on taking ultra-high doses of vitamins and minerals, sweating in the sauna for extensive periods of time, and running, was a contrast to both medical narcology and the Christian twelve-step program. As mentioned in Chapter 1, at some point the Russian Ministry of Health approved this technique as a medical program, but later it was once again downgraded to "informal healthcare".[183]

In general, the contribution of religious social work to healthcare is not as straightforward as it seems. On the one hand, charity appears to be a natural and legitimate way of cooperating with medical institutions. Donations, volunteer work, and the establishment of in-house medical facilities compliant with general rules—all this is beyond the scope of "informal healthcare". On the other hand, the social work of religious organizations is subordinated to the task of expanding their influence, thus determining the priorities—who and how to help, and that may stimulate them to work as informal healthcare providers.

We saw two different strategies on the examples of the Russian Orthodox Church and Pentecostal churches. In the first case, social work with sick people is not a priority (it is carried out, but on an insignificant scale when compared to the other social activities of the Church), and the

---

183  Currently, the Narconon and Narconon-Standard network of rehab centers for drug addicts is legally functioning in Russia. It provides social rehabilitation on a fee basis. The services are quite expensive. Occasionally, criminal cases are opened in Russian regions against the management of such centers. They are suspected of illegal entrepreneurship and engagement in medical activity without an appropriate license. Their activities are suspended or banned by court orders; however, the program is not completely prohibited.

participation in maintaining people's health is realized mainly in the form of direct religious practices. In the second case, social service to the sick, by contrast, is one of the key ways to win new adherents; however, instead of contributing additional resources to the "bottlenecks" of official healthcare, the churches establish their own alternative structures, where Jesus helps the patient instead of a professional narcologist.

## 5.4. Religious associations in the markets for health products

In our basic classification of "informal healthcare", religious associations are the main agents in the segment of providing ideas to customers. They are also partially involved in the industry of information on alternative therapies (primarily through publishing and trade activities—Chapter 6 will focus on that) and work in the markets for health products and natural remedies. This concerns the immediate business activities of religious organizations and their affiliated entities—both commercial and non-profit—engaged in manufacturing and trade.

Along with agriculture and production of church supplies and ceremonial objects, beekeeping and processing gifts of nature are the most common occupations in the economy of Russian Orthodox monasteries. Their products are used for both in-house needs and sold. Based on information obtained in the Perm Territory, we can say that the monasteries engage not so much in harvesting, as in intermediary activities and processing. They buy honey, berries, and herbs from villagers, thus partly replacing the long gone Soviet procurement agencies. Healing products are sold in the refectory or church shop in the form of packaged jars of honey, herbal combinations, oils, tinctures, herbal liqueurs, and ointments. Such remedies cost from one hundred to three hundred rubles (three to nine dollars), which is less than the price of similar products of MLM companies and more than the price of tinctures, for example, in pharmacies.

Tinctures and oils of the same brand sold in large quantities in church shops throughout Russian regions are most probably produced by ordinary enterprises affiliated with religious organizations rather than by monasteries. We saw shops at major monasteries in Moscow and Perm selling remedies for external and internal use, which were obviously industrially produced and simply placed there for sale. This concerns products under the brand name *Monastic Pharmacy* from the Sverdlovsk Region. According to information from publicly available sources, their producer is a company of from Nizhny Tagil bearing the same name and incorporated in 2011. The founder of the company is presented as a pediatrician, Orthodox phytotherapist, and homeopath. These same herbal oil tinctures prepared "in conformity with ancient monastic recipes" used to be made and sold at one of the monasteries in the Tyumen Region. The remedies are on sale in some church shops (including in the surveyed localities of the Perm Territory), online stores, and Orthodox fairs throughout Russia. An inscription "Consecrated product" is the only information on the label indicating the conformity and quality of the goods. The oils are produced quite legally—in 2012 they were entered in Rospotrebnadzor's Register of State Registration Certificates as "cosmetic products for external use". Poplar-aspen oil was even patented as a product of plant origin with preventive and healing properties.

In other cases, however, the church shops were selling obvious artisanal products manufactured by amateurs—priests and monastery staff keen on folk medicine. Following is a description of the production process in one of the convents:

> The church shop is selling medicinal flower honey, home-made jams, gingerbread cakes, and, most interestingly—herbal oil tinctures and ointments produced by a woman at the convent. Previously, she used to sell "Altai herbs" in the city. She takes the recipes from the *HLS Bulletin* and experiments a lot herself. The oil production facility is a cellar next to the refectory. Three-liter glass jars line the walls. They are standing on wooden shelves covered with a clean oilcloth. Something is filtering, settling or flowing from one jar to another. The herbs come from a field adjacent to the convent, the pinecones—"from three pines". Tinctures are stored down in the cellar. Naturally, the priest blesses them all.[184]

Both the Church community and the society perceive such activity favorably as being socially important, because it's result is aimed at preserving people's health. The association between Orthodox traditions and folk medicine, present in public opinion, is implemented in practice here.

For customers, such bee products and church-made remedies have a dual healing effect—coming from the nature itself and from contact

---

184 Field notes of Olga Makarova, participant of fieldwork in the Kama area (September 2013).

with the sacred. This combination gives Orthodox healing products a competitive edge in the "informal healthcare" market. In addition, for the customer, the producer's affiliation with a religious organization somehow automatically means its utmost reliability, a guarantee that there is no fraud. In other words, this business is built on trust, implying that a consecrated product cannot be fake or substandard. This explains why ordinary consumer logic urging to be wary of goods with an unconfirmed quality does not work in this case.

Orthodox remedies are marketed as folk medicines. Their therapeutic properties are emphasized by enclosed instructions imitating the style of patient information leaflets (with "indications", "contraindications" and other sections). A specific feature is reference to consecrated components in the composition of the remedy, which determines special application and storage requirements. For example, the leaflet inserted in the package of Turpentine liniment sold at an Orthodox fair in Moscow informs: "For any of the below mentioned ailments, apply the liniment to the sore spot crosswise and then rub it in reciting the Lord's Prayer; Rejoice, O Virgin Theotokos; I Believe, or any other Orthodox canonical prayer with the grace to heal."

Orthodox artisanal "pharmaceutical products" are sanctified but completely excluded from the state system of quality control and product safety. They are not certified and have no sanitary approvals; generally, neither their composition, nor even the manufacturer is indicated. In other words, this segment of health products is definitely a shadow one in terms of the regulatory environment. Nevertheless, such potions are openly sold within the walls of church institutions raising no questions from the regulatory authorities.

Trade under the auspices of Orthodoxy is not limited to church shops and retail outlets. Temporary Orthodox exhibition fairs are currently widespread throughout Russia. They are a venue for exhibiting sacred objects; holding cultural and religious events; taking orders for prayer services and rites at monasteries and churches; selling candles, books, church supplies, as well as household items and foodstuffs that are usually attributed to the Russian folk tradition (crafts and peasant farming). Major national, interregional, and regional exhibition sites have the fairs listed in their calendar of events. In Perm, the annual exhibition *Orthodox Rus'* has now been held for eleven consecutive years. It lasts for seven days and receives about thirty thousand visitors. Under a single socio-ecclesial project, exhibitions with the same title are held in eight other major Russian cities, including Moscow.

As part of fieldwork, our team conducted observations at the above exhibition in Perm in August 2013, and, for comparison, at a similar exhibition in Moscow—*Christmas Gift*, December 2013—which took place at the All-Russian Exhibition Center, where such events were held almost monthly. Before sharing the findings of these observations, I will briefly outline the policy of the Russian Orthodox Church on exhibition activities.

Regulations on holding Orthodox exhibition fairs were introduced in Russia quite recently. The Synodal Commission for the Coordination of Exhibition Activities was established only in 2011; subsequently, the Regulation on the Exhibition Activity of the Russian Orthodox Church was adopted. In 2013, the leadership of the ROC stated that many events were not in conformity with their designation. They were organized by secular companies, and the proportion of participants representing the ROC reached only thirty percent; the consumer goods offered for sale were often of poor quality; and, finally, they "had become a favorite venue for the activities of pseudo-Orthodox sects." The Moscow Patriarchate denounced a fraudulent group—followers of "God Kuzya" (Andrey Popov)—that was living off such fairs. Posing as representatives of the lesser-known temples and monasteries, they took orders from the visitors for prayer services and rites, which were naturally never performed.[185]

To counteract this, *Requirements for Organizers and Participants of Orthodox Exhibition Events of the Russian Orthodox Church* were adopted. Patriarch Kirill approved these rules on 30 April 2013. The document states that an exhibition event may be called Orthodox, if the proportion of church organizations or Orthodox exhibits is at least seventy percent of the total number. The rules include a restriction on the volume of associated trade and a ban for representatives of temples and monasteries to display price tags for the performed rites and advertise their icons as miracle-working ones. Books and other media products disseminated at the fair must bear the seal of the Publishing Council of the ROC. The sale of "prescription-only medicines, dietary supplements, personal hy-

---

185 The Moscow Patriarchate (website).
URL: http://www.patriarchia.ru/db/text/2904478.html.

giene items, contraceptives and other pharmaceuticals", as well as alcoholic beverages is prohibited. Food products must have all the required permits.

However, as in the case of book trade in church shops, the practice of Orthodox exhibition fairs significantly differs from the regulatory requirements of the centralized religious organization. Monasteries and temples display price tags for prayer services in their booths. Among the Orthodox literature, one can find publications without the seal of the Publishing Council of the ROC, and even books that address topics unrelated to religion, such as alternative therapies and healers. Regardless of the ban on alcoholic beverages, "monastery made" Kagor wine and herbal liqueurs are on sale; moreover, they are advertised here as health products. In one case, a counter with alcohol was adorned with information sheets "The Healing Power of Wine" and folk medicine recipes based on Kagor. Finally, Orthodox fairs are de-facto a popular sales channel for dietary supplements and other health products (balms, oils, and medicinal herbs) originating both from monastic sources and quite secular businesses, including MLMs.

At the August exhibition titled *Orthodox Rus'* in Perm, about half of all booths selling consumer goods belonged to religious organizations—monasteries and temples. The remaining ones represented secular businesses (mainly in the status of sole proprietor). About thirty participants were selling honey and bee products. The rest were offering medicinal herbs, oils, herbal liqueurs, tinctures, wine, magnetic bracelets and chains, dietary supplements and vitamins, creams, onyx water cups "that lower the blood pressure", and other products intended to improve health.

A lot of exhibitors are regulars at such events. Sellers of health products roam the country, taking part in various fairs dedicated to different themes (healthy lifestyle, folk crafts, religion). Visitors here are more set on buying than at regular stores, thus guaranteeing the vendors robust sales of their goods and services. Women "over 50" are typical visitors of Orthodox fairs (although the organizers of the Perm exhibition noted the growing number of young people in recent years). It is the same audience that is interested in health products. And like the sellers, many of them are regulars. They systematically attend temporary trade events always purchasing the same products.

Poor control of the organizers over who is selling what at such fairs under the auspices of the Orthodox faith is observable not only in terms of compliance with the above-mentioned rules of trade. The ideological filter is also lacking. Consequently, companies openly affiliated with religious movements that the ROC considers to be sects or occult teachings take part in Orthodox exhibitions under the banner of folk medicine and healthy lifestyle. Among others, this concerns entities affiliated with the Anastasians, Hare Krishnas, and proponents of Chinese medicine.

Situations where the production and sale of health products go hand in hand with the activity of religious organizations are typical not only of Orthodoxy, but also of other religious institutions and spiritual teachings. As mentioned earlier, many NRMs that oppose modern civilization urge their adherents to turn to traditional medicine. Respectively, business in health goods and services is more than pure commerce for them—it is a socially and spiritually important affair. For teachings with a strong health component, the strategy of expanding their sphere of influence through secular commercial and social structures serves as an additional incentive to develop such businesses. And, finally, work in the market for health products is a source of income in those cases when the adherents' voluntary contributions, donations, and proceeds from the sale of literature do not raise enough funds for the sustenance of the organization. Following are some examples from our Kama area field records.

To contact the followers of Vladimir Megre in person, there is no need to search for their scattered family homesteads in the remote areas of the region. Four shopping centers in Perm had small shops selling products under the brand name Ringing Cedars of Russia. A clerk in one of them said their product range came from the Novosibirsk Region, where "production is based on an ancient technology, without any contact with metal, that is on wooden equipment", and from family homesteads. Megre's books and the movement's newspaper can be purchased here as well. Megre LLC—a company founded by Vladimir Megre's daughter and son-in-law—is developing a dealer network throughout Russia under a franchise agreement. They offer for sale under a single brand cosmetics, foodstuffs based on the healing gifts of nature, and household items produced in conformity with Anastasian teachings. The Megre company from Novosibirsk supplies the core product range made from the Siberian cedar (from nuts and oil to toothpaste and wooden dishware), which is supposed to have "a special healing power for man", hence its curative effect. In addition, the shop sells goods for health and eco-friendly life (presented as the produce of family homesteads) made by various sole proprietors and LLCs. A female distributor of the Ringing Cedars of Russia is convinced that these goods are a product of the new economy, the principles of which are set out in Anastasian teachings:

> See, for example, the ointments from the Sverdlovsk Region. They are made from aloe. This aloe grows on a windowsill in a private house on a family homestead, where a loving family lives in their environment of love. They are not static; they also progress and develop their business.[186]

Promed—one of the few companies in Perm producing registered dietary supplements from bee products—is closely linked with the Neo-Christian movement Family of the Children of God founded by Vladimir Beloded. A former follower communicated that the leadership of the company sustained Beloded's teaching after his death, and former members of the closed community were among the core staff.

The small group of devotees of the Neo-Hindu preacher Sri Chinmoy in Perm is engaged in direct sales—distribution of Ojas bio-energetic devices that are intended to "structure water" and "harmonize the environment" in order to protect oneself from geopathic stress, get rid of insomnia and chronic fatigue, improve the health and rejuvenate.

The fast-growing chain of Lakshmi healthy food stores in Perm is another example of how trade in health products turns out to be one of the most suitable occupations for people sharing certain religious beliefs. Its owners also operate the Aurama Ayurvedic massage salon. The stores sell vegetarian foods, farm milk to order, herbal combinations, dietary supplements from different producers, Ayurvedic cosmetics and remedies, and books about the East, including religious Vedic literature. A representative of Perm's Hare Krishnas explained, "This is not directly linked with the Society for Krishna Consciousness. It just so happens that people practicing Ayurveda observe the principles of Krishna. It is impossible otherwise."[187]

Summarizing the above, we can say that organizations representing religious and spiritual teachings are quite successful in the markets for health products and natural remedies. They get a competitive advantage over secular players, because the useful qualities of their products have an additional ideological foundation based on faith. This is most evident

---

186 Informant: female, 30–35 years old, distributor of health products, Perm.
187 Informant: female, about 25 years old, member of the Society for Krishna Consciousness, Perm.

on the example of the Russian Orthodox Church whose moral authority allows the agents selling healing potions in its name to ignore government control over health products.

\*\*\*

The information presented in this Chapter demonstrates that even a cursory glance at the participation of religions in maintaining the health of the population requires an extended description of a variety of practices, rules, and ideas, as the current Russian religious landscape is very diverse, despite the dominant position of the Russian Orthodox Church. We were considering the same topic from different angles, so certain repetitions in presenting the facts were inevitable. However, this highlighted the ambiguity and inconsistency of religious institutions acting as "informal healthcare" agents.

When the leading Russian religious organizations articulate their attitude to healthcare, they pose as allies of conventional medicine and opponents of alternative therapies. However, their doctrines and religious community practices demonstrate an opposition to the health system rather than solidarity with it. The declared non-interference in the competence of secular science is combined with the firm belief of the sinful cause of disease, and, consequently, the inability to cure it by scientific methods only. Moreover, the religious community produces its own knowledge of health issues and a respective infrastructure to apply such knowledge, including businesses engaged in manufacturing and selling health products.

In today's secular world (including Russia), the religious organizations, on the one hand, live "according to the Statutes" developed by the secular state. Any attempts of the churches to establish a completely alternative way of life are fraught with accusations of extremism, a sign of which is denying believers access to healthcare. On the other hand, by its very nature the religious organization is a social regulator, which dominates and determines every aspect of the believer's life, including physical health. And this causes a latent conflict with conventional medicine, which has monopolized care for the human body.

Besides, the fact that health issues were and remain one of the principal incentives for turning to faith encourages religious associations to participate in "informal healthcare". According to Berger (1967), religious pluralism is a global consequence of secularization in the modern world. This means that religion is no longer imposed but becomes a matter of marketing, and religious groups must develop such forms of organization that will help them win customers in competition with other groups pursuing the same goal. Based on the concept of the religious market, we can say that the promise of healing is a successful strategy for gaining new supporters and expanding the influence of religions and spiritual teachings, even if it contradicts the established church principles of interacting with secular public institutions.

# 6 The "informal healthcare" framework: Information markets

The segment of "informal healthcare" discussed in this chapter occupies a special place and addresses specific tasks. It is exchange of information on the ways and sources of maintaining health that ensures the existence and development of this sphere.

In formal healthcare, information, just as medical services, is within the competence of professionals. Legislation and official medicine assign the primary role in health education to doctors. The Law *On the Fundamentals of Public Healthcare in the Russian Federation* requires that medical organizations participating in the Guarantee Package Program on free healthcare "promote healthy living and provide health information to the population" (Art. 79.2.4). As one of our interviewees pointed out, even promoting healthy living in the media should be undertaken under the guidance of professionals, "A TV program must be with the participation of a doctor; a newspaper—with the participation of a doctor; even a newsletter must be written specifically by a doctor."[188]

In practice, however, awareness-raising is one of the activities which is most often neglected in clinics and hospitals due to the high workload. At the level of health facilities education is limited to two formats: information boards and posters in the clinic hallways, and lectures of medical professionals at schools and colleges. At best, they are supplemented by presentations and articles in the local media. However, none of our medical informants had personally engaged even in this—they mentioned holding preventive conversations only with their patients.

Therefore, people who for whatever reason have no wish to go to hospital seek answers to their health questions in the media, where information is provided not only and not so much by doctors as by a variety of alternative agents.

In the context of the study it is important to distinguish between sources of information that: 1) either are recognized by official medicine as reliable for self-medication or encourage early diagnosis and timely recourse to treatment at a medical facility; 2) advocate "irresponsible" self-

---

188 Informant: female, about 50 years old, oncologist, Perm.

medication and recourse to the help of alternative agents. The first group of sources is not part of "informal healthcare". The second, on the contrary, forms its integral part. This group includes not only periodicals with folk recipes and numerous online forums, but also specialized information sources for doctors (handbooks of diseases and medicines, research papers, and the results of clinical trials) that the public uses for self-medication.

In addition to the media industry, various non-profit and business entities are involved in the exchange of health information. They perform the function of intermediaries between the agents and customers of "informal healthcare"—aggregate the data and help to disseminate it in the interest of their audience or for profit. What can be classified as information intermediaries? These are platforms enabling regular exchange of treatment knowledge and skills (social organizations, hobby clubs); sources of free access to printed matter (libraries); entities offering preselection and delivery of "informal healthcare" products (specialty stores, shops); companies arranging tours to treatment sites (travel agencies and pilgrimage services). Formal promotion of healthy living is also impossible without them, so sometimes they serve the interests of both the health system and alternative agents.

The selected methods of empirical research do not allow us to present herein a complete and detailed description of information providers in Russian "informal healthcare". Obviously, one needs other methods than interviews and observations in selected localities to study the agents operating in the Russian markets for broadcast and digital content. The more so that regular statistical studies of the domestic media market do not distinguish the segment of health information intended for non-professionals. Therefore, below we will consider primarily those agents whose operations can be captured and depicted using the available field records. The first part of the chapter focuses on information providers (media and others); the second—on selected information intermediaries.

## 6.1. Mass media

Internet resources have clearly the best prospects among providers of health information. The proliferation of digital technology is accompanied by a rapid development of self-medication, which relies on the recommendations published by numerous websites devoted to medical and associated topics.

According to the liveinternet.ru rating (performance counters), the total audience of websites in the Russian language in the "medicine" category amounted to 63.5 million people in March 2013, rising to 85.8 million in March 2015.[189] Of them, women constitute approximately sixty percent. The daily audience averages about 6 million people (March 2015). BabyBlog.ru—a website dedicated to pregnancy and baby care—is the absolute leader of the rating. The top thirty Internet resources in the "medicine" category include seven websites on women's and children's health; online pharmacies; reference resources on healthcare institutions and medicines; and websites with recommendations offering medical consultations on health issues or promoting methods of folk medicine. Forums on websites for women are a real treasure trove of information on alternative therapies. Moms and housewives discuss various health devices; weight loss remedies; search for a *babushka* healer; exchange self-medication experiences; and consult each other. The statistics of Yandex search queries show that mostly middle-aged and elderly women browse the Internet for health and wellness information (Yandex Users, 2013).

In search of information for self-medication patients are increasingly turning to online resources rather than other media. Our physician informants regard this as a major trend. However, despite the growing popularity, by its impact on the audience the Internet still lags behind television and radio, which offer a wide selection of broadcasts on health. Such radio shows are usually broadcast in the middle of the day when pensioners are the main audience. The program schedule of the leading federal TV channels also without fail includes a show dedicated to health issues. With the help of medical professionals, the moderators teach the audience responsible self-medication practices, explain how healthcare institutions operate, and urge not to neglect disease prevention. Such shows indirectly advertise dietary supplements, "health" devices, and non-conventional therapies.

In addition, considering the audience's passion for miracles, TV and radio channels in pursuit of ratings often directly promote "informal

---

189  Please note that these statistics concern specialized websites only; they cover neither relevant social network web pages, nor news or other online resources of a broader focus.

healthcare" agents. The most striking example is the already closed show *Malakhov Plus* on TV Channel One, thanks to which the country learned about original methods of treatment and healers. One of the highest rated entertainment show on Russian TV—Andrey Malakhov's talk show *Let Them Talk* on Channel One—from time to time includes stories about psychics, faith healing, etc. The *Battle of Psychics*—a record-breaking show broadcast by the TNT TV channel sixteen seasons in a row—boosted interest in paranormal methods of treatment. Participation in the project became an opportunity for business-focused healers to raise the price of their services. Even an entire market of fake show participants emerged. A separate genre are documentaries about miraculous faith healing that promote Orthodox health practices based on prayers, recourse to elders, veneration of the saints, etc. (for example, the films *Saint Matrona of Moscow* broadcast by NTV and *Wonderworkers of the XX Century* broadcast by Channel One).

Thanks to the electronic media, markets for information on self-medication have become truly nationwide. They ensure swift and mass dissemination of such knowledge and make it universally available, even to people not interested in alternative therapies. However, it is the market for printed matter that serves as a classifier and conductor of ideas. Figuratively speaking, it is a framework that ensures their integrity, continuity, and development. It is a vehicle for disseminating original doctrines, systems, and methods of self-healing; creating trends; and establishing opinion leaders.

Periodicals addressing health topics are among the leaders of the Russian press market. The most popular one is the *Healthy Lifestyle Bulletin (Vestnik Zdorovogo Obraza Zhizhni)*, in conversation usually referred to simply as *HLS (ZOZh)*. Its content largely consists of readers' letters, where they share experiences in using folk remedies. Before the 2008-2009 economic crisis, the *HLS Bulletin*'s declared circulation (without inserts) exceeded 3 million copies, and was later estimated tentatively at 2.5 million copies.

This periodical has become the symbol of uncontrolled self-medication of Russian senior citizens and an alternative to formal healthcare. For its readers, it is not simply another source of information, but a good friend and mentor. "The *HLS* is everything to me! I have been subscribed to it since 1992," exclaims an elderly female informant.[190] "I test everything I read in the *HLS* on myself," says another one.[191]

*HLS Bulletin* sets trends in the health efforts pursued by Russian pensioners. An article in this periodical triggers a surge of interest in a specific technique or folk recipe. Thus, the promotion of one of the popular "cure-alls"—Dorogov's antiseptic stimulant (ASD)—was launched in 2006 with the publication of an article titled *Healing Antiseptic*.

Besides providing recommendations and recipes of folk medicine, the *HLS Bulletin* also serves as a communication platform for the elderly and builds a certain readers' community. One of the informants who had been buying it for the past thirteen years said she was cautious about using the actual recipes and health tips but appreciated the paper in general. She remarked that the publication had changed in recent years: it now had a page with the readers' poetry, letters-stories about domestic animals and life in the village, as well as articles written by physicians. She liked this, because "no one is writing anything about the village nowadays."[192]

For the periodicals market, *HLS Bulletin* may serve as an example of a unique and quite successful business model: the publisher makes money on subscription and retail sales of the paper rather than on advertising. The cost of such publications is very low: they are printed on the cheapest paper and the expenses of maintaining an editorial office are minimized, because the content is generated mainly from the readers' letters. The readers request recipes of remedies for ailments they are suffering from, give tips on self-medication and health maintenance, or simply share their stories and approaches to life. The volume of advertising in such periodicals is insignificant, with the advertisers being mainly producers of dietary supplements and other health products. Generally, popular periodicals of this kind are great advertising media not only for major pharmaceutical companies but also for small "informal healthcare" agents that use them to develop sales channels for their products. Some informants reported ordering goods from healers by phone, using the numbers listed in such publications.

---

190  Informant: female, 60–70 years old, health club activist, village.
191  Informant: female, about 60 years old, newsstand vendor, district center.
192  Informant: female, 50–60 years old, newsstand vendor, medium-sized town.

It is noteworthy that the readership of mass health periodicals is not limited to proponents of alternative medicine and poorly educated elderly people; it also includes representatives of formal healthcare. About half of the medical professionals we interviewed mentioned reading such publications and sometimes using their recommendations; some were even their subscribers.

There is another aspect to the interaction of physicians and such "informal healthcare" agents. Virtually all health-related periodicals secure the involvement of doctors (preferably distinguished) as authors of articles or interviewees. The advice of representatives of scientific societies and medical associations, holders of academic degree, is often published next to the recommendations of psychics, healers, etc.

We shall now consider the range of health periodicals and reading preferences at the local level.

The three main distribution channels of periodicals in Russia are subscription, retail sales in post offices and at newsstands. Sometimes one can buy printed press in urban supermarkets. Village shops offer newspapers and magazines for sale only if they cooperate with the Russian Post. Press distribution market experts estimate the number of retail press sales outlets in Russia at 68,300. There is on average one sales outlet per 2,100 inhabitants, and one newsstand—per 4,770 people. About 300 newsstands operate in Perm, and retail press sales outlets total about 400.[193]

Newsstands are the main providers of health press in the cities and, partially, in the district centers. Each newsstand sells on average about a dozen publications on health. Here three categories are distinguishable: cheap "folk" magazines devoted entirely to treatment issues,[194] popular collected universal tips for the home,[195] and dedicated glossy magazines, selling much worse, especially in rural areas. In addition, there are special thematic supplements to women's publications and

---

193   Guild of Press Publishers (website).
      URL: http://www.gipp.ru/viewer.php?id=47607.
194   They are similar by title and design and look like clones in the display window exploiting the "folk" periodical model successfully developed by *HLS Bulletin*. *Grandma's Recipes* lie next to *Grandma's Tips*. *Healing Letters* are alongside *Healing News* and *Letters to Aybolit*. *People's Doctor* challenges *Your Family Doctor* and *Aybolit*; *100 Health Recipes* competes with *Health Recipes*.
195   For example, *Popular Tips, 1000 Tips*.

newspapers of general interest: *Boudoir Health, Vesta Health, Lisa—First Aid, AiF Health,* and others.

According to newsstand vendors, health periodicals are second in popularity only to the local press. *HLS Bulletin* is the unquestionable leader here (it is also among the subscription leaders). It is published every two weeks, and each issue is bought up very quickly. It is usually delivered in abundance—the double or triple of any other health publication—but it is the first to be sold out. *Healing Letter, Popular Tips, Prevention, One's Own Doctor,* and *Kind Doctor* are also in demand. All popular publications cost about 20 rubles (less than $1). "In fact, they are inexpensive," sums up the newsstand vendor. "The expensive ones just lie around for ages."

Russian periodicals have a specific category of buyers, which consists primarily of retired people. Therefore, in summer, when they move to their cottages in the countryside, the demand for "healing" press in the cities drops. Popular media has its own audience, which is committed to the favorite periodical. Such readers keep track of the days when the publications are issued and purposefully come for them. On the days when the newsstand receives the latest press releases (usually twice per week), an average of five to ten people come to purchase health publications.

In rural areas, post offices are usually the only place where one can buy printed matter. Postal clerks estimate the share of health publications at ten to thirty percent of the total product range. The windows in the surveyed post offices displayed from three to ten magazines in this category.

Our overview would be incomplete without local (municipal, urban) newspapers. Along with other media, they perform the function of health education and promotion of healthy living under the supervision of professionals. Especially because "medicine is generally the most popular topic, the most widely read one; by the number of requests it is the most popular topic."[196] On the other hand, it is the local media that is the main marketing channel for "informal healthcare" goods and services in the localities. If the federal media advertises mainly dietary supplements and, to a lesser extent, portable physiotherapy devices, local publications are accessible for healers, psychics, and vendors of herbal liqueurs and hearing aids. Local newspapers are indispensable in the work of visiting vendors, psychotherapists, and healers, who, in fact, work illegally. The reason is, local

---

196  Informant: male, 30–40 years old, newspaper editor, medium-sized town.

media charges minimum rates on advertising,[197] it accepts classifieds from individuals, and the editors are not interested in diligently filtering the ads and verifying the information submitted by the advertiser.

Just like the administrators of municipal cultural institutions that lease out premises, the local media editors usually do not probe into the matter of who their advertisers are and what they are doing. When interviewed, they insisted that they accepted only advertisements compliant with the Law *On Advertising*,[198] and that all the advertised goods and services had the necessary permits, licenses, and certificates. However, the newspaper ads themselves indicate that legal provisions are observed only in every second case. Moreover, most of them emphasize the therapeutic effect of goods and services that are formally not medical. The fact that the Federal Antimonopoly Service pays no attention to such deceptive advertisements can be explained only by the magnitude of the violations. Although sometimes local media editors are subjected to exemplary punishment.

Concluding the overview of the media industry supplying information for "informal healthcare", we shall consider the market for health-related literature. Along with cook books, brochures on treatment with herbs or incantations, bestsellers written by trendy doctors, collected *Health Tips for Every Day*, medical encyclopedias, and other books of this kind are a must in the home libraries of Russian housewives; they can be found in almost every home.

It is impossible to determine the exact size of the market for the production and sale of such books, because official statistics and business ratings do not distinguish it as a separate segment; it is either presented in the same category as professional medical literature or in the general non-fiction section.

The bulk of this book market segment is literature of which official medicine does not approve. For example, as of 20 August 2015, the

---

197 A standard advertisement for "comprehensive computer-aided diagnosis" or a session of "coding" from alcoholism cost from 500 to 1,000 rubles ($15–$30), and if it was published in the general "Classifieds" section on behalf of an individual—even less (30 rubles or $1 per line).

198 This concerns the requirement set forth in Article 24.7 of the Law *On Advertising*: Any advertisement of drugs, medical services or medical products must contain a warning about the existing contraindications for their use or application and inform about the need to read carefully the patient information leaflet or consult a specialist.

Ozon.ru online store's catalog of books in the "Medical Literature" section contained about 23,500 modern printed books in Russian. Of these, approximately two-thirds (15,700 books) relate to the "popular and alternative medicine" subsection.

Often, the authors of such books claim to be healers and developers of "systems", but in fact offer the reader a compilation of methods of treatment drawn from various sources, mainly from folk medicine. The publication of Gennady Malakhov's books in the early 1990s was perhaps the most successful project in this field. Their total circulation is estimated at twenty to thirty million copies; thus, Malakhov's books can be found in every second Russian family. For comparison: the circulation of books written by folk healer Nikolay Maznev is five million copies; those by Valentina Travinka, a popularizer of treating with clay—over a million copies. The popularity of such literature peaked in the 1990s.

Judging by sales in metropolitan bookstores (they form the basis for the Pro-Books.ru rating[199]), other genres have become especially popular in recent years: self-actualization concepts which can be used to improve health, and the recommendations of extensively promoted representatives of conventional medicine. Thus, besides literature on diets and slimming, the list of 50 top-selling non-fiction publications regularly includes books by Vadim Zeland—author of the "reality transurfing" idea—and doctors Alexander Myasnikov and Evgeny Komarovsky. Looking ahead, I will say that the preferences of readers in metropolitan areas and in the Russian province vary significantly.

"Healing" magic is also popular today: collected incantations, prayers, rites, and herbal recipes, the authorship of which is attributed to hereditary healers. The absolute leader in this category is Natalia Stepanova from the Novosibirsk Region. Her *Incantations of a Siberian Healer* comprises already thirty-nine editions; each edition was issued with a circulation ranging from 30,000 to 100,000 copies. *The Book of the Siberian Healer's Answers*, *The Big Book of Incantations*, and others are also published under her name, as well as special postcard talismans and amulets (a total of over three hundred different items). In addition, Stepanova publishes the magazine *Magic and Life*. Ripol Classic Publishing House releases this variety of products, marking the cover with a certain

---

199 The rating of the Pro-Books.ru website is generated based on automated processing of data on bestsellers in eleven bookstores (mainly in Moscow and Saint Petersburg).

"sign of authenticity"—this suggests that other publishers are printing Stepanova's works in violation of copyright. "Healer Stepanova" may be a very successful business project, which exploits the obsession with the supernatural. Online women's and occult forums are debating whether Stepanova actually exists or whether this is an artificially created brand.

Our group inspected book shops outside Perm.[200] We wanted to understand what kind of literature was available to residents of the provinces and what was the thematic variety of the printed matter dedicated to health issues. The product range indirectly reflects the popularity of various ideas, methods, and health improvement areas.

Shop owners and administrators build the product range primarily based on specific consumer demand ("they ask—we order"), except when they themselves are keen on health or spiritual teachings. Demand, in turn, is determined by two factors: the readers' commitment to particular authors and the promotion of certain books on television and the Internet.

The general trend is clear—the bigger the locality, the larger and more varied the book range, and the more often it includes esoteric and "psychological" literature. The prevailing subjects are:

- Original "healing systems" and universal health techniques developed by Russian popular health teachers (usually entire series of books and brochures)
- Naturopathy: collected folk herbal recipes and publications on monotherapy devoted to a plant or natural factor, which is declared to be a cure-all[201]
- Home magic and healing for housewives (the absolute leader here are collected incantations by Natalia Stepanova)

A special group is literature on health improvement areas not linked to one Russian "guru": publications about body cleansing, fasting therapy, raw foodism, breathing therapy, and water therapy. In total, such books constitute an impressive part of the range.

Literature falling in the category of approved by conventional medicine (home medical handbooks and first aid manuals), is lost among self-

---

200 District centers had one sales outlet (a combined stationery, toy, and printed matter shop); medium-sized towns—two-three bookstores each, including representatives of regional retail chains.

201 Examples of titles: *Tibetan Mushroom—the Magic Potion; The Good Doctor Blue Iodine and Its Aides; Leech—Your Family Doctor; Beetroot Instead of Drugs; Treatment with Oats.*

study tutorials on alternative therapies. In addition to esoteric literature, there are also a few books on Eastern health practices (qigong, yoga). Books outlining spiritual teachings (Osho, Vladimir Megre, meditation handbooks, etc.) and popular self-actualization concepts (Vadim Zeland and others) can be found only in the cities.

For readers enthusiastic about spiritual endeavors and alternative ways of maintaining health, a full-fledged book service exists only in Perm, but not in medium-sized towns. Customers from other towns of the region regularly visit esoteric salons in Perm to find out about new arrivals and buy trendy novelties. Readers in medium-sized cities also use the potential of the Internet to order books online with home delivery.

According to the vendors, pensioners are the main buyers of publications on health. They prefer cheap books and brochures (up to 100 rubles each)—mostly collections of folk medicine recipes or self-healing techniques. The latter are especially popular—they are the most diverse, have the highest circulation, and are sold out the fastest. They can be divided into two groups:

- Original health theories and universal health doctrines with an element of esoteric knowledge and expressed opposition to official medicine. An alternative understanding of the nature of disease is inherent in them. According to the vendors, the most popular authors in this category are B. Bolotov, G. Malakhov, V. Sinelnikov, and S. Konovalov. Books by G. Sytin, I. Neumyvakin, M. Norbekov, A. Nekrasov, A. Tartak, and others are less popular, but also quite common.
- Handbooks by manual therapists following in the steps of legendary Soviet *manual'shchiks* Valentin Dikul' and Nikolay Kasian—such literature successfully "monetizes" the problems elderly people have with the musculoskeletal system. The most prominent authors are S. Bubnovsky and A. Sittel, who have created their own "unique techniques" to achieve flexibility of the spine and joints through exercise.

Where else besides book stores can one buy literature that is of interest to us? It is available in small boutiques selling health products or esoteric goods, church shops, and MLM offices.

The first category (they are often called souvenir and talisman shops) offer literature corresponding to the eclectic worldview of their owners. The range of products in this case targets like-minded, "thinking" people. Books on Eastern health practices (yoga, Ayurveda, qigong, Reiki, acupuncture), spiritual teachings, psychic studies and practice, and self-understanding prevail. Such publications cost on average RUB 200–RUB 300 ($6–$10), but there are also more expensive ones—RUB 1,000–RUB 1,500 ($30–$50). Amulets, talismans, icons, healing minerals, dietary supplements, and healthy foods complement the book range.

Literature on spiritual teachings is distributed mainly through associations uniting the followers of such teachings and through religious communities. Orthodox printed matter has the most extensive distribution network. It is sold at church shops and temporary Orthodox fairs. Since church bookselling is associated with liturgical, theological, and spiritual and educational literature, the appearance of other books in a church shop may be perceived as a violation of rules. Is that the case?

About seven hundred entities in Russia publish Orthodox literature. They include both the publishers of religious organizations and secular companies, among which are many supporters of the specific "Orthodox medicine" and other alternative methods of treatment. The current system of controlling the range of book products emerged in the ROC quite recently, in 2010, with the introduction of mandatory review of all publications intended for distribution through the church bookselling channels by the Publishing Council of the Russian Orthodox Church.[202] However, the ban on selling unreviewed literature is observed not always and not everywhere. In the inspected church shops and especially at the visiting Orthodox fairs, we saw books without the required seal (instead, there could be some printed blessing of a Church hierarch from a CIS country). The shop vendors and priests insisted they were selling only literature supplied by the diocesan administration. However, in different temples and localities of the same diocese, the number and content of the books varied. This allows assuming that the personal position of the parish priest is the determining factor in shaping the product range.

Based on the facts obtained through observation, we can distinguish two categories of Orthodox literature informing the reader on ways to maintain health. The first is directly linked to the religious activities:

---

202 *See Resolution of the Holy Synod of the Russian Orthodox Church of 25 December 2009 on Publishing.* The Publishing Council of the Russian Orthodox Church (website). URL: http://izdatsovet.ru/catalog/stamps/.

- Collections of prayers, akathists, and canons to read in disease
- Educational brochures that in plain language explain the basic principles and rules of behavior of an Orthodox Christian; tell about the appropriate attitude to physical ailments and the ways to overcome them; provide guidance on special cases (childhood diseases, etc.); and explicitly clarify the danger of alternative methods (resorting to sorcerers, psychics, yoga, etc.)
- Methodological publications for priests on organizing social work, which help to explain to parishioners the attitude of the ROC to medicine (for example, regarding preventive vaccination, schools of sobriety, etc.)

Books of the second category are beyond the actual religious competence, offering readers recommendations on maintaining physical health and dealing with disease. The most common ones at the points of sale of Orthodox literature are:

- Themed books-calendars with collected prayers for certain ailments, folk medicine recipes, and recommendations (*Healing Book (Tselebnik), God's Healer, Health-Giver (Zdravushka)*, etc.)
- Collections of recipes for treatment with herbs or bee products (the undisputed leader here is a series of booklets *God's Pharmacy* published by the Orthodox Brotherhood of St. John the Theologian)
- Didactic literature on the expected special Orthodox behavior of patients (the most common books in this category are those written by Konstantin Zorin, "an Orthodox therapist and clinical psychologist", where he promotes his original aromatherapy technique)
- Books and brochures on alternative "Orthodox medicine": methods of the Ukrainian herbalist and healer Evgeny Lebedev, as well as handbooks on special Orthodox homeopathy, presented in the heritage of the Holy Martyr Metropolitan Seraphim (Chichagov) and his contemporary follower Ksenia Kravchenko. In 2013, Kravchenko's book was even entered in the black list of publications not recommended for distribution through the church bookselling network.

Just as in ordinary bookselling, the range of literature on health issues is broader in large church shops and can be represented by only a couple of books (prayer books and akathists) in small shops, although there are exceptions. As internal church censorship becomes increasingly strict, the number of such books sold in temple shops might be reduced to a minimum.

Finally, offices of MLM companies specializing in health products sell mainly the writings of their respective founders or authors of concepts supporting the use of their products. If the distributor is interested in other health doctrines and concepts, the offered range of printed matter may be broader.

At the beginning of this chapter I mentioned that information markets occupied a special place in "informal healthcare", because they ensured its stability, supported other segments and facilitated their development. We see that they shape the demand for certain products and services and create a positive or negative image of health ideas and practices. Moreover, information is the most popular product. Apart from healthcare institutions, the media is where Russians turn to in the first place when they have health problems. This is obvious, although the media itself portrays "informal healthcare" primarily as the domain of sorcerers and psychics. The important role played by the providers of information for self-medication was one of the reasons we abandoned the idea of designating the field of our study as "alternative medicine". Finally, compared with the other segments of "informal healthcare", the media are poorly controlled by the state. Even the existing restrictions (in terms of advertisement content requirements) are violated on a massive scale, since the authorities do not possess the adequate resources to monitor and punish the offenders; moreover, they have other priorities in the media sphere.

## 6.2. Information intermediaries

*Libraries*
According to Rosstat data for 2013, there are about forty thousand public libraries in Russia. Most of them are under the competence of the Russian Ministry of Culture; however, the municipalities are responsible for their functioning and stocking. About a third of Russians are registered library users. Approximately 76.3 percent of the libraries are in rural areas where a quarter of Russia's population resides (*Government Report of the Russian Ministry of Culture*, 2013). In other words, the predominant type of Russian libraries is the rural municipal (inter-settlement) library. Not all of

them have access to the Internet (slightly more than a half in 2013), which means that they continue to fulfill their primary function—to provide free access to books and periodicals. A library in the village replaces the sales outlets of printed matter (newsstands, book shops, and, recently, post offices), the number of which outside urban settlements and district centers tends to zero. In recent years, there has been a gradual curtailment of library services: libraries are optimized through consolidation and the establishment of branches; there is not enough funding to develop library collections; working hours are reduced, especially in the rural settlements. In 2014, about 27 percent of the municipal libraries in the Perm Territory had reduced working hours (*Report on the implementation..*, 2015).

Based on information obtained in the Kama area, we can distinguish several healthcare functions of libraries.

First, libraries provide free access to books and periodicals containing useful information. There is no official statistics as to the share of books on health and medicine in library holdings. The libraries themselves keep no such records either. An inspection of the shelves in the surveyed libraries did not reveal a single trend—the amount and proportion of this literature vary considerably. It is safe to assume that these parameters depend above all on the vital interests and preferences of the librarians themselves. The common feature is the availability of both books approved by official medicine (educational literature for physicians and home handbooks) and publications advocating alternative methods of maintaining health.

The wide variety of themes as well as the worn state of many books is due to the irregular development of library collections. Often, the readers themselves donate books. Librarians strive to retain publications acquired in the Soviet times. When procuring new literature, they are guided by the readers' requests, which largely include sources of information on self-medication: "wellness medicine, therapeutic exercises, breathing exercises, specific diseases."[203]

The list of health periodicals in municipal libraries usually includes from two to five titles. Their number and range are also determined by reader demand and personal preferences of the librarians. Therefore, one can find not only the *School Health* journal in children's libraries, but also

---

[203] Informant: female, 40–50 years old, librarian, medium-sized town.

*HLS Bulletin*, for example. Due to the lack of funding, some library directors cut subscription at the expense of "health" periodicals; others, on the contrary, strive to keep such publications, because "the people are asking" and "these are all magazines that help people, and are always in high demand."[204]

Health literature is in less demand than other genres of popular literature (detective stories, novels for women, or books for children): "Children's books top the list followed by romance novels, detective stories, and books on health."[205] However, it also has its readers. They are, naturally, people over forty, mainly pensioners, although young mothers are also interested in books on child health. Magazines as well as encyclopedias (*2000 Diseases*, *Encyclopedia of Home Medicine*, etc.) and specialized books on folk medicine are popular with middle-aged and elderly persons. According to a librarian informant, people nowadays get folk medicine recipes mainly from the Internet, "but we have some readers who copy pages from books on medicinal herbs."[206]

Second, libraries are an element of the public health education system. Such work focuses mainly on children and young people—a target audience that can be brought to the library in an organized manner to attend a lecture or another event. But judging by the comments of the informants, such activity is more of a formality and is often carried out for the sake of appearance.

Third, as repeatedly mentioned herein, libraries—along with palaces of culture and rural clubs—lease their premises to "informal healthcare" agents. According to informants, until the end of the 2000s, libraries were a venue for meetings with visiting esoterics and healers, lectures and presentations of MLM companies, sales of health products and "computer-aided diagnosis". However, in 2013, such lease arrangements were no longer allowed by the directors, and were a rare case. Premises are often provided without any formalized arrangements and without lease payments.

Fourth (this is a resulting function), libraries promote exchange of information between the consumers of "informal healthcare" goods and services. This happens where the employees themselves are keen on alternative medicine, and their personal priorities facilitate the organization

---

204   Informant: female, 50–60 years old, librarian, village.
205   Informant: female, 50–60 years old, librarian, medium-sized town.
206   Informant: female, 50–60 years old, librarian, district center.

of education and communication platforms for the local community on the basis of the libraries. Given the demographic profile of the average Russian librarian (woman over 40), this happens often. In small settlements, the library remains a real cultural center of local life. Observations in the Perm Territory show that it often promotes not only a love of reading but also an attentive attitude to health; for the elderly people, who are more likely to visit the library, this topic is important.

The library's role of an "information hub" is reflected both in its reported events and the activities that remain invisible to the superior authorities. The first category includes: lectures by authors of health literature and their meetings with the readers; book exhibitions timed to the Day of the Elderly People or other festive occasions with such indicative names as *We Are Fit Beyond Our Years*, *Age Is Not an Obstacle in Life*, *Health from the Garden*, etc. The second category includes: exchange of opinions on the application of recipes and practices gleaned from the read literature; selection of books for the library collection based on the readers' requests; and the librarian's recommendations to readers about books on health issues.

The exchange of knowledge on the methods of treatment between the staff and the readers occurs during regular meetings of senior citizens organized by the library in the context of dedicated health clubs or other hobby groups—from sessions of the local council of veterans to embroidery group meetings or even a simple discussion of journal articles.

*Health clubs and groups for socializing*

Despite the indifference of most Russians to their own health, small communities always have a self-organized group of five to twenty people, who seek to maintain a healthy lifestyle and spend their leisure time together. Most of them are women—retired and of pre-retirement age. According to the leader of such a club, their members are "people who want to be fit and active at any age." Heads of the local council of veterans, retired doctors, and librarians usually initiate such associations. Health clubs and groups meet at the premises of cultural institutions and leisure facilities. The members share useful information and provide psychological support to each other, which adds value to the work of the groups.

According to our observations, there are two kinds of such associations. The "library" option is a platform for holding thematic literature discussions, practicing needlework, and spending leisure time. In Orda village, for example, the library hosts a club called *Socializing and Health*.

In Kormovishche, the library jointly with the local council of veterans founded a club called *Cheerful Hearts*. It unites people who like socializing. Among other activities, the members practice Nordic walking. In Ust-Kishert, this function is performed by the *Inspiration* club organized under the auspices of the council of veterans.

The second option is when the group meets for sports: exercising in the gym or Nordic walking, which became popular quite recently. Health groups were established with the assistance of the municipal authorities, which in recent years had to promote healthy living among the population. In Suksun district, budgetary funds are allocated to support the work of health groups, and grants—to purchase equipment for them. A representative of the district administration said health groups were emerging in those localities where there were proactive senior citizens as well as certified fitness instructors.

This type of social associations is not typical of major cities. MLM companies selling health products and religious associations play a somewhat similar role in the urban environment.

In general, health clubs and groups may be considered an example of real grassroots self-organization and social activity of the Russian people. However, they are not in line with the government's idea of the role social associations should play in promoting healthy living—the idea underlying the development and implementation of public policy in this area.

*Esoteric shops and salons*
In contrast to the rural health groups, where enthusiastic senior citizens share medicinal herbs, health recipes, etc. with the like-minded, esoteric salons focus on urban youth and middle-aged people interested in mysticism. In other words, they are not designed for a mass audience. Besides selling esoteric books and exotic goods, such salons serve as a platform for exchanging information. This turns them into specific fairs of ideas and services, where followers of completely different—sometimes competing—spiritual, occult, and health teachings are presented. The ideological diversity and variety of advertising opportunities distinguishes them from ordinary shops selling health products or "oriental goods" established by the adherents of one or another healthy lifestyle movement.[207]

---

[207] Ordinary shops selling health products are associated with another interesting type of business activity. Owners of such sales outlets often launch associated micro businesses covering all aspects of healthy living (per their understanding). The activities vary: "spiritual" seminars and psychological trainings; club for

Such entities are rare and emerge somewhat spontaneously, since they depend not only on the intentions of their owners, but also on the activity of the agents of esoteric services and communities in the city. In Perm, three shops fell into this category with great reserve, of them only one could be considered a full-fledged information intermediary.

This shop sells: esoteric literature (new arrivals and a wide range of very different ideological and spiritual teachings), amulets, healing minerals, various appliances for rituals from different traditions and cultures, etc. Part of the shop may be leased for lectures, seminars, presentations, and meetings with potential customers or associates. With varying intervals, followers of Sri Chinmoy, Carlos Castaneda, and others gathered there in a small enclosed space (a long table and ten to fifteen chairs); in-between, a manual therapist and an astrologer consulted clients. Furthermore, the owner of the salon displays against payment promotional posters and large color notices on a special stand or for free allows to spread out flyers, booklets, and business cards on certain shelves. Various centers and agents whose practice is too small to resort to other marketing channels use this opportunity. Anyone may leave information about their activity if it is in line with the shop's business, promising in exchange to display the salon's business cards in their offices. Hence, a wide range of advertised services, most of them health-related—here one can find the ads of healers, psychics, yoga studios, massage parlors, health food stores, and MLM companies.

*Health tourism agencies*
Intermediaries providing travel arrangements to places where clients can get informal medical care form a separate group. Currently, both holidays at health resorts organized by regular travel agencies and trips to alternative medicine and esoteric centers (Ayurveda tours, yoga tours, trips to the so-called power places, and pilgrimages to holy places) are popular in Russia. In the latter case, social and business entities that associate themselves with the relevant ideas usually take care of the travel arrangements. For them, such a trip is an opportunity to introduce clients to their

---

children and parents; fitness/yoga center; direct selling of health products; salt chamber; own production of ecologically clean foods and medicinal herbs; networks for purchasing gifts of nature in the villages and processing them; tourist travel and hiking, etc. However, the information intermediary function of such entities is limited, because the owners select goods and services according to their own preferences and beliefs.

values. Therefore, the geography of the proposed tours can be virtually global. Thus, subject to availability of sufficient funds, a resident of some remote settlement in the Perm Territory can go to Hawaii to acquire local healing and self-medication skills. The Center for Polynesian Practices representing Aloha International will be happy to assist with the travel arrangements.

This intermediary market offers relatively mass destinations (tours to Southeast Asia for treatment and spiritual self-actualization and Orthodox pilgrimages) and specialized tours. For example, small businesses have recently emerged that arrange health tours to farms in Egypt (Marsa Matrouh), where diseases of the digestive system (including hepatitis B and C) are treated "according to Sunnah" with camel milk and urine. Medical tours are also arranged to the traditional Filipino healers. In the Kama area, tourists are invited to visit a Komi-Permyak shaman and the local "power places": the Perm anomalous zone, Kungur ice cave, and Plakun waterfall.

A stalker from a large city comes to Molebka on the weekends to organize paid walking tours for visitors. He leads small groups of tourists into the Perm anomalous zone to improve their health. The organizer and his clients believe that certain places in the forest help treating various diseases (from infertility to cancer). The stalker has worked out the itinerary based on his personal experience, "I have already helped myself; so, if a person comes to me with problems of the musculoskeletal system, I now know where to take him."

\* \* \*

Information intermediaries are perhaps the least visible of the "informal healthcare" agents we have considered. They often emerge to serve the specific requirements of focused communities and are part of the overall infrastructure that meets the needs of such communities in terms of maintaining health and intellectual life. Municipal libraries, on the contrary, are an example of social institutions, whose participation in "informal healthcare" is at variance with their main functions aimed at serving the interests of formal healthcare.

# Afterword

The format of sociographic essays does not imply far-reaching generalizations. However, there is a recurring feature in the material presented in the different chapters of this book, which I would nevertheless like to highlight.

I mentioned in the Author's note that sociographic work was useful and necessary as preparation for the scientific problematization of social phenomena, since a reliable factual basis allows avoiding distortions in interpretations. Although qualitative methods make it impossible to measure accurately the depicted phenomena on a national scale, they nevertheless provide a general understanding that helps to assess whether the cases are frequent or sporadic, the practices mass or isolated, widespread or typical only of major cities.

We see that the resulting "informal healthcare" landscape significantly differs from the dominant public perceptions of the arrangement and magnitude of alternative healthcare practices and the economic agents serving them. Yet, such perceptions are transmitted and reproduced in the media. For example, homeopathy is presented in the media as the flagship of alternative medicine. Perhaps, this is because the opponents of this therapy are part of the active segment of the Russian scientific community fighting pseudoscience. Homeopathy, along with the anti-vaccination movement and GMO opponents, has been one of the main targets of their criticism in recent years. However, as we have seen, classical homeopathy is a rare practice throughout the country and virtually non-existent outside of major cities, and the prospects of integrating this CAM area into formal healthcare look bleak.

In general, the media focuses primarily on those characters that grasp the imagination—sorcerers and psychics, major fraudsters and scams. In addition, alternative health practices are considered against the background of the unsatisfactory state of affairs in formal healthcare. Consequently, a village sorcerer or witch doctor is presented as the central figure of "informal healthcare" to whom the people are forced to turn because Russian medicine is underfunded by the state.

The healer's appealing image overshadows routine health practices, which are left out of the discussion. Truly mass agents serving millions of patients remain behind the scenes. First and foremost, these are the mass media themselves, pharmacies, religious organizations, as well as all kinds of illegal vendors of health products. The activities of such "informal healthcare" agents are routine and daily, and the consumers rarely perceive them as something alternative.

# Appendices

**Appendix 1. Characteristics of the fieldwork in the Perm Territory**

*Methods of fieldwork*
With some exceptions, we surveyed each locality according to the following scenario. First we collected information from publicly available sources (websites of the municipalities, local community groups in the social networks, local online forums, etc.). Then we visited the localities. The program of each field visit included:
- Inspection of the main public places presumably associated with "informal healthcare" (marketplace, central streets and squares, sports and recreation facilities, large shopping centers, medical facilities, pharmacies, cultural institutions and leisure facilities, and religious institutions)
- Semi-structured interviews with the experts[208] and "informal healthcare" agents (we tried to interview all the agents we identified during the visit)
- Informal conversations with the agents and local residents
- Participant observations (under the guise of customers or visitors) in places providing health services or selling health products
- Collection of statistics and other information from the local authorities, as well as purchase and study of local press

For Perm we adopted another pattern due to the large size of the city. We used publicly available sources to collect as much information as possible about the "informal healthcare" agents operating in the regional center (legal entities and individuals). A quantitative analysis of this data array provided a general understanding of the "informal healthcare" markets in the city. Then, from the obtained database, we selected for further interviewing one or two representatives of each agent category. In Perm, we also interviewed representatives of public authorities (Rospotrebnadzor's regional office for the Perm Territory, Ministry of Health of the Perm Terri-

---

[208] As experts we considered members of the local community who due to their occupation or status were presumably informed as to where the local residents turn to (in addition to healthcare institutions) in case of health problems.

tory, and Permstat) and parent organizations operating in the region (regional branches and central offices of religious organizations and MLM companies). We requested from them statistics and other information on the subject of our research.

In addition, we selectively visited the sites in Perm where we expected to encounter "informal healthcare" agents: unauthorized sales points, cultural centers, large shopping centers, medical facilities, churches and other places of worship. Without exception, we surveyed all the legal food markets in the city. Instead of making a round of all the pharmacies (like in the other localities), in Perm we organized a monitoring of customer behavior in one pharmacy in October 2013. During two shifts—one on Saturday and one on Monday—the pharmacists recorded for us all customer requests and purchases. Separately, I would like to mention participant observations at public events related to the topic of research: the VIII Interregional Exhibition *Orthodox Rus'—2013* and the XIX International Exhibition *Medicine and Health—2013*, as well as at the events held by visiting representatives of health doctrines at urban cultural centers (Rushel Blavo's session and the presentation of Mirzakarim Norbekov's system).

Although the geography of fieldwork was limited to the Perm Territory, we also monitored several sites and events in Moscow and the Moscow Region to compare the situation in the regional center with that in the capital. Observations were conducted at the Trinity Lavra of St. Sergius; Pokrovsky Convent; Orthodox Christmas Exhibition *Christmas Gift* (at the All-Russian Exhibition Center), International Exhibition *Healthy Lifestyle—2013* (at the Expocentre), as well as several Orthodox churches in Moscow.

*Design of interviews*
For the semi-structured interviews, we developed a general guide consisting of eighteen questions, which allowed to determine what "informal healthcare" agents and practices were represented in the locality. Besides, we prepared additional sets of personal questions for the main groups of informants (doctors, officials, healers, pharmacists, clergy, journalists, etc.) enabling us to collect information about the individual segments of this sector and assess the informants' involvement in them. All interviews were conducted on condition of anonymity in the form of a free discussion. Depending on the situation, the interviewer could change the

wording of the questions, their sequence, and level of detail. The interviews were held in person, except for a few phone calls.

In the event of informal conversations, the researchers posing as visitors or potential customers checked out certain specific facts (prices, range of goods and services, demand for them, etc.). This category also included communications when the participants were aware of the purpose of our research, but no interview guide was used for the conversation.

The interviews and informal conversations lasted from ten–fifteen minutes to two hours, depending on how busy the informant was. The average duration was thirty minutes. In all, we held about 370 conversations (not counting short situational dialogues with "informal healthcare" agents when surveying public places, such as markets or exhibition fairs, as well as discussions during observations in Moscow and the Moscow Region). Of these, 191 interviews were recorded on tape. Sixty-seven interviews were held without audio recording, mainly because the respondents refused to speak on the record; in several cases, there was no physical opportunity to record the conversation. The remaining discussions were informal.

*Profile of the respondents*

Table 7 presents the breakdown of informants from the Perm Territory by principal categories. Some informants appear in two categories (e.g., CAM doctor and distributor of health products), so the total number of interviews and informal conversations exceeds the above figure of about 370.

## Table 7. Composition and number of informants in the Perm Territory (2013)

| № | Informant category | Total interviews and informal conversations | Including interviews |
|---|---|---|---|
| 1. | Medical professionals: doctors and nursing staff, including: | 49 | 46 |
|  | Personnel of health resort facilities | 14 | 11 |
| 2. | Pharmacy personnel | 29 | 22 |
| 3. | Representatives of public and municipal authorities | 20 | 20 |
| 4. | Social activists involved in health issues (in health groups, councils of veterans, societies of the disabled, and other NPOs) | 13 | 12 |
| 5. | Clergy, church staff, and activists of religious organizations, including: | 54 | 38 |
|  | Orthodox | 31 | 27 |
|  | Muslim | 3 | 3 |
|  | Protestants and Neo-Protestants | 16 | 13 |
|  | Other | 4 | 3 |
| 6. | Participants of the market for health information, including: | 52 | 42 |
|  | Local media staff | 10 | 10 |
|  | Staff of retail outlets selling printed products (newsstands and bookstores) | 16 | 8 |
|  | Post office staff | 12 | 12 |
|  | Library staff | 14 | 12 |
| 7. | Representatives of organizations forming the healthy living infrastructure, including: | 36 | 23 |
|  | Cultural and leisure facilities | 16 | 13 |
|  | Sports and recreation facilities | 8 | 4 |
|  | Beauty salons | 8 | 2 |
|  | Travel agencies | 4 | 4 |
| 8. | Sellers of industrial health products, including: | 46 | 29 |
|  | Direct sellers | 28 | 18 |

| № | Informant category | Total interviews and informal conversations | Including interviews |
|---|---|---|---|
| 9. | Agents in the segment of procuring and selling healing gifts of nature, including: | 33 | 14 |
| | Beekeepers and honey vendors | 14 | 5 |
| | Hunters | 5 | 5 |
| | Herbalists and medicinal herb dealers | 14 | 4 |
| 10. | Teachers (instructors) of Eastern health practices | 5 | 4 |
| 11. | Agents providing treatment services, including: | 22 | 13 |
| | Healers, bonesetters | 9 | 7 |
| | Doctors of complementary and alternative medicine (medical professionals) | 5 | 3 |
| | Psychotherapists | 2 | 1 |
| | Other | 6 | 2 |
| 12. | Local residents | 35 | 10 |
| | **TOTAL** | **394** | **273** |

Our initial classification of interviewees into experts and non-experts turned out to be rather nominal for two reasons. First, the experts themselves were often involved in the social and economic relations of "informal healthcare" as service providers or ordinary consumers. This affected the objectivity of their expert judgments. Second, practice showed that the providers of health products and services were generally fully aware of what was happening in the other segments of the sector, since they were interested in various kinds of health practices and could therefore act as experts. For example, some distributors of dietary supplements are keen on esoteric knowledge, deal with healers, are integrated into religious structures, and willingly share information on these issues.

In addition, the range of people that we initially designated as experts, turned out to be quite heterogeneous. Unexpectedly, employees of libraries—for both children and adults —proved to be valuable informants. In most cases, they possessed the fullest information and willingly shared it. After the first expedition, visiting the local library in the settlements became a priority item of our research agenda. Interviews with doctors and officials proved to be less meaningful than we expected. Many of them preferred to voice the official position (like "alternative medicine is unacceptable", "I know nothing about dietary supplements", "we don't have such healers") rather than describe the actual situation in the locality. We found the clergy, especially Orthodox clerics, to be an unexpectedly difficult category. In some cases, they flatly refused to be interviewed; in many others, they did not give permission to record the conversation.

**Appendix 2. The religious landscape in the field research area**

With some exceptions, the religious landscape in the area where we conducted fieldwork on "informal healthcare" is in line with the situation for Russia in general. The official figures on the number of registered religious organizations in the Kama area and the surveyed municipalities are presented in Table 8. However, we should keep in mind that the actual number of active communities is higher. This concerns especially various Protestant communities, many of which exist in the form of religious groups.

Table 8. Number of local religious organizations (LROs) in the surveyed municipalities of the Perm Territory[209]

| Registered religious organizations | Total in the PT | Perm | Lysva urban district | Chusovoy district | Kungur urban district | Kungur district | Suksun district | Kishert district | Orda district |
|---|---|---|---|---|---|---|---|---|---|
| ROC parishes (communities) | 242 | 40 | 6 | 11 | 6 | 18 | 3 | 3 | 7 |
| Including ROC monasteries and convents | 15 | 4 | 0 | 2 | 1 | 2 | 0 | 0 | 0 |
| Old Believer LROs | 15 | 3 | 2 | 0 | 0 | 0 | 0 | 0 | 0 |
| Muslim LROs | 106 | 8 | 4 | 1 | 2 | 5 | 3 | 1 | 3 |
| LROs of Evangelical Christian Baptists | 7 | 3 | 0/1 | 0 | 0/1 | 0 | 0/1 | 0 | 0 |
| LROs of Christians of Evangelical Faith (Pentecostals) | 42 | 9 | 2 | 1 | 1 | 0 | 1 | 0 | 1 |
| LROs of the Christian Presbyterian Church | 4 | 0 | 0 | 0 | 0 | 0 | 0 | 0 | 0 |
| LROs of the Evangelical Christians | 3 | 1 | 2 | 0 | 0 | 0 | 0 | 0 | 0 |
| LROs of the Evangelical Lutheran Church | 4 | 2 | 0 | 0 | 0 | 0 | 0 | 0 | 0 |
| LROs of the Seventh Day Adventists Church | 6 | 2 | 0/1 | 0 | 0/1 | 0 | 0 | 0 | 0 |
| LROs of Jehovah's Witnesses | 4 | 1 | 1 | 0 | 0/1 | 0 | 0 | 0 | 0 |
| Other | 10 | 7 | 0 | 0 | 0 | 0 | 0 | 0 | 0 |

[209] According to the Russian Ministry of Justice as of 10 March 2015. In some cells, the figure after the slash shows the number of unregistered religious communities identified during fieldwork.

**Orthodoxy** is the prevailing religion in the Perm Territory. About half of the total 443 registered religious organizations pertained to the Russian Orthodox Church (Moscow Patriarchate) in March 2015. However, the number of ROC parishes, as well as the share and activity of practicing Orthodox believers differs significantly even in the surveyed districts. This may be related to the local cultural and historical traditions, the social environment, and the specific work of the local hierarchs. Thus, the activity of the ROC is much more noticeable in Kungur and the Kungur district than in the Lysva urban district and the neighboring Chusovoy district. The commercial town of Kungur and the agricultural Kungur district historically have been and still remain the major centers of Orthodoxy in the region. According to the Russian Ministry of Justice, twenty-four ROC parishes (communities) are registered there. The Dean—Archpriest Shirinkin—estimated the number of active parishioners in the four functioning temples of Kungur at about one thousand people. At the same time, Lysva—a typical industrial town—and its district have only six parishes; Lysva itself has only one. In Chusovoy, where two small temples are currently functioning and a new one is under construction, elderly residents in an informal conversation speculated that the old church might be closed, because "there are not enough churchgoers" in town.

Any attempt by an outsider, a researcher, to find out the exact number of active parishioners is doomed to failure. Note that this concerns not only Orthodox parishes but all the others as well. There are several reasons for this—from the unwillingness of the community leaders to disclose information to the fact that such records are not kept in principle. Many Orthodox priests told us that the size of the parish depended on the season and on festive occasions (i.e., by the number of parishioners they meant the number of people attending church service), for example: "Depending on the religious holidays, from 100–150 to 300 on average. You see, we're in the countryside here. A spring day feeds a year. In summer, usually, there is no time for anything but the garden. But in winter we can have up to 300 people."[210] In response to questions about the core of the parish, we were given numbers from 30 to 70–100 people. Our observations revealed 20–30 churchgoers regularly attending Sunday worship service outside of religious holidays. It is noteworthy that these figures did

---

210  Informant: male, about 40 years old, Orthodox priest, district center.

not vary depending on the size of the settlement and the number of churches in it. A typical Orthodox parishioner is an elderly woman. Outside of major religious holidays, young people go to church mainly when preparing for special events (wedding, baptism), or when they are family members of the priest or church workers. Parishes with a constant flow of visiting churchgoers form a separate group. In our case, such was the church in Klyuchi village. Its priest provided spiritual guidance to holidaymakers and the surrounding monasteries. Even the schedule of services in Klyuchi was adapted to the needs of such visitors.

The Perm Territory is one of the regions where **Old Belief** was traditionally popular. Currently, there is a community of the Russian Orthodox Old Believers Church (Belokrinitskoe Soglasie) in Perm, as well as several priestless Old Believer communities. A representative of the former community mentioned having about 800 members, with 200–250 people attending religious services weekly. They have virtually no *zakhozhane* ("we know everyone by sight"), and since the faith is transmitted "through the family", the congregation includes people of different ages and social status. Developed Old Believer communities exist also in the southwestern part of the Kama area, which was outside the geography of our fieldwork.

The region's **Muslim** communities are located in large towns and the rural areas densely populated by Tatars and Bashkirs. Urban mosques are attended largely by migrants from Central Asia. In Perm, there are two mosques and three–four prayer houses, where people gather for prayer and other rituals. The regional center has only two shops selling Islamic spiritual literature, cosmetics and accessories for Muslims—at the mosque and at the Central Market. Up to 800 worshippers gather on weekends at the congregation mosque in Perm. In Lysva, the congregation does not exceed a dozen people; moreover, they can hardly be called very religious, according to the Imam: "They come, so to say, the Imam recites, so to say, they offer their prayers, and that's it, off they go home."

Most of the regional Muslim organizations are subordinated to the Regional Muslim Spiritual Directorate (Perm muftiyat). However, in 2013, due to disagreements between the leader of the Perm muftiyat and the Imam heading the Kungur muhtasibat, Muslim associations that were part of the latter (in Lysva, Beryozovka, Kishert, Suksun, and Kungur districts, and in the towns of Kungur and Lysva) were transferred to the jurisdiction of the Central Muslim Spiritual Directorate.[211] The conflict between the two leaders, among others, has an ideological aspect—the Perm Mufti considers the Kungur Imam to be an apostate, because his views differ from traditional Islam.

**Protestant** churches and denominations are third in the Kama area by the number of registered organizations. Some of them have more than a century-long history of presence in the region (Evangelical Christian Baptists, Lutherans, and Adventists). Others, Pentecostals-reformers, have appeared quite recently, and they are more often referred to as NRMs. On the one hand, Protestant associations are a large group of heterogeneous and independent movements, which are usually classified into traditionalists with small but sustainable communities dating back to the Soviet times and liberals,[212] whose organizations in the region have been growing in numbers and developing over the past decade. On the other hand, amid constant accusations of sectarianism on the part of the Russian Orthodox Church and endless inspections by the authorities, they are trying if not to unite, then to organize some sort of interaction to look more impressive in the overall religious picture on the local and national level.

Pentecostalism is the most actively developing movement in the region. The media often calls Perm the capital of Russian Pentecostalism. Edward Grabovenko, senior pastor of the New Testament church in Perm, is the senior bishop of the Russian Church of Christians of Evangelical Faith (RC HVE). According to him, Pentecostal services were held in 380 localities in March 2013, with the communities rapidly growing—sixty-four new churches opened in 2012.[213]

Extensive involvement of the believers in the life of the congregation is characteristic of Protestant communities. Consequently, the total number of their active adherents in a locality may be comparable or even

---

211 *"Dissenting" Imam Came into CMSD.* Islam News. 24.07.2013.
URL: http://www.islamnews.ru/news-140859.html.
212 It is common practice to distinguish within Russian Pentecostalism conservatives, whose illegal communities already existed in Soviet times, and reformers, often called Neo-Pentecostals or Charismatics. This classification is popular in Orthodox sectology; Russian sociologists of religion also use it (e.g., Kormina, 2013). However, some scholars of religion believe it to be somewhat artificial (e.g., Lunkin, 2006).
213 Protestant.ru (website).
URL: http://www.protestant.ru/news/church/ofchrist/article/149572.

exceed the number of practicing Orthodox believers. Lysva has five Pentecostal communities, which, according to their representatives, differ by "the degree of emotionality of the service" and "the manner of praying". Over 500 people regularly participate in community life.

In small towns, the presence of such organizations is visually noticeable due to their active missionary policy,[214] even if the local authorities deny them any opportunity for this. They use all available means—outdoor advertising, graffiti, cultural and social events, and the work of charity foundations. Urban Protestant organizations are extensively involved in missionary work in the villages, where there are no registered communities. They hold services at the homes of the few adherents. Thus, the influence of these religious movements is not limited to the urban environment only.

In addition to being religious associations, Pentecostal communities also serve as social and family leisure clubs. This is particularly noticeable in small towns, where the infrastructure for leisure time activities and socializing is underdeveloped. Festive clothing and attending service with the whole family; sobriety; a differentiated approach to parishioners of different ages; opportunities to develop small businesses with fellow believers; additional social and cultural programs—for the adherent, all this shapes a way of life, which is somewhat like the pictures from American soap operas and has an obvious advantage over the everyday reality of the Russian outback. Protestants include representatives of different social groups—there are many employees, social workers, students, and small entrepreneurs.

The other world religions are poorly represented in the Kama area. **Catholicism** has a distinct ethno-national reference. Historically, exiled Poles and their descendants formed the congregation in Perm, and Germans deported during WWII—in Berezniki. Currently there are two registered organizations. The pastor of the Perm congregation estimated the number of worshippers regularly attending Sunday service at about 100,

---

214 Their presence was most visible in Lysva: billboards, banners, and leaflets at bus stops. The central street of the town uses a special promotional medium—benches with backs, into which advertising boards are mounted. One of the benches was carrying the following poster: "I will hear your prayers. I will answer!!!!! The Lord". Here and there one could read spray-painted inscriptions on the pavement: "Jesus loves you", etc.

and the total size of the congregation—at 200—300 people.[215] There are also several pastoral posts in the cities with small Catholic communities, but there were none in the field research area. Followers of **Buddhism** can be found only in the regional capital, where there is a center related to the Russian Association of Diamond Way Buddhists of Karma Kagyu Tradition. The community is small and engages mainly in cultural projects. Some other Buddhist branches and schools are represented in Perm by several small groups of followers.[216]

By far not all **new religious movements** existing in Russia are represented in the Perm Territory. Not more than a dozen NRMs have registered organizations there. Note that the region has followers of at least one movement of local origin. It is the Neo-Christian association Family of the Children of God led by Vladimir Beloded. The movement was popular in the 1990s among Perm's intellectuals. Their closed community at the Tchaikovskaya station in the Nytva district functioned till the end of the 2000s; after the death of the leader, it effectively ceased to exist.

Perm scholars of religion (e.g., Goryunov, 2013) indicate that in recent years, the population has been losing interest in most of the new religious teachings that were popular in the region in the 1990s. This concerns first and foremost orientalist NRMs (the Perm Society for Krishna Consciousness, as well as followers of Osho, Sri Chinmoy, Maharishi, Sathya Sai Baba, etc.) and syncretic movements (Baha'i Faith, the Unification Church, and Scientology). Consequently, the number of their followers and active groups is decreasing; however, they are still present in the region, especially in the regional center.

Among the NRMs (besides the Neo-Protestants), followers of Jehovah's Witnesses and various Neo-Hindu movements were most frequently represented in the surveyed localities. They were rarely functioning as registered organizations, and their groups were small. Jehovah's Witnesses and the Hare Krishnas have been present in the region since the early 1990s, and they have developed quite sustainable communities. The total number of Jehovah's Witnesses in Perm is estimated at about 1,000 people (Goryunov, 2010). Representatives of the Perm Society for

---

215  *Finding the Father.* Business Class. 01.04.2013.
    URL: http://www.business-class.su/news/2013/04/01/79868.
216  Representatives of the Ural Buddhist Monastery Shad Tchup Ling of the National Center for Far Eastern Mahayana Buddhism, the Perm Dhammapada Buddhist Association (Tibetan Gelug School).

Krishna Consciousness indicated about 400 regular followers as of 2013 (which is less than half as compared to the beginning of the 2000s). At the time of the interview, they had neither temple nor permanent office; for their meetings, the organization rented premises in a residential district. The sign on the door read "Family Education Support Center".

The followers of Vladimir Megre's teachings (Anastasians) are worth mentioning among the movements dissimilar from classic religious associations that have received certain development in the region in the 2000s. They have founded about a dozen isolated settlements of one-two families each, including in the Chusovoy, Kishert, and Kungur districts. Perm followers of neo-paganism[217] manifest themselves publicly by cultural and ethnographic initiatives, such as festivals of Slavic culture (Day of Perun and other) organized in Perm and throughout the region. Finally, Olga Skrypnik, an energy therapist from Perm, launched in the early 2010s the syncretic Interregional Public Movement of Spiritual Unity Rule of God (*BogoDerjavie*) in the region. It is a New Age movement, which relies on the spiritual teaching developed by Muscovite Leonid Maslov.[218] In 2011–2012, Olga Skrypnik held regular lectures and seminars in virtually all the districts of the Perm Territory.

The diversity of NRMs represented in the Perm Territory is mainly due to the developments in the regional center. The rural population is immune to new spiritual teachings which can be trendy in the urban environment, even if NRM followers establish communities or hold field events near their settlements. The locals consider such events as something exotic, a whim of the townsfolk, or sectarianism.

This attitude ensuring the absolute priority of Orthodoxy in the provinces, despite the low parish activity of the population, is upheld by the obvious inequality of religious associations in the public space. In most surveyed localities, the activity of religious associations, other than the traditional ones, received no support whatsoever from the local authorities or their subordinated media, as well as healthcare and social institutions.

---

217 In Perm, there is a registered organization of the Ancient Russian Ynglist Church of the Orthodox Old Believers—Ynglings. Since the Ministry of Justice has declared the organization extremist, the group engages in no public activity, except for holding cultural events in line with the "Russian Vedic tradition".

218 Leonid Maslov also heads the All-Russian Public Movement for the Spiritual Development of the Population "For Statehood and the Spiritual Revival of Holy Rus".

Furthermore, representatives of such bodies at times demonstrated their willingness to protect the interests of traditional religions using the administrative resource, and perceived it as their duty.

# References

Bailey R. L. et al. (2013) Why US Adults Use Dietary Supplements. *JAMA Internal Medicine*, 173 (5), pp. 355–361.

Barnes P. M. et al. (2004) Complementary and Alternative Medicine Use Among Adults: United States, 2002. *Seminars in Integrative Medicine. WB Saunders*, 2 (2), pp. 54–71.

Barry C. A. (2006) The Role of Evidence in Alternative Medicine: Contrasting Biomedical and Anthropological Approaches. *Social Science & Medicine*, 62 (11), pp. 2646–57.

Berger P. (1967) *The Social Reality of Religion*. London: Faber.

Berlant J. L. (1975) *Profession and Monopoly: A Study of Medicine in the United States and Great Britain*. Berkeley: University of California Press.

Biggart N. (1989) *Charismatic Capitalism: Direct Selling Organizations in America*. University of Chicago Press.

Bradley C. and Blenkinsopp A. (1996) Over the Counter Drugs. The Future for Self-Medication. *British Medical Journal*, 312 (7034), pp. 835–837.

Brodie S., Stanworth J. and Wotruba T. (2002) Comparisons of Salespeople in Multilevel vs. Single Level Direct Selling Organizations. *The Journal of Personal Selling and Sales Management*, 22 (2), pp. 67–75.

Brown J. V. and Rusinova N. L. (2002) "Curing and Crippling": Biomedical and Alternative Healing in Post-Soviet Russia. *Annals of the American Academy of Political and Social Science*, vol. 583, pp. 160–172.

Burgess E. A., Stoner S. S. and Foley K. E. (2014) *Brought to Bear: An Analysis of Seizures across Asia (2000—2011)*. TRAFFIC, Petaling Jaya, Selangor, Malaysia.

Cahn P. S. (2009) Using and Sharing: Direct Selling in the Borderlands. In: McCrossen A. (ed.) *Land of Necessity: Consumer Culture in the United States–Mexico Borderlands*. Duke University Press, pp. 274–297.

Droney D. (2016) Networking Health: Multi-Level Marketing of Health Products in Ghana. *Anthropology & Medicine*, 23 (1), pp. 1–13.

Eisenberg D. M. et al. (1993) Unconventional Medicine in the United States—Prevalence, Costs, and Patterns of Use. *New England Journal of Medicine*, 328 (4), pp. 246–252.

Gale N. (2014) The Sociology of Traditional, Complementary and Alternative Medicine. *Sociology Compass*, 8 (6), pp. 805–822

Gil A. et al. (2009) Availability and Characteristics of Nonbeverage Alcohols Sold in 17 Russian Cities in 2007. *Alcoholism—Clinical and Experimental Research*, 33 (1), pp. 79–85.

Gu C.-J. (2004) Disciplined Bodies in Direct Selling. In: *The Minor Arts of Daily Life: Popular Culture in Taiwan*, University of Hawai`i Press, pp. 150–174.

Guallar E. et al. (2013) Enough Is Enough: Stop Wasting Money on Vitamin and Mineral Supplements. *Annals of Internal Medicine*, 159 (12), pp. 850–851.

Hahn R. and Kleinman A. (1983) Biomedical Practice and Anthropological Theory: Framework and Directions. *Annual Review of Anthropology*, vol. 12, pp. 305–333.

Homes V. (ed.) (2004) *No Licence to Kill: the Population and Harvest of Musk Deer and Trade in Musk in the Russian Federation and Mongolia*. TRAFFIC Europe.

Hughes B. M. (2006) Regional Patterns of Religious Affiliation and Availability of Complementary and Alternative Medicine. *Journal of Religion and Health*, 45 (4), pp. 549–557.

Iarskaia-Smirnova E. and Romanov P. (2008) Culture Matters: Integration of Folk Medicine in Health Care in Russia // In: Kuhlmann E. and Saks M. (eds.) *Rethinking professional governance: International directions in health care*, Bristol: The Policy Press, pp. 41–154.

Koenig H., King D. and Carson V. B. (2012) *Handbook of Religion and Health*. Oxford University Press.

Larkin G. (1983) *Occupational Monopoly and Modern Medicine*. Tavistok Publications. London and N-Y.

Lan P. C. (2002) Networking capitalism: Network construction and control effects in direct selling. *The Sociological Quarterly*, 43 (2), pp. 165–184.

Lindquist G. (2001) Transforming Signs. Iconicity and Indexicality in Russian Healing and Magic. *Ethnos*, 66:2, pp. 181–206.

Madsen M. V., Gøtzsche P. C, Hróbjartsson A. (2009) Acupuncture Treatment for Pain: Systematic Review of Randomised Clinical Trials with Acupuncture, Placebo Acupuncture, and No Acupuncture Groups. *British Medical Journal*, 338:a3115.

Merton R. K. (1957) *Social Theory and Social Structure*. Glencoe, IL: Free Press.

Osho (Bhagwan Shree Rajneesh) (2000) *From Medication to Meditation*. Beekman Publishers.

Peterson R. A. and Wotruba Th. R. (1996) What is Direct Selling?—Definition, Perspectives, and Research Agenda. *Journal of Personal Selling & Sales Management*, 16 (Fall), pp. 1–16.

Sackett D. L. et al. (1996) Evidence Based Medicine: What It Is and What It Isn't. *British Medicine Journal*, 312: 7023, pp. 71–72.

Saks M. (2003) *Orthodox and Alternative Medicine: Politics, Professionalization, and Health Care*. SAGE.

Scott R. W. (2004) Competing Logics in Health Care: Professional, State, and Managerial. In: Dobbin F. (ed.) *The Sociology of the Economy*, N.Y.: Russell Sage Foundation, pp. 267–287.

Shang A. et al. (2005) Are the Clinical Effects of Homoeopathy Placebo Effects? Comparative Study of Placebo-Controlled Trials of Homoeopathy and Allopathy. *The Lancet*, 366: 9487, pp. 726–732.

Smith J. C. (2010) *Pseudoscience and Extraordinary Claims of the Paranormal: A Critical Thinker's Toolkit*.

Stickley A. et al. (2013) Prevalence and Factors Associated with the Use of Alternative (Folk) Medicine Practitioners in 8 Countries of the former Soviet Union. *BMC Complementary and Alternative Medicine*, 13:83.

Timmermans St. and Kolker E. S. (2004) Evidence-Based Medicine and the Reconfiguration of Medical Knowledge. *Journal of Health and Social Behavior*, vol. 45, pp. 177–193.

Villanueva-Russell Y. (2005) Evidence-Based Medicine and its Implications for the Profession of Chiropractic. *Social Science & Medicine*, 60 (3), pp. 545–561.

Александров А. А., Королев К. Ю., Айзберг О. Р. (2008) «Код Да'Вженко», или ещё раз к вопросу о так называемой стрессопсихотерапии. *Психиатрия: научно-практический журнал*. № 2. С. 121–127.

Aleksandrov A. A., Korolev K. Yu. and Aizberg O. R. (2008) "Da'Vzhenko Code", or Once More to the Issue of the So-Called Stress Psychotherapy. *Psikhiatriya: nauchno-prakticheskiy zhurnal*, no 2. C. 121–127.

Александров Е. Б. (2006) Проблемы экспансии лженауки. *В защиту науки. Бюллетень №1 Комиссии по борьбе с лженаукой и фальсификацией научных исследований при Президиуме РАН*. С. 8–16.

Aleksandrov E. B. (2006) The Expansion of Pseudoscience. *V zaschitu nauki. Byulleten' №1 Komissii po bor'be s lzhenaukoy i fal'sifikatsiey nauchnykh issledovaniy pri Prezidiume RAN*, pp. 8–16.

Архимандрит Герман (Чесноков) (2006) *Проповедь перед чином изгнания злых духов из человека*. М.

Archimandrite Herman (Chesnokov) (2006) *Sermon Before the Rite of Exorcising Evil Spirits from Man*. Moscow.

Астафьева Н. Г., Кобзев Д. Ю. (2012) Между верой и знанием: официальная, альтернативная и комплементарная медицина в лечении астмы и аллергии. *Лечащий врач. Медицинский научно-практический журнал*. № 6. URL: http://www.lvrach.ru/2012/06/15435453.

Astafieva N. G. and Kobzev D. Yu. (2012) Between Faith and Knowledge: Conventional, Alternative, and Complementary Medicine in Treating Asthma and Allergy. *Lechaschiy vrach. Meditsinskiy nauchno-prakticheskiy zhurnal*, no 6. URL: http://www.lvrach.ru/2012/06/15435453.

Автономов Д. А. Вклад А. Р. (2014) Довженко в мифологизацию отечественной наркологии. Предпосылки, практика, анализ и последствия. *Наркология*. № 10. С. 94–102.

Avtonomov D. A. (2014) A. R. Dovzhenko's Contribution to Mythologizing Russian Narcology. Background, Practice, Analysis, and Implications. *Narkologiya*, no 10, pp. 94–102.

Балагушкин Е. Г., Шохин В. К. (2006) Религиозный плюрализм в современной России: новые религиозные движения на постсоветском этапе. *Мир России*. № 2. С. 62–78.

Balagushkin E. G. and Shokhin V. K. (2006) Religious Pluralism in Contemporary Russia: New Religious Movements at the Post-Soviet Stage. *Mir Rossii*, no 2. pp. 62–78.

Барсукова С. Ю. (2003) Неформальная экономика: понятие, структура. *Экономическая социология*. Т. 4. № 4. С. 15–36.

Barsukova S. Yu. (2003) Informal Economy: Concepts and Structure. *Ekonomicheskaya sotsiologiya*, vol. 4, no 4, pp. 15–36.

Белоногова В. Д. (2009) *Ресурсы, экологическая безопасность и фитохимические исследования дикорастущих лекарственных растений Пермского края*. Автореферат диссертации на соискание ученой степени доктора фармацевтических наук. Пермь.

Belonogova V. D. (2009) *Resources, Environmental Safety and Phytochemical Studies of Wild Medicinal Plants of the Perm Territory*. Abstract of the dissertation for a doctoral degree in pharmaceutical sciences. Perm.

Беляев Д. О. (2009) Опыт эмпирического исследования гетеродоксальной религиозности в современной России. *Социологические исследования*. № 11. С. 78–88.

Belyaev D. O. (2009) An Empirical Study of Heterodox Religiosity in Contemorary Russia. *Sotsiologicheskie issledovaniya*, no 11, pp. 78–88.

Беребин М. А. (2012) О статусе медицинского психолога в системе здравоохранения, недостатках системы подготовки клинических психологов и связанных с ними проблемами и перспективах. *Медицинская психология в России*: электрон. науч. журн. № 2. URL: http:// medpsy.ru.

Berebin M. A. (2012) On the Status of Clinical Psychologist in the Healthcare System, the Shortcomings of the System of Training Clinical Psychologists, and the Associated Problems and Prospects. *Meditsinskaya psikhologiya v Rossii*: *elektron. nauch. zhurn*, no 2. URL: http:// medpsy.ru.

Бурдяк А. Я., Селезнева Е. В., Шишкин С. В. (2008) Различия в доступности медицинской помощи для населения России . *SPERO. Социальная политика: экспертиза, рекомендации, обзоры*. № 8. С. 135—158.

Burdyak A. Ya., Selezneva E. V. and Shishkin S. V. (2008) Differences in Access to Healthcare for the Russian Population. *SPERO. Sotsial'naya politika: ekspertiza, rekomendatsii, obzory*, no 8. pp. 135—158.

Чепурная О., Эткинд А. (2006) Инструментализация смерти. Уроки антиалкогольной терапии. *Отечественные записки*. № 2.
URL: http://www.strana-oz.ru/2006/2/instrumentalizaciya-smerti-uroki-antialkogolnoy-terapii.

Chepurnaya O. and Etkind A. (2006) Instrumentalization of Death. Lessons of Anti-Alcohol Therapy. *Otechestvennye zapiski*, no 2. URL: http://www.strana-oz.ru/2006/2/instrumentalizaciya-smerti-uroki-antialkogolnoy-terapii.

Черкашина Т. Ю. (2014) Оценка неравенства населения по потреблению медицинских услуг. В кн.: *XIV Апрельская международная научная конференция по проблемам развития экономики и общества*. Книга 3 / Отв. ред.: Е. Г. Ясин. М.: Издательский дом НИУ ВШЭ. С. 718–729.

Cherkashina T. Yu. (2014) Estimating Inequality by the Consumption of Medical Services. In: Yasin E. G. (ed.) *XIV Aprel'skaya mezhdunarodnaya nauchnaya konferentsiya po problemam razvitiya ekonomiki i obschestva*. Book 3. Moscow: NRU HSE, pp. 718–729.

Чеснокова В. Ф. (2005) *Тесным путём: процесс воцерковления населения России в конце XX века*. М.: Академический Проект.

Chesnokova V. F. (2005) *The Narrow Path: The Process of Churching Russia's Population in the Late XX Century*. Moscow: Akademicheskiy Proekt.

Эдельштейн М. (2000) Церковная экономика Центральной России: приход, монастырь, епархия. *Экономическая деятельность Русской Православной Церкви и ее теневая составляющая*. М.: Изд. РГГУ.

Edelstein M. (2000) The Church Economy of Central Russia: Parish, Monastery, Diocese. In: *Ekonomicheskaya deyatel'nost' Russkoy Pravoslavnoy Tserkvi i ee tenevaya sostavlyayuschaya*. Moscow: Izd. RGGU.

*Эпическое наследие и духовные практики в прошлом и настоящем. Памяти В.Н. Басилова* (2013) Сборник статей / Отв. ред. В. И. Харитонова. М.: ИЭА РАН (Этнологические исследования по шаманству и иным традиционным верованиям и практикам. Т. 15, ч. 1 и 2).

*Epic Heritage and Spiritual Practices of the Past and Present. In Memory of V.N. Basilov* (2013) Collected Papers. Ed. by Kharitonova V. I. Moscow: IEA RAN (Etnologicheskie issledovaniya po shamanstvu i inym traditsionnym verovaniyam i praktikam. Vol. 15, parts. 1 and 2).

Филатов С. Б. (2005) Христианские религиозные сообщества России как субъект гражданского общества. *Отечественные записки*. № 6. URL: http://old.strana-oz.ru/?numid=27&article=1187.

Filatov S. B. (2005) Christian Religious Communities in Russia as a Subject of Civil Society. *Otechestvennye zapiski*, no 6. URL: http://old.strana-oz.ru/?numid=27&article=1187.

Филатов С. Б., Лункин Р. Н. (2005) Статистика российской религиозности: магия цифр и неоднозначная реальность. *Социологические исследования*. № 6. С. 35–45.

Filatov S. B. and Lunkin R. N. (2005) Statistics of Russian Religiosity: Magic Numbers and Mixed Reality. *Sotsiologicheskie issledovaniya*, no 6. pp. 35–45.

*Фитотерапия. Методические рекомендации № 2000/63* (2006) Утв. Минздравом России 26.04.2000. Авторы: Карпеев А.А., Киселева Т.Л., Коршикова Ю.И., Лесиовская Е.Е., Саканян Е.И. Организации - разработчики: ФНКЭЦ ТМДЛ, Санкт-Петербургская химико-фармацевтическая академия // В кн.: Фитотерапия: нормативные документы/ Под общ. ред. А.А. Карпеева, Т.Л. Киселевой. М.: Изд-во ФНКЭЦ ТМДЛ Росздрава. С. 9–42.

*Phytotherapy. Methodology Guide № 2000/63* (2006) Approved by the Russian Ministry of Health on 26 April 2000. Authors: Karpeev A. A., Kiseleva T. L., Korshikova Yu. I., Lesiovskaya E. E., Sakanyan E. I. Developers: FCTRC TDTM, Saint-Petersburg Chemical and Pharmaceutical Academy. In: Fitoterapiya: normativnye dokumenty. Ed. by Karpeev A. A., Kiseleva T. L. Moscow: FCTRC TDTM Roszdrava, pp. 9–42.

Горюнов Д. (2013) Новые религии Пермского края. Человеческое измерение. *Журнал Уполномоченного по правам человека в Пермском крае*. № 5. С. 10–13.

Goryunov D. (2013) New Religions of the Perm Territory. Chelovecheskoe izmerenie. *Zhurnal Upolnomochennogo po pravam cheloveka v Permskom krae*, no 5, pp. 10–13.

Горюнов В. (2010) Религиозная карта Прикамья. Детали. *Мир религий*. 27.04.2010. URL: http://religo.ru/journal/7398.

Goryunov V. (2010) The Religious Map of the Kama Area. Details. *Mir religiy.* 27.04.2010. URL: http://religo.ru/journal/7398.

Готовский М. Ю., Москалева О. В. (2007) Традиционная медицинская деятельность: ее возможности и проблемы в современных условиях. В кн.: Тезисы и доклады XIII международной конференции "Теоретические и клинические аспекты применения биорезонансной и мультирезонансной терапии". М.:"ИМЕДИС". Ч. 1. С. 3–9.

Gotovskiy M. Yu., Moskaleva O. V. (2007) Traditional Medical Activity: Current Opportunities and Challenges. In: *Tezisy i doklady XIII mezhdunarodnoy konferentsii "Teoreticheskie i klinicheskie aspekty primeneniya biorezonansnoy i mul'tirezonansnoy terapii"*. Moscow: "IMEDIS", part 1. pp. 3–9.

*Государственный доклад о состоянии культуры в Российской Федерации в 2013 году* (2014). Министерство культуры Российской Федерации.

*Government Report on the State of Culture in the Russian Federation in 2013* (2014). Ministry of Culture of the Russian Federation.

Григорьева Е. (2009) Гомеопатия есть, специальности нет. *Медицинский вестник.* № 27 (496).

Grigorieva E. (2007) Homeopathy Exists, the Specialty Does Not. *Meditsinskiy vestnik*, no 27 (496).

Иваничев Г. А., Левит К. (2010) Техническая идентичность и терминологическая некорректность в мануальной (манипулятивной) медицине. Мануальная терапия. № 1 (37). С. 3–9.

Ivanichev G. A. and Lewit K. (2010) Technical Identity and Incorrect Terminology in Manual (Manipulative) Medicine. *Manual'naya terapiya*, no 1 (37), pp. 3–9.

Камушкина Л. В. (2003) Об адаптационных возможностях населения в системе сетевого маркетинга. *Социологические исследования*. № 11. С. 142–145.

Kamushkina L. V. (2003) On the Adaptability of the Population in Network Marketing. *Sotsiologicheskie issledovaniya*, no 11, pp. 142–145.

Карпеев А. А., Киселева Т. Л. (2003) *Лицензионные требования и условия работ и услуг по применению методов традиционной медицины*. Методические указания. Утв. Минздравом России 14.11.2003. Организация—разработчик: ФНКЭЦ ТМДЛ.

Karpeev A. A. and Kiseleva T. L. (2003) *Licensing Requirements and the Preconditions for Work and Services Using Methods of Traditional Medicine*. Practical Guidance. Approved by the Russian Ministry of Health on 14 November 2003. Developer: FCTRC TDTM.

Казаков А. С. (2008) Опыт Росздравнадзора по организации систем добровольной сертификации услуг в здравоохранении. *Вестник Росздравнадзора.* № 1. С. 51–57.

Kazakov A. S. (2008) The Experience of Roszdravnadzor on Organizing the System of Voluntary Certification of Services in Healthcare. *Vestnik Roszdravnadzora*, no 1, pp. 51–57.

Харитонова В. И. (1999) *Заговорно-заклинательное искусство восточных славян: проблемы традиционных исследований и возможности новых интерпретаций*. М.: ИЭА РАН. Часть 1 (Этнологические исследования по шаманству и иным традиционным верованиям и практикам. Т. 3, ч. 1–2).

Kharitonova V. I. (1999) *The Charms and Spells Art of the Eastern Slavs: Problems of Traditional Studies and Potential New Interpretations*. Moscow: IEA RAN. Part 1 (Etnologicheskie issledovaniya po shamanstvu i inym traditsionnym verovaniyam i praktikam. Vol. 3, parts 1–2).

Христофорова О. Б. (2010) *Колдуны и жертвы: Антропология колдовства в современной России*. М.: ОГИ, РГГУ.

Khristoforova O. B. (2010) *Sorcerers and Victims: The Anthropology of Sorcery in Contemporary Russia*. Moscow: OGI, RGGU.

Кнорре Б. К. (2012) Социальное служение современной Русской православной церкви Московского патриархата как отражение поведенческих стереотипов церковного социума. В кн.: *Православная церковь при новом патриархе*. М.: РОССПЭН.

Knorre B. K. (2012) The Social Service of the Contemporary Russian Orthodox Service of the Moscow Patriarchate as a Reflection of Behavioral Stereotypes of the Church Society. In: *Pravoslavnaya tserkov' pri novom patriarkhe*. Moscow: ROSSPEN.

Кофанова Е. Н., Мчедлова М. М. (2010) Религиозность россиян и европейцев. *Мониторинг общественного мнения*. № 4 (98). С. 201–230.

Kofanova E. N. and Mchedlova M. M. (2010) The Religiosity of Russians and Europeans. *Public Opinion Monitoring*, no 4 (98), pp. 201–230.

Колонуто А. Е., Крашенинникова Ю. А. (2012) Целители на селе: образ жизни и роль в местном сообществе. *Крестьяноведение. Теория. История. Современность. Ученые записки*. Выпуск 7. М.: ИД "Дело". С. 361–374.

Kolonuto A. E. and Krasheninnikova Yu. A. (2012) Rural Healers: Way of Life and Role in the Local Community. *Krest'yanovedenie. Teoriya. Istoriya. Sovremennost'. Uchenye zapiski*. Issue 7. Moscow: Delo Pub., pp. 361–374.

Кордонский С. Г., Плюснин Ю. М., Крашенинникова Ю. А., Тукаева А. Р., Моргунова О. М., Ахунов Д. Э., Бойков Д. В. (2011) Российская провинция и ее обитатели (опыт наблюдения и попытка описания). *Мир России*. № 1. С. 3–33.

Kordonsky S. G. et al. (2011) The Russian Province and its Inhabitants (Observation and Attempted Description. *Mir Rossii*, no 1. pp. 3–33.

Кормина Ж. В. (2013) "Гигиена сердца": дисциплина и вера "заново рожденных" харизматических христиан. *Антропологический форум*. Т. 18. С. 300–320.

Kormina Zh. V. (2013) "Hygiene of the Heart": Discipline and Faith of the "Newly Born" Charismatic Christians. *Antropologicheskiy forum*, vol. 18, pp. 300–320.

Крашенинникова Ю. А. (2011) Медицинская статистика как способ легитимации распределения ресурсов в российской системе здравоохранения. *Вопросы государственного и муниципального управления*. № 4. С. 28–42.

Krasheninnikova Yu. A. (2011) Medical Statistics as a Means of Legitimizing Resource Allocation in Russian Healthcare. *Voprosy gosudarstvennogo i munitsipal'nogo upravleniya*, no 4, pp. 28–42.

Крашенинникова Ю. А. (2015) «Неформальное здравоохранение» в современной России и факторы его развития (по материалам пилотного исследования). *Мир России*. № 4. С. 99–122.

Krasheninnikova Yu. A. (2015) "Informal Healthcare" in Contemporary Russia and Its Drivers (Based on a Pilot Study). *Mir Rossii*, no 4, pp. 99–122.

Куровский В., Куровская Л. (2010) *Жива—энергия Жизни. Уникальная система духовного целительства. Сила Родосвета*. М.: Изд. "Центрполиграф".

Kurovskiy V. and Kurovskaya L. (2010) *Jiva—the Life Energy. A Unique System of Spiritual Healing. The Power of Rodosvet*. M.: Centrepolygraph Pub.

Кузнецова Т. Е. (2012) Возрождение промыслового хозяйства в современной России—важнейшее направление использования её пространственного потенциала. В кн.: *Вторая Россия: дифференциация и самоорганизация*. Сборник научных статей / Под общ.ред. А. М. Никулина. М.: ИД "Дело". С. 182—201.

Kuznetsova T. E. (2012) Revival of Hunting and Fishing in Contemporary Russia as a Major Trend in Using Its Territorial Potential. In: *Vtoraya Rossiya: differentsiatsiya i samoorganizatsiya*. Sbornik nauchnykh statey. Ed. by Nikulin A. M. Moscow: Delo Pub., pp. 182–201.

Лункин Р. (2006) Пятидесятники и харизматы: единство в многообразии. *Russian Review*. № 11.
URL: http://www.keston.org.uk/_russianreview/edition11/02Charismatics.html.

Lunkin R. (2006) Pentecostals and Charismatics: Unity in Diversity. *Russian Review*, no 11.
URL: http://www.keston.org.uk/_russianreview/edition11/02Charismatics.html.

Мазалова Н. Е. (2012) Современные целительницы: статус, функции в социуме. *Вестник ЛГУ им. А. С. Пушкина*. № 4. С. 21–28.

Mazalova N. E. (2012) Contemporary Female Healers: Status and Functions in Society. *Vestnik LGU im. A. S. Pushkina*, no 4, pp. 21–28.

Мегре В. (2009) *Анастасия. Книга первая. Звенящий кедр*. Серия: Звенящие кедры России. СПб.: Изд. "Диля".

Megre V. (2009) *Anastasia. Book One. The Ringing Cedar*. Series: The Ringing Cedars of Russia. SPb: Dilya Pub.

Мерсиянова И. В., Корнеева И. Е. (2013) *Благотворительность и участие россиян в практиках гражданского общества: региональное измерение*. Научный редактор: М. С. Рождественская. Вып. VIII. М.: НИУ ВШЭ.

Mersiyanova I. V., Korneeva I. E. (2013) *Charity and the Participation of Russians in Civil Society Practices: the Regional Dimension*. Science Editor: M. S. Rozhdestvenskaya. Issue VIII. Moscow: NRU HSE.

Митрохин Н. (2001) Экономика Русской православной церкви. *Отечественные записки*. № 1. URL: http://www.strana-oz.ru/2001/1/ekonomika-russkoy-pravoslavnoy-cerkvi.

Mitrokhin N. (2001) The Economy of the Russian Orthodox Church . *Otechestvennye zapiski*, no 1. URL: http://www.strana-oz.ru/2001/1/ekonomika-russkoy-pravoslavnoy-cerkvi.

*Новые религии в России: двадцать лет спустя* (2013) Материалы Международной научно-практической конференции. Москва, Центральный дом журналиста, 14 декабря 2012 г. М.

New Religions in Russia: Twenty Years Later (2013) Materialy Mezhdunarodnoy nauchno-prakticheskoy konferentsii. Moskva, Tsentral'nyy dom zhurnalista, 14 dekabrya 2012 g. Moscow.

Орешина Д. А., Пруцкова Е. В., Забаев И. В. (2013) Специфика социальной работы на приходах Русской православной церкви: проблема концептуализации. *Журнал исследований социальной политики*. № 3. С. 355–368.

Oreshina D. A., Prutskova E. V., Zabaev I. V. (2013) Specifics of Social Work in the Parishes of the Russina Orthodox Church: Conceptualization Challenge. *Zhurnal issledovaniy sotsial'noy politiki*, no 3, pp. 355–368.

Осипов А. (2000) Что такое "отчитка" или что необходимо знать об отчитке (экзорцизме), чтобы на нее не идти. *Православная беседа*. № 1.

Osipov A. (2000) What is "Otchitka", or What Should One Know About Otchitka (Exorcism) to Avoid It. *Pravoslavnaya beseda*, no 1.

Паченков О. (2001) Рациональное "заколдовывание мира": современные российские "маги". В кн.: *Невидимые грани социальной реальности*. Сборник статей по материалам полевых исследований / Под ред. Воронкова В., Паченкова О., Чикадзе Е. СПб.: Труды ЦНСИ. Вып. 9.

Pachenkov O. (2001) "Bewitching the World" Rationally: Contemporary Russian "Magicians". In: *Nevidimye grani sotsial'noy real'nosti*. Sbornik statey po materialam polevykh issledovaniy. Ed. by Voronkov V., Pachenkov O., Chikadze E. Saint-Petersburg: Trudy TSNSI. Issue 9.

Плетт Л. (2008) *Духовные болезни*. Издание религиозной организации "Христианское общество "Библия для всех" Российского союза евангельских христиан-баптистов". Издательство "Миссия "Живые воды".

Plett L. (2008) *Spiritual Disease*. Izdanie religioznoy organizatsii "Khristianskoe obschestvo "Bibliya dlya vsekh" Rossiyskogo soyuza evangelicheskikh khristian-baptistov". Izdatel'stvo "Missiya "Zhivye vody".

Попова И. П. (2013) Профессиональные ассоциации: тенденции исследований в западной социологии профессий. В кн.: *Профессионалы в эпоху реформ: динамика идеологии, статуса и ценностей* / под ред. Мансурова В. А. М.: ИС РАН, РОС. С. 64–75.

Popova I. P. (2013) Professional Associations: Research Trends in the Western Sociology of Professions. In: *Professionaly v epokhu reform: dinamika ideologii, statusa i tsennostey*. Ed. by Mansurov V. A. Moscow: IS RAN, ROS, pp. 64–75.

Пруцкова Е. (2012) Операционализация понятия «религиозность» в эмпирических исследованиях. *Государство, религия, церковь в России и за рубежом*. № 2. С. 268–293.

Prutskova E. (2012) Operationalizing the Concept of "Religiosity" in Empirical Research. *Gosudarstvo, religiya, tserkov' v Rossii i za rubezhom*, no 2, pp. 268–293.

*Отчет о выполнении государственной программы Пермского края «Культура Пермского края» за 2015 год* (2016) Министерство культуры Пермского края.

*Report on the Implementation of the Perm Regional Government Program "Culture of the Perm Territory" for the year 2015* (2016) Ministry of Culture of the Perm Territory.

*Итоги Всероссийской сельскохозяйственной переписи 2006 года* (2008) Федеральная служба гос. статистики. М.: ИИЦ «Статистика России». Т. 4: Посевные площади сельскохозяйственных культур и площади многолетних насаждений и ягодных культур: кн. 1.: Площади сельскохозяйственных культур и многолетних насаждений.

*Results of the 2006 All-Russian Agricultural Census* (2008) Federal State Statistics Service. Moscow: IITS «Statistika Rossii». Vol. 4: The Acreage of Crops and the Area of Perennial Plants and Berries: Book 1.: Ploschadi sel'sko-khozyaystvennykh kul'tur i mnogoletnikh nasazhdeniy.

*Итоги Всероссийской сельскохозяйственной переписи 2006 года* (2008) Федеральная служба гос. статистики. М.: ИИЦ «Статистика России». Т. 5: Поголовье сельскохозяйственных животных: кн. 1.: Поголовье сельскохозяйственных животных. Структура поголовья сельскохозяйственных животных.

*Results of the 2006 All-Russian Agricultural Census* (2008) Federal State Statistics Service. Moscow: IITS «Statistika Rossii». Vol. 5: Livestock: Book 1.: Pogolov'e sel'skokhozyaystvennykh zhivotnykh. Struktura pogolov'ya sel'skokhozyaystvennykh zhivotnykh.

Романов П., Ярская-Смирнова Е. (2007) Социальное как иррациональное? (Диагнозы 1990 года). *Новое литературное обозрение.* № 3. С. 205–226.

Romanov P., Iarskaya-Smirnova E. (2007) Social as Irrational? (Diagnoses of 1990). *Novoe literaturnoe obozrenie*, no 3, pp. 205–226.

Русина Н. А. (2011) Проблемы клинического психолога в системе здравоохранения. Bulletin of Medical Internet Conferences. Vol. 1. Issue 7. С. 24–28.

Rusina N. A. (2011) Challenges Facing a Clinical Psychologist in the Health System. *Bulletin of Medical Internet Conferences*, vol. 1, issue 7, pp. 24–28.

*Регионы России. Социально-экономические показатели. 2014* (2014) Р32. Стат. сб. / М.: Росстат.

*Russian Regions. Socio-Economic Indicators. 2014* (2014): R32. Statistical Handbook / Moscow: Rosstat.

Садыков Р. А. (2013а) *Особенности социального положения и профессионализации врачей альтернативной медицины (на примере врачей-гомеопатов).* Диссертация на соискание ученой степени кандидата социологических наук. М.

Sadykov R. A. (2013a) *Particularities of the Social Status and Professionalization of Doctors of Alternative Medicine (On the Example of Homeopaths).* Dissertation for a doctoral degree in sociology. Moscow.

Садыков Р. А. (2013b) Практики и перспективы профессионализации гомеопатии в России. В кн.: *Профессии социального государства/* Под ред. П. В. Романова и Е. Р. Ярской-Смирновой. М.: Вариант, ЦСПГИ. С. 116–136.

Sadykov R. A. (2013b) Practices and Prospects for Professionalizing Homeopathy in Russia. In: *Professii sotsial'nogo gosudarstva*. Ed. by Romanov P. V. and Iarskaya-Smirnova E. R. Moscow: Variant, TSSPGI, pp. 116–136.

Сакс М., Олсоп Дж. (2003) Социология профессий: государство, медицина и рынок в Великобритании. В кн.: *Профессиональные группы интеллигенции /* Отв. ред. В. А. Мансуров. М.: Изд-во Института социологии РАН. С. 79–104.

Saks M. and Allsop J. (2003) Sociology of Professions: State, Medicine and Market in Great Britain. In: *Professional Groups of Intellectuals*. Ed. by Mansurov V. A. Moscow: Izd-vo Instituta sotsiologii RAN, pp. 79–104.

Сало Е. П. (2008) Опыт изучения социального статуса специалистов традиционной медицины. *Социология: 4М*. № 26. С. 139–167.

Salo E. P. (2008) A Study of the Social Status of a Specialist in Traditional Medicine. *Sotsiologiya: 4M*, no 26, pp. 139–167.

Сало Е. П. (2009) *Социальный статус специалистов традиционной медицины в России: социологический анализ*. Автореферат диссертации на соискание ученой степени кандидата социологических наук. М.

Salo E. P. (2009) *The Social Status of Specialists in Traditional Medicine in Russia: Sociological Analysis*. Abstract of the dissertation for a doctoral degree in sociology. Moscow.

Самарская Т. А., Тепер Г. А. (2007) Альтернативная медицина российской провинции. *Журнал исследований социальной политики*. № 1. С. 87–103.

Samarskaya T. A., Teper G. A. (2007) Alternative Medicine of the Russian Provinces. *Zhurnal issledovaniy sotsial'noy politiki*, no 1, pp. 87–103.

Савельева Н. В. (2013a) Корпоративная культура, стигматизация и карьеры дистрибьюторов в организациях прямых продаж в России. *Мониторинг общественного мнения*. № 7 (113). С. 114–126.

Savelieva N. V. (2013a) Corporate Culture, Stigmatization, and Careers of Distributors in Direct Selling Companies in Russia. *Public Opinion Monitoring*, no 7 (113), pp. 114–126.

Савельева Н. В. (2013b) Практики «заботы о себе» в организациях прямых продаж. *Социологический журнал*. № 3. С. 22–38.

Savelieva N. V. (2013b) "Taking Care of Yourself" Practices in Direct Selling Companies. *Sotsiologicheskiy zhurnal*, no 3, pp. 22–38.

Щелокова Л. Г., Глумов С. Г. (2009) *Атлас лекарственных растений Пермского края. Применение в медицине и ветеринарии*. Пермь.

Shchelokova L. G., Glumov S. G. (2009) *Atlas of Medicinal Plants of the Perm Territory*. Application in Medicine and Veterinary. Perm.

Синелина Ю. Ю. (2005) Воцерковленность и суеверное поведение жителей Ярославской области. *Социологические исследования*. № 3. С. 96–107.

Sinelina Yu. Yu. (2005) Church-Going and the Superstitious Behavior of the Inhabitants of the Yaroslavl Region. *Sotsiologicheskie issledovaniya*, no 3, pp. 96–107.

Синелина Ю. Ю. (2013) О динамике религиозности россиян и некоторых методологических проблемах его изучения (религиозное сознание и поведение православных и мусульман). *Социологические исследования*. № 10. С. 104–115.

Sinelina Yu. Yu. (2013) On the Changes in the Religiosity of Russians and Some Methodological Challenges of Its Study (Religious Consciousness and Behavior of Orthodox Christians and Muslims). *Sotsiologicheskie issledovaniya*, no 10, pp. 104–115.

Сошников С. С., Владимиров С. К., Сосунов Р. А., Власов В. В., Граница А. С., Смирнов А. А. (2011) Контент-анализ запатентованных методов лечения наркологических расстройств в России. *Неврологический вестник*. № 4. С. 3–7.

Soshnikov S. S. et al (2011) Content analysis of Patented Methods for Treating Addiction Disorders in Russian. *Nevrologicheskiy vestnik*, no 4, pp. 3–7.

*Государственный реестр новых медицинских технологий* (2002). Выпуск 3. Официальное издание. Под ред. А. Я. Вялкова. М.: Минздрав России.

*State Register of New Medical Technologies* (2002) Issue 3. Official edition. Ed. by Vyalkov A. Ya. Moscow: Minzdrav Rossii.

*Система поддержания здоровья в современной России* (2012) Сборник статей и материалов полевых исследований / Под ред. И. В. Кошкаровой. М.: Страна Оз.

*System for Maintaining Health in Contemporary Russia* (2012) Collected Papers and Field Records. Ed. by Koshkarova I. V. Moscow: Strana Oz.

Темплинг В. Я. (2014) Жизненный путь и формирование индивидуального магико-медицинского опыта в практике народного целительства. *Вестник археологии, антропологии и этнографии*. № 1 (24). С. 157—162.

Templing V. Ya. (2014) The Life Journey and the Development of the Personal Magic-Medical Experience in Traditional Healing Practice. *Vestnik arkheologii, antropologii i etnografii*, no 1 (24), pp. 157–162.

*Основы православной веры* (2010) Пермь: Издательский отдел Пермской и Соликамской Епархии РПЦ.

*The Foundations of the Orthodox Faith* (2010) Perm: Publications Office of the Perm and Solikamsk Diocese of the Russian Orthodox Church.

*Традиционная медицина: политика и практика профессионализации* (2011) Под ред. Е. Р. Ярской-Смирновой. М.: ООО «Вариант», ЦСПГИ.

*Traditional Medicine: Professionalization Policy and Practice* (2011) Ed. by Iarskaya-Smirnova E. R. Moscow: OOO «Variant», TSSPGI.

*Применение терминов натуротерапии и натурофармации в практическом здравоохранении. Методические рекомендации № 2000/154* (2000) Утв. Минздравом России 01.11.2000. Организация—разработчик: Науч.-практ. центр традиц. медицины и гомеопатии Минздрава России.

*Using the Terms Natural Therapy and Natural Pharmacy in Healthcare Practice. Methodology Guide No. 2000/154* (2000) Approved by the Russian Ministry of Health on 1 November 2000. Developer: Nauch.-prakt. tsentr tradits. meditsiny i gomeopatii Minzdrava Rossii.

Власов В. В. (2014) Терпимость к обману в русской медицине. В кн.: *Гуманитарные ориентиры научного познания.* ИД "Навигатор". С. 221–225.

Vlassov V. V. (2014) Tolerance of Cheating in Russian Medicine. In: *Gumanitarnye orientiry nauchnogo poznaniya.* Izdatel'skiy dom "Navigator", pp. 221–225.

Волкова О. А. (2007) Целители как специфическая социальная группа. *Социологические исследования.* № 3. С. 86–88.

Volkova O. A. (2007) Healers as a Specific Social Group. *Sotsiologicheskie issledovaniya,* no 3, pp. 86—88.

*Когда поставлен диагноз: О науке болеть и выздоравливать* (2012) Сборник. М.: Издательство Московской Патриархии Русской Православной Церкви.

*When Diagnosed: The Science of Being Ill and Recovering* (2012) Collected Works. M.: Publishing House of the Moscow Patriarchate of the Russian Orthodox Church.

*"Благодеяния записывай на меди, а обиды на воде..." Жизнеописание протоиерея Николая Рогозина. Воспоминания. Письма* (2011) Верхне-Чусовская Казанская Трифонова женская пустынь.

*"Write down good deeds on copper, but resentment on water…" The Life of Archpriest Nikolai Rogozin. Memoirs. Letters* (2011) Verkhnechusovskaya Kazanskaya Trifonova Convent.

*Пользователи Яндекса: интересы и поисковое поведение* (2013) Яндекс. Исследования.
URL: https://yandex.ru/company/researches/2013/ya_search_interests_2013.

*Yandex Users: Interests and Search Behavior* (2013). Yandex. Research.
URL: https://yandex.ru/company/researches/2013/ya_search_interests_2013.

Забаев И. В., Пруцкова Е. В. (2013) Факторы формирования общины на основе прихода православного храма в начале XXI в. по данным опроса священнослужителей, социальных работников и активных прихожан храмов г. Москвы. *Вестник Московского университета. Серия 18. Социология и политология.* № 1. С. 114–215.

Zabaev I. V., Prutskova E. V. (2013) Factors Underlying the emergence of Communities on the Basis of an Orthodox Parish in the Early XXI Century According to the Survey of Clergy, Social Workers, and Active Church-Goers in Moscow. *Vestnik Moskovskogo universiteta. Series 18. Sotsiologiya i politologiya,* no 1, pp. 114–215.

Зуева Д. С. (2005) Сетевой маркетинг как нетрадиционная форма хозяйственной деятельности. *Экономическая социология.* Т. 6. № 4. С. 67–92.

Zueva D. S. (2005) Network Marketing as a Non-Traditional Form of Business Activity. *Ekonomicheskaya sotsiologiya,* vol. 6, no 4, pp. 67–92.

# SOVIET AND POST-SOVIET POLITICS AND SOCIETY

Edited by Dr. Andreas Umland

ISSN 1614-3515

1   Андреас Умланд (ред.)
    Воплощение Европейской
    конвенции по правам человека в
    России
    Философские, юридические и
    эмпирические исследования
    ISBN 3-89821-387-0

2   Christian Wipperfürth
    Russland – ein vertrauenswürdiger
    Partner?
    Grundlagen, Hintergründe und Praxis
    gegenwärtiger russischer Außenpolitik
    Mit einem Vorwort von Heinz Timmermann
    ISBN 3-89821-401-X

3   Manja Hussner
    Die Übernahme internationalen Rechts
    in die russische und deutsche
    Rechtsordnung
    Eine vergleichende Analyse zur
    Völkerrechtsfreundlichkeit der Verfassungen
    der Russländischen Föderation und der
    Bundesrepublik Deutschland
    Mit einem Vorwort von Rainer Arnold
    ISBN 3-89821-438-9

4   Matthew Tejada
    Bulgaria's Democratic Consolidation
    and the Kozloduy Nuclear Power Plant
    (KNPP)
    The Unattainability of Closure
    With a foreword by Richard J. Crampton
    ISBN 3-89821-439-7

5   Марк Григорьевич Меерович
    Квадратные метры, определяющие
    сознание
    Государственная жилищная политика в
    СССР. 1921 – 1941 гг
    ISBN 3-89821-474-5

6   Andrei P. Tsygankov, Pavel
    A. Tsygankov (Eds.)
    New Directions in Russian
    International Studies
    ISBN 3-89821-422-2

7   Марк Григорьевич Меерович
    Как власть народ к труду приучала
    Жилище в СССР – средство управления
    людьми. 1917 – 1941 гг.
    С предисловием Елены Осокиной
    ISBN 3-89821-495-8

8   David J. Galbreath
    Nation-Building and Minority Politics
    in Post-Socialist States
    Interests, Influence and Identities in Estonia
    and Latvia
    With a foreword by David J. Smith
    ISBN 3-89821-467-2

9   Алексей Юрьевич Безугольный
    Народы Кавказа в Вооруженных
    силах СССР в годы Великой
    Отечественной войны 1941-1945 гг.
    С предисловием Николая Бугая
    ISBN 3-89821-475-3

10  Вячеслав Лихачев и Владимир
    Прибыловский (ред.)
    Русское Национальное Единство,
    1990-2000. В 2-х томах
    ISBN 3-89821-523-7

11  Николай Бугай (ред.)
    Народы стран Балтии в условиях
    сталинизма (1940-е – 1950-е годы)
    Документированная история
    ISBN 3-89821-525-3

12  Ingmar Bredies (Hrsg.)
    Zur Anatomie der Orange Revolution
    in der Ukraine
    Wechsel des Elitenregimes oder Triumph des
    Parlamentarismus?
    ISBN 3-89821-524-5

13  Anastasia V. Mitrofanova
    The Politicization of Russian
    Orthodoxy
    Actors and Ideas
    With a foreword by William C. Gay
    ISBN 3-89821-481-8

14 Nathan D. Larson
Alexander Solzhenitsyn and the
Russo-Jewish Question
ISBN 3-89821-483-4

15 Guido Houben
Kulturpolitik und Ethnizität
Staatliche Kunstförderung im Russland der
neunziger Jahre
Mit einem Vorwort von Gert Weisskirchen
ISBN 3-89821-542-3

16 Leonid Luks
Der russische „Sonderweg"?
Aufsätze zur neuesten Geschichte Russlands
im europäischen Kontext
ISBN 3-89821-496-6

17 Евгений Мороз
История «Мёртвой воды» – от
страшной сказки к большой
политике
Политическое неоязычество в
постсоветской России
ISBN 3-89821-551-2

18 Александр Верховский и Галина
Кожевникова (ред.)
Этническая и религиозная
интолерантность в российских СМИ
Результаты мониторинга 2001-2004 гг.
ISBN 3-89821-569-5

19 Christian Ganzer
Sowjetisches Erbe und ukrainische
Nation
Das Museum der Geschichte des Zaporoger
Kosakentums auf der Insel Chortycja
Mit einem Vorwort von Frank Golczewski
ISBN 3-89821-504-0

20 Эльза-Баир Гучинова
Помнить нельзя забыть
Антропология депортационной травмы
калмыков
С предисловием Кэролайн Хамфри
ISBN 3-89821-506-7

21 Юлия Лидерман
Мотивы «проверки» и «испытания»
в постсоветской культуре
Советское прошлое в российском
кинематографе 1990-х годов
С предисловием Евгения Марголита
ISBN 3-89821-511-3

22 Tanya Lokshina, Ray Thomas, Mary
Mayer (Eds.)
The Imposition of a Fake Political
Settlement in the Northern Caucasus
The 2003 Chechen Presidential Election
ISBN 3-89821-436-2

23 Timothy McCajor Hall, Rosie Read
(Eds.)
Changes in the Heart of Europe
Recent Ethnographies of Czechs, Slovaks,
Roma, and Sorbs
With an afterword by Zdeněk Salzmann
ISBN 3-89821-606-3

24 Christian Autengruber
Die politischen Parteien in Bulgarien
und Rumänien
Eine vergleichende Analyse seit Beginn der
90er Jahre
Mit einem Vorwort von Dorothée de Nève
ISBN 3-89821-476-1

25 Annette Freyberg-Inan with Radu
Cristescu
The Ghosts in Our Classrooms, or:
John Dewey Meets Ceauşescu
The Promise and the Failures of Civic
Education in Romania
ISBN 3-89821-416-8

26 John B. Dunlop
The 2002 Dubrovka and 2004 Beslan
Hostage Crises
A Critique of Russian Counter-Terrorism
With a foreword by Donald N. Jensen
ISBN 3-89821-608-X

27 Peter Koller
Das touristische Potenzial von
Kam''janec'-Podil's'kyj
Eine fremdenverkehrsgeographische
Untersuchung der Zukunftsperspektiven und
Maßnahmenplanung zur
Destinationsentwicklung des „ukrainischen
Rothenburg"
Mit einem Vorwort von Kristiane Klemm
ISBN 3-89821-640-3

28 Françoise Daucé, Elisabeth Sieca-
Kozlowski (Eds.)
Dedovshchina in the Post-Soviet
Military
Hazing of Russian Army Conscripts in a
Comparative Perspective
With a foreword by Dale Herspring
ISBN 3-89821-616-0

29  Florian Strasser
Zivilgesellschaftliche Einflüsse auf die
Orange Revolution
Die gewaltlose Massenbewegung und die
ukrainische Wahlkrise 2004
Mit einem Vorwort von Egbert Jahn
ISBN 3-89821-648-9

30  Rebecca S. Katz
The Georgian Regime Crisis of 2003-
2004
A Case Study in Post-Soviet Media
Representation of Politics, Crime and
Corruption
ISBN 3-89821-413-3

31  Vladimir Kantor
Willkür oder Freiheit
Beiträge zur russischen Geschichtsphilosophie
Ediert von Dagmar Herrmann sowie mit
einem Vorwort versehen von Leonid Luks
ISBN 3-89821-589-X

32  Laura A. Victoir
The Russian Land Estate Today
A Case Study of Cultural Politics in Post-
Soviet Russia
With a foreword by Priscilla Roosevelt
ISBN 3-89821-426-5

33  Ivan Katchanovski
Cleft Countries
Regional Political Divisions and Cultures in
Post-Soviet Ukraine and Moldova
With a foreword by Francis Fukuyama
ISBN 3-89821-558-X

34  Florian Mühlfried
Postsowjetische Feiern
Das Georgische Bankett im Wandel
Mit einem Vorwort von Kevin Tuite
ISBN 3-89821-601-2

35  Roger Griffin, Werner Loh, Andreas
Umland (Eds.)
Fascism Past and Present, West and
East
An International Debate on Concepts and
Cases in the Comparative Study of the
Extreme Right
With an afterword by Walter Laqueur
ISBN 3-89821-674-8

36  Sebastian Schlegel
Der „Weiße Archipel"
Sowjetische Atomstädte 1945-1991
Mit einem Geleitwort von Thomas Bohn
ISBN 3-89821-679-9

37  Vyacheslav Likhachev
Political Anti-Semitism in Post-Soviet
Russia
Actors and Ideas in 1991-2003
Edited and translated from Russian by Eugene
Veklerov
ISBN 3-89821-529-6

38  Josette Baer (Ed.)
Preparing Liberty in Central Europe
Political Texts from the Spring of Nations
1848 to the Spring of Prague 1968
With a foreword by Zdeněk V. David
ISBN 3-89821-546-6

39  Михаил Лукьянов
Российский консерватизм и
реформа, 1907-1914
С предисловием Марка Д. Стейнберга
ISBN 3-89821-503-2

40  Nicola Melloni
Market Without Economy
The 1998 Russian Financial Crisis
With a foreword by Eiji Furukawa
ISBN 3-89821-407-9

41  Dmitrij Chmelnizki
Die Architektur Stalins
Bd. 1: Studien zu Ideologie und Stil
Bd. 2: Bilddokumentation
Mit einem Vorwort von Bruno Flierl
ISBN 3-89821-515-6

42  Katja Yafimava
Post-Soviet Russian-Belarussian
Relationships
The Role of Gas Transit Pipelines
With a foreword by Jonathan P. Stern
ISBN 3-89821-655-1

43  Boris Chavkin
Verflechtungen der deutschen und
russischen Zeitgeschichte
Aufsätze und Archivfunde zu den
Beziehungen Deutschlands und der
Sowjetunion von 1917 bis 1991
Ediert von Markus Edlinger sowie mit einem
Vorwort versehen von Leonid Luks
ISBN 3-89821-756-6

44  *Anastasija Grynenko in Zusammenarbeit mit Claudia Dathe*
Die Terminologie des Gerichtswesens der Ukraine und Deutschlands im Vergleich
Eine übersetzungswissenschaftliche Analyse juristischer Fachbegriffe im Deutschen, Ukrainischen und Russischen
Mit einem Vorwort von Ulrich Hartmann
ISBN 3-89821-691-8

45  *Anton Burkov*
The Impact of the European Convention on Human Rights on Russian Law
Legislation and Application in 1996-2006
With a foreword by Françoise Hampson
ISBN 978-3-89821-639-5

46  *Stina Torjesen, Indra Overland (Eds.)*
International Election Observers in Post-Soviet Azerbaijan
Geopolitical Pawns or Agents of Change?
ISBN 978-3-89821-743-9

47  *Taras Kuzio*
Ukraine – Crimea – Russia
Triangle of Conflict
ISBN 978-3-89821-761-3

48  *Claudia Šabić*
"Ich erinnere mich nicht, aber L'viv!"
Zur Funktion kultureller Faktoren für die Institutionalisierung und Entwicklung einer ukrainischen Region
Mit einem Vorwort von Melanie Tatur
ISBN 978-3-89821-752-1

49  *Marlies Bilz*
Tatarstan in der Transformation
Nationaler Diskurs und Politische Praxis 1988-1994
Mit einem Vorwort von Frank Golczewski
ISBN 978-3-89821-722-4

50  *Марлен Ларюэль (ред.)*
Современные интерпретации русского национализма
ISBN 978-3-89821-795-8

51  *Sonja Schüler*
Die ethnische Dimension der Armut
Roma im postsozialistischen Rumänien
Mit einem Vorwort von Anton Sterbling
ISBN 978-3-89821-776-7

52  *Галина Кожевникова*
Радикальный национализм в России и противодействие ему
Сборник докладов Центра «Сова» за 2004-2007 гг.
С предисловием Александра Верховского
ISBN 978-3-89821-721-7

53  *Галина Кожевникова и Владимир Прибыловский*
Российская власть в биографиях I
Высшие должностные лица РФ в 2004 г.
ISBN 978-3-89821-796-5

54  *Галина Кожевникова и Владимир Прибыловский*
Российская власть в биографиях II
Члены Правительства РФ в 2004 г.
ISBN 978-3-89821-797-2

55  *Галина Кожевникова и Владимир Прибыловский*
Российская власть в биографиях III
Руководители федеральных служб и агентств РФ в 2004 г.
ISBN 978-3-89821-798-9

56  *Ileana Petroniu*
Privatisierung in Transformationsökonomien
Determinanten der Restrukturierungs-Bereitschaft am Beispiel Polens, Rumäniens und der Ukraine
Mit einem Vorwort von Rainer W. Schäfer
ISBN 978-3-89821-790-3

57  *Christian Wipperfürth*
Russland und seine GUS-Nachbarn
Hintergründe, aktuelle Entwicklungen und Konflikte in einer ressourcenreichen Region
ISBN 978-3-89821-801-6

58  *Togzhan Kassenova*
From Antagonism to Partnership
The Uneasy Path of the U.S.-Russian Cooperative Threat Reduction
With a foreword by Christoph Bluth
ISBN 978-3-89821-707-1

59  *Alexander Höllwerth*
Das sakrale eurasische Imperium des Aleksandr Dugin
Eine Diskursanalyse zum postsowjetischen russischen Rechtsextremismus
Mit einem Vorwort von Dirk Uffelmann
ISBN 978-3-89821-813-9

60  Олег Рябов
«Россия-Матушка»
Национализм, гендер и война в России XX века
С предисловием Елены Гощило
ISBN 978-3-89821-487-2

61  Ivan Maistrenko
Borot'bism
A Chapter in the History of the Ukrainian Revolution
With a new introduction by Chris Ford
Translated by George S. N. Luckyj with the assistance of Ivan L. Rudnytsky
ISBN 978-3-89821-697-5

62  Maryna Romanets
Anamorphosic Texts and Reconfigured Visions
Improvised Traditions in Contemporary Ukrainian and Irish Literature
ISBN 978-3-89821-576-3

63  Paul D'Anieri and Taras Kuzio (Eds.)
Aspects of the Orange Revolution I
Democratization and Elections in Post-Communist Ukraine
ISBN 978-3-89821-698-2

64  Bohdan Harasymiw in collaboration with Oleh S. Ilnytzkyj (Eds.)
Aspects of the Orange Revolution II
Information and Manipulation Strategies in the 2004 Ukrainian Presidential Elections
ISBN 978-3-89821-699-9

65  Ingmar Bredies, Andreas Umland and Valentin Yakushik (Eds.)
Aspects of the Orange Revolution III
The Context and Dynamics of the 2004 Ukrainian Presidential Elections
ISBN 978-3-89821-803-0

66  Ingmar Bredies, Andreas Umland and Valentin Yakushik (Eds.)
Aspects of the Orange Revolution IV
Foreign Assistance and Civic Action in the 2004 Ukrainian Presidential Elections
ISBN 978-3-89821-808-5

67  Ingmar Bredies, Andreas Umland and Valentin Yakushik (Eds.)
Aspects of the Orange Revolution V
Institutional Observation Reports on the 2004 Ukrainian Presidential Elections
ISBN 978-3-89821-809-2

68  Taras Kuzio (Ed.)
Aspects of the Orange Revolution VI
Post-Communist Democratic Revolutions in Comparative Perspective
ISBN 978-3-89821-820-7

69  Tim Bohse
Autoritarismus statt Selbstverwaltung
Die Transformation der kommunalen Politik in der Stadt Kaliningrad 1990-2005
Mit einem Geleitwort von Stefan Troebst
ISBN 978-3-89821-782-8

70  David Rupp
Die Rußländische Föderation und die russischsprachige Minderheit in Lettland
Eine Fallstudie zur Anwaltspolitik Moskaus gegenüber den russophonen Minderheiten im „Nahen Ausland" von 1991 bis 2002
Mit einem Vorwort von Helmut Wagner
ISBN 978-3-89821-778-1

71  Taras Kuzio
Theoretical and Comparative Perspectives on Nationalism
New Directions in Cross-Cultural and Post-Communist Studies
With a foreword by Paul Robert Magocsi
ISBN 978-3-89821-815-3

72  Christine Teichmann
Die Hochschultransformation im heutigen Osteuropa
Kontinuität und Wandel bei der Entwicklung des postkommunistischen Universitätswesens
Mit einem Vorwort von Oskar Anweiler
ISBN 978-3-89821-842-9

73  Julia Kusznir
Der politische Einfluss von Wirtschaftseliten in russischen Regionen
Eine Analyse am Beispiel der Erdöl- und Erdgasindustrie, 1992-2005
Mit einem Vorwort von Wolfgang Eichwede
ISBN 978-3-89821-821-4

74  Alena Vysotskaya
Russland, Belarus und die EU-Osterweiterung
Zur Minderheitenfrage und zum Problem der Freizügigkeit des Personenverkehrs
Mit einem Vorwort von Katlijn Malfliet
ISBN 978-3-89821-822-1

75　*Heiko Pleines (Hrsg.)*
　　Corporate Governance in post-
　　sozialistischen Volkswirtschaften
　　ISBN 978-3-89821-766-8

76　*Stefan Ihrig*
　　Wer sind die Moldawier?
　　Rumänismus versus Moldowanismus in
　　Historiographie und Schulbüchern der
　　Republik Moldova, 1991-2006
　　Mit einem Vorwort von Holm Sundhaussen
　　ISBN 978-3-89821-466-7

77　*Galina Kozhevnikova in collaboration*
　　*with Alexander Verkhovsky and*
　　*Eugene Veklerov*
　　Ultra-Nationalism and Hate Crimes in
　　Contemporary Russia
　　The 2004-2006 Annual Reports of Moscow's
　　SOVA Center
　　With a foreword by Stephen D. Shenfield
　　ISBN 978-3-89821-868-9

78　*Florian Küchler*
　　The Role of the European Union in
　　Moldova's Transnistria Conflict
　　With a foreword by Christopher Hill
　　ISBN 978-3-89821-850-4

79　*Bernd Rechel*
　　The Long Way Back to Europe
　　Minority Protection in Bulgaria
　　With a foreword by Richard Crampton
　　ISBN 978-3-89821-863-4

80　*Peter W. Rodgers*
　　Nation, Region and History in Post-
　　Communist Transitions
　　Identity Politics in Ukraine, 1991-2006
　　With a foreword by Vera Tolz
　　ISBN 978-3-89821-903-7

81　*Stephanie Solywoda*
　　The Life and Work of
　　Semen L. Frank
　　A Study of Russian Religious Philosophy
　　With a foreword by Philip Walters
　　ISBN 978-3-89821-457-5

82　*Vera Sokolova*
　　Cultural Politics of Ethnicity
　　Discourses on Roma in Communist
　　Czechoslovakia
　　ISBN 978-3-89821-864-1

83　*Natalya Shevchik Ketenci*
　　Kazakhstani Enterprises in Transition
　　The Role of Historical Regional Development
　　in Kazakhstan's Post-Soviet Economic
　　Transformation
　　ISBN 978-3-89821-831-3

84　*Martin Malek, Anna Schor-*
　　*Tschudnowskaja (Hrsg.)*
　　Europa im Tschetschenienkrieg
　　Zwischen politischer Ohnmacht und
　　Gleichgültigkeit
　　Mit einem Vorwort von Lipchan Basajewa
　　ISBN 978-3-89821-676-0

85　*Stefan Meister*
　　Das postsowjetische Universitätswesen
　　zwischen nationalem und
　　internationalem Wandel
　　Die Entwicklung der regionalen Hochschule
　　in Russland als Gradmesser der
　　Systemtransformation
　　Mit einem Vorwort von Joan DeBardeleben
　　ISBN 978-3-89821-891-7

86　*Konstantin Sheiko in collaboration*
　　*with Stephen Brown*
　　Nationalist Imaginings of the
　　Russian Past
　　Anatolii Fomenko and the Rise of Alternative
　　History in Post-Communist Russia
　　With a foreword by Donald Ostrowski
　　ISBN 978-3-89821-915-0

87　*Sabine Jenni*
　　Wie stark ist das „Einige Russland"?
　　Zur Parteibindung der Eliten und zum
　　Wahlerfolg der Machtpartei
　　im Dezember 2007
　　Mit einem Vorwort von Klaus Armingeon
　　ISBN 978-3-89821-961-7

88　*Thomas Borén*
　　Meeting-Places of Transformation
　　Urban Identity, Spatial Representations and
　　Local Politics in Post-Soviet St Petersburg
　　ISBN 978-3-89821-739-2

89　*Aygul Ashirova*
　　Stalinismus und Stalin-Kult in
　　Zentralasien
　　Turkmenistan 1924-1953
　　Mit einem Vorwort von Leonid Luks
　　ISBN 978-3-89821-987-7

90　*Leonid Luks*
　　Freiheit oder imperiale Größe?
　　Essays zu einem russischen Dilemma
　　ISBN 978-3-8382-0011-8

91　*Christopher Gilley*
　　The 'Change of Signposts' in the
　　Ukrainian Emigration
　　A Contribution to the History of
　　Sovietophilism in the 1920s
　　With a foreword by Frank Golczewski
　　ISBN 978-3-89821-965-5

92　*Philipp Casula, Jeronim Perovic
　　(Eds.)*
　　Identities and Politics
　　During the Putin Presidency
　　The Discursive Foundations of Russia's
　　Stability
　　With a foreword by Heiko Haumann
　　ISBN 978-3-8382-0015-6

93　*Marcel Viëtor*
　　Europa und die Frage
　　nach seinen Grenzen im Osten
　　Zur Konstruktion ‚europäischer Identität' in
　　Geschichte und Gegenwart
　　Mit einem Vorwort von Albrecht Lehmann
　　ISBN 978-3-8382-0045-3

94　*Ben Hellman, Andrei Rogachevskii*
　　Filming the Unfilmable
　　Casper Wrede's 'One Day in the Life
　　of Ivan Denisovich'
　　Second, Revised and Expanded Edition
　　ISBN 978-3-8382-0044-6

95　*Eva Fuchslocher*
　　Vaterland, Sprache, Glaube
　　Orthodoxie und Nationenbildung
　　am Beispiel Georgiens
　　Mit einem Vorwort von Christina von Braun
　　ISBN 978-3-89821-884-9

96　*Vladimir Kantor*
　　Das Westlertum und der Weg
　　Russlands
　　Zur Entwicklung der russischen Literatur und
　　Philosophie
　　Ediert von Dagmar Herrmann
　　Mit einem Beitrag von Nikolaus Lobkowicz
　　ISBN 978-3-8382-0102-3

97　*Kamran Musayev*
　　Die postsowjetische Transformation
　　im Baltikum und Südkaukasus
　　Eine vergleichende Untersuchung der
　　politischen Entwicklung Lettlands und
　　Aserbaidschans 1985-2009
　　Mit einem Vorwort von Leonid Luks
　　Ediert von Sandro Henschel
　　ISBN 978-3-8382-0103-0

98　*Tatiana Zhurzhenko*
　　Borderlands into Bordered Lands
　　Geopolitics of Identity in Post-Soviet Ukraine
　　With a foreword by Dieter Segert
　　ISBN 978-3-8382-0042-2

99　*Кирилл Галушко, Лидия Смола
　　(ред.)*
　　Пределы падения – варианты
　　украинского будущего
　　Аналитико-прогностические исследования
　　ISBN 978-3-8382-0148-1

100　*Michael Minkenberg (ed.)*
　　Historical Legacies and the Radical
　　Right in Post-Cold War Central and
　　Eastern Europe
　　With an afterword by Sabrina P. Ramet
　　ISBN 978-3-8382-0124-5

101　*David-Emil Wickström*
　　Rocking St. Petersburg
　　Transcultural Flows and Identity Politics in
　　the St. Petersburg Popular Music Scene
　　With a foreword by Yngvar B. Steinholt
　　Second, Revised and Expanded Edition
　　ISBN 978-3-8382-0100-9

102　*Eva Zabka*
　　Eine neue „Zeit der Wirren"?
　　Der spät- und postsowjetische Systemwandel
　　1985-2000 im Spiegel russischer
　　gesellschaftspolitischer Diskurse
　　Mit einem Vorwort von Margareta Mommsen
　　ISBN 978-3-8382-0161-0

103　*Ulrike Ziemer*
　　Ethnic Belonging, Gender and
　　Cultural Practices
　　Youth Identitites in Contemporary Russia
　　With a foreword by Anoop Nayak
　　ISBN 978-3-8382-0152-8

104 Ksenia Chepikova
,Einiges Russland' - eine zweite KPdSU?
Aspekte der Identitätskonstruktion einer postsowjetischen „Partei der Macht"
Mit einem Vorwort von Torsten Oppelland
ISBN 978-3-8382-0311-9

105 Леонид Люкс
Западничество или евразийство? Демократия или идеократия?
Сборник статей об исторических дилеммах России
С предисловием Владимира Кантора
ISBN 978-3-8382-0211-2

106 Anna Dost
Das russische Verfassungsrecht auf dem Weg zum Föderalismus und zurück
Zum Konflikt von Rechtsnormen und -wirklichkeit in der Russländischen Föderation von 1991 bis 2009
Mit einem Vorwort von Alexander Blankenagel
ISBN 978-3-8382-0292-1

107 Philipp Herzog
Sozialistische Völkerfreundschaft, nationaler Widerstand oder harmloser Zeitvertreib?
Zur politischen Funktion der Volkskunst im sowjetischen Estland
Mit einem Vorwort von Andreas Kappeler
ISBN 978-3-8382-0216-7

108 Marlène Laruelle (ed.)
Russian Nationalism, Foreign Policy, and Identity Debates in Putin's Russia
New Ideological Patterns after the Orange Revolution
ISBN 978-3-8382-0325-6

109 Michail Logvinov
Russlands Kampf gegen den internationalen Terrorismus
Eine kritische Bestandsaufnahme des Bekämpfungsansatzes
Mit einem Geleitwort von Hans-Henning Schröder
und einem Vorwort von Eckhard Jesse
ISBN 978-3-8382-0329-4

110 John B. Dunlop
The Moscow Bombings of September 1999
Examinations of Russian Terrorist Attacks at the Onset of Vladimir Putin's Rule
Second, Revised and Expanded Edition
ISBN 978-3-8382-0388-1

111 Андрей А. Ковалёв
Свидетельство из-за кулис российской политики I
Можно ли делать добро из зла?
(Воспоминания и размышления о последних советских и первых послесоветских годах)
With a foreword by Peter Reddaway
ISBN 978-3-8382-0302-7

112 Андрей А. Ковалёв
Свидетельство из-за кулис российской политики II
Угроза для себя и окружающих
(Наблюдения и предостережения относительно происходящего после 2000 г.)
ISBN 978-3-8382-0303-4

113 Bernd Kappenberg
Zeichen setzen für Europa
Der Gebrauch europäischer lateinischer Sonderzeichen in der deutschen Öffentlichkeit
Mit einem Vorwort von Peter Schlobinski
ISBN 978-3-89821-749-1

114 Ivo Mijnssen
The Quest for an Ideal Youth in Putin's Russia I
Back to Our Future! History, Modernity, and Patriotism according to Nashi, 2005-2013
With a foreword by Jeronim Perović
Second, Revised and Expanded Edition
ISBN 978-3-8382-0368-3

115 Jussi Lassila
The Quest for an Ideal Youth in Putin's Russia II
The Search for Distinctive Conformism in the Political Communication of Nashi, 2005-2009
With a foreword by Kirill Postoutenko
Second, Revised and Expanded Edition
ISBN 978-3-8382-0415-4

116 Valerio Trabandt
Neue Nachbarn, gute Nachbarschaft?
Die EU als internationaler Akteur am Beispiel ihrer Demokratieförderung in Belarus und der Ukraine 2004-2009
Mit einem Vorwort von Jutta Joachim
ISBN 978-3-8382-0437-6

117 Fabian Pfeiffer
Estlands Außen- und Sicherheitspolitik I
Der estnische Atlantizismus nach der
wiedererlangten Unabhängigkeit 1991-2004
Mit einem Vorwort von Helmut Hubel
ISBN 978-3-8382-0127-6

118 Jana Podßuweit
Estlands Außen- und Sicherheitspolitik II
Handlungsoptionen eines Kleinstaates im
Rahmen seiner EU-Mitgliedschaft (2004-2008)
Mit einem Vorwort von Helmut Hubel
ISBN 978-3-8382-0440-6

119 Karin Pointner
Estlands Außen- und Sicherheitspolitik III
Eine gedächtnispolitische Analyse estnischer
Entwicklungskooperation 2006-2010
Mit einem Vorwort von Karin Liebhart
ISBN 978-3-8382-0435-2

120 Ruslana Vovk
Die Offenheit der ukrainischen
Verfassung für das Völkerrecht und
die europäische Integration
Mit einem Vorwort von Alexander
Blankenagel
ISBN 978-3-8382-0481-9

121 Mykhaylo Banakh
Die Relevanz der Zivilgesellschaft
bei den postkommunistischen
Transformationsprozessen in mittel-
und osteuropäischen Ländern
Das Beispiel der spät- und postsowjetischen
Ukraine 1986-2009
Mit einem Vorwort von Gerhard Simon
ISBN 978-3-8382-0499-4

122 Michael Moser
Language Policy and the Discourse on
Languages in Ukraine under President
Viktor Yanukovych (25 February
2010–28 October 2012)
ISBN 978-3-8382-0497-0 (Paperback edition)
ISBN 978-3-8382-0507-6 (Hardcover edition)

123 Nicole Krome
Russischer Netzwerkkapitalismus
Restrukturierungsprozesse in der
Russischen Föderation am Beispiel des
Luftfahrtunternehmens "Aviastar"
Mit einem Vorwort von Petra Stykow
ISBN 978-3-8382-0534-2

124 David R. Marples
'Our Glorious Past'
Lukashenka's Belarus and
the Great Patriotic War
ISBN 978-3-8382-0574-8 (Paperback edition)
ISBN 978-3-8382-0675-2 (Hardcover edition)

125 Ulf Walther
Russlands "neuer Adel"
Die Macht des Geheimdienstes von
Gorbatschow bis Putin
Mit einem Vorwort von Hans-Georg Wieck
ISBN 978-3-8382-0584-7

126 Simon Geissbühler (Hrsg.)
Kiew – Revolution 3.0
Der Euromaidan 2013/14 und die
Zukunftsperspektiven der Ukraine
ISBN 978-3-8382-0581-6 (Paperback edition)
ISBN 978-3-8382-0681-3 (Hardcover edition)

127 Andrey Makarychev
Russia and the EU
in a Multipolar World
Discourses, Identities, Norms
With a foreword by Klaus Segbers
ISBN 978-3-8382-0629-5

128 Roland Scharff
Kasachstan als postsowjetischer
Wohlfahrtsstaat
Die Transformation des sozialen
Schutzsystems
Mit einem Vorwort von Joachim Ahrens
ISBN 978-3-8382-0622-6

129 Katja Grupp
Bild Lücke Deutschland
Kaliningrader Studierende sprechen über
Deutschland
Mit einem Vorwort von Martin Schulz
ISBN 978-3-8382-0552-6

130 Konstantin Sheiko, Stephen Brown
History as Therapy
Alternative History and Nationalist
Imaginings in Russia, 1991-2014
ISBN 978-3-8382-0665-3

131 Elisa Kriza
Alexander Solzhenitsyn: Cold War
Icon, Gulag Author, Russian
Nationalist?
A Study of the Western Reception of his
Literary Writings, Historical Interpretations,
and Political Ideas
With a foreword by Andrei Rogatchevski
ISBN 978-3-8382-0589-2 (Paperback edition)
ISBN 978-3-8382-0690-5 (Hardcover edition)

132  Serghei Golunov
     The Elephant in the Room
     Corruption and Cheating in Russian
     Universities
     ISBN 978-3-8382-0570-0

133  Manja Hussner, Rainer Arnold (Hgg.)
     Verfassungsgerichtsbarkeit in
     Zentralasien I
     Sammlung von Verfassungstexten
     ISBN 978-3-8382-0595-3

134  Nikolay Mitrokhin
     Die "Russische Partei"
     Die Bewegung der russischen Nationalisten in
     der UdSSR 1953-1985
     Aus dem Russischen übertragen von einem
     Übersetzerteam unter der Leitung von Larisa Schippel
     ISBN 978-3-8382-0024-8

135  Manja Hussner, Rainer Arnold (Hgg.)
     Verfassungsgerichtsbarkeit in
     Zentralasien II
     Sammlung von Verfassungstexten
     ISBN 978-3-8382-0597-7

136  Manfred Zeller
     Das sowjetische Fieber
     Fußballfans im poststalinistischen
     Vielvölkerreich
     Mit einem Vorwort von Nikolaus Katzer
     ISBN 978-3-8382-0757-5

137  Kristin Schreiter
     Stellung und Entwicklungspotential
     zivilgesellschaftlicher Gruppen in
     Russland
     Menschenrechtsorganisationen im Vergleich
     ISBN 978-3-8382-0673-8

138  David R. Marples, Frederick V. Mills
     (eds.)
     Ukraine's Euromaidan
     Analyses of a Civil Revolution
     ISBN 978-3-8382-0660-8

139  Bernd Kappenberg
     Setting Signs for Europe
     Why Diacritics Matter for
     European Integration
     With a foreword by Peter Schlobinski
     ISBN 978-3-8382-0663-9

140  René Lenz
     Internationalisierung, Kooperation
     und Transfer
     Externe bildungspolitische Akteure in der
     Russischen Föderation
     Mit einem Vorwort von Frank Ettrich
     ISBN 978-3-8382-0751-3

141  Juri Plusnin, Yana Zausaeva, Natalia
     Zhidkevich, Artemy Pozanenko
     Wandering Workers
     Mores, Behavior, Way of Life, and Political
     Status of Domestic Russian Labor Migrants
     Translated by Julia Kazantseva
     ISBN 978-3-8382-0653-0

142  Matthew Kott, David J. Smith (eds.)
     Latvia – A Work in Progress?
     100 Years of State- and Nation-building
     ISBN 978-3-8382-0648-6

143  Инна Чувычкина (ред.)
     Экспортные нефте- и газопроводы
     на постсоветском пространстве
     Анализ трубопроводной политики в свете
     теории международных отношений
     ISBN 978-3-8382-0822-0

144  Johann Zajaczkowski
     Russland – eine pragmatische
     Großmacht?
     Eine rollentheoretische Untersuchung
     russischer Außenpolitik am Beispiel der
     Zusammenarbeit mit den USA nach 9/11 und
     des Georgienkrieges von 2008
     Mit einem Vorwort von Siegfried Schieder
     ISBN 978-3-8382-0837-4

145  Boris Popivanov
     Changing Images of the Left in
     Bulgaria
     The Challenge of Post-Communism in the
     Early 21st Century
     ISBN 978-3-8382-0667-7

146  Lenka Krátká
     A History of the Czechoslovak Ocean
     Shipping Company 1948-1989
     How a Small, Landlocked Country Ran
     Maritime Business During the Cold War
     ISBN 978-3-8382-0666-0

147  Alexander Sergunin
     Explaining Russian Foreign Policy
     Behavior
     Theory and Practice
     ISBN 978-3-8382-0752-0

148  Darya Malyutina
     Migrant Friendships in
     a Super-Diverse City
     Russian-Speakers and their Social
     Relationships in London in the 21st Century
     With a foreword by Claire Dwyer
     ISBN 978-3-8382-0652-3

149  Alexander Sergunin, Valery Konyshev
     Russia in the Arctic
     Hard or Soft Power?
     ISBN 978-3-8382-0753-7

150  John J. Maresca
     Helsinki Revisited
     A Key U.S. Negotiator's Memoirs
     on the Development of the CSCE into the
     OSCE
     With a foreword by Hafiz Pashayev
     ISBN 978-3-8382-0852-7

151  Jardar Østbø
     The New Third Rome
     Readings of a Russian Nationalist Myth
     With a foreword by Pål Kolstø
     ISBN 978-3-8382-0870-1

152  Simon Kordonsky
     Socio-Economic Foundations of the
     Russian Post-Soviet Regime
     The Resource-Based Economy and Estate-
     Based Social Structure of Contemporary
     Russia
     With a foreword by Svetlana Barsukova
     ISBN 978-3-8382-0775-9

153  Duncan Leitch
     Assisting Reform in Post-Communist
     Ukraine 2000–2012
     The Illusions of Donors and the Disillusion of
     Beneficiaries
     With a foreword by Kataryna Wolczuk
     ISBN 978-3-8382-0844-2

154  Abel Polese
     Limits of a Post-Soviet State
     How Informality Replaces, Renegotiates, and
     Reshapes Governance in Contemporary
     Ukraine
     With a foreword by Colin Williams
     ISBN 978-3-8382-0845-9

155  Mikhail Suslov (ed.)
     Digital Orthodoxy in the Post-Soviet
     World
     The Russian Orthodox Church and Web 2.0
     With a foreword by Father Cyril Hovorun
     ISBN 978-3-8382-0871-8

156  Leonid Luks
     Zwei „Sonderwege"? Russisch-
     deutsche Parallelen und Kontraste
     (1917-2014)
     Vergleichende Essays
     ISBN 978-3-8382-0823-7

157  Vladimir V. Karacharovskiy, Ovsey I.
     Shkaratan, Gordey A. Yastrebov
     Towards a New Russian Work Culture
     Can Western Companies and Expatriates
     Change Russian Society?
     With a foreword by Elena N. Danilova
     Translated by Julia Kazantseva
     ISBN 978-3-8382-0902-9

158  Edmund Griffiths
     Aleksandr Prokhanov and Post-Soviet
     Esotericism
     ISBN 978-3-8382-0903-6

159  Timm Beichelt, Susann Worschech
     (eds.)
     Transnational Ukraine?
     Networks and Ties that Influence(d)
     Contemporary Ukraine
     ISBN 978-3-8382-0944-9

160  Mieste Hotopp-Riecke
     Die Tataren der Krim zwischen
     Assimilation und Selbstbehauptung
     Der Aufbau des krimtatarischen
     Bildungswesens nach Deportation und
     Heimkehr (1990-2005)
     Mit einem Vorwort von Swetlana
     Czerwonnaja
     ISBN 978-3-89821-940-2

161  Olga Bertelsen (ed.)
     Revolution and War in
     Contemporary Ukraine
     The Challenge of Change
     ISBN 978-3-8382-1016-2

162  Natalya Ryabinska
     Ukraine's Post-Communist
     Mass Media
     Between Capture and Commercialization
     With a foreword by Marta Dyczok
     ISBN 978-3-8382-1011-7

163   *Alexandra Cotofana,*
      *James M. Nyce (eds.)*
      Religion and Magic in Socialist and
      Post-Socialist Contexts
      Historic and Ethnographic Case Studies of
      Orthodoxy, Heterodoxy, and Alternative
      Spirituality
      With an afterword by Catherine Wanner
      ISBN 978-3-8382-0989-0

164   *Nozima Akhrarkhodjaeva*
      The Instrumentalisation of Mass
      Media in Electoral Authoritarian
      Regimes
      Evidence from Russia's Presidential Election
      Campaigns of 2000 and 2008
      ISBN 978-3-8382-1013-1

165   *Yulia Krasheninnikova*
      Informal Healthcare in Contemporary
      Russia
      Sociographic Essays on the Post-Soviet
      Infrastructure for Alternative Healing
      Practices
      ISBN 978-3-8382-0970-8

*ibidem*-Verlag
Melchiorstr. 15
D-70439 Stuttgart
info@ibidem-verlag.de

www.ibidem-verlag.de
www.ibidem.eu
www.edition-noema.de
www.autorenbetreuung.de